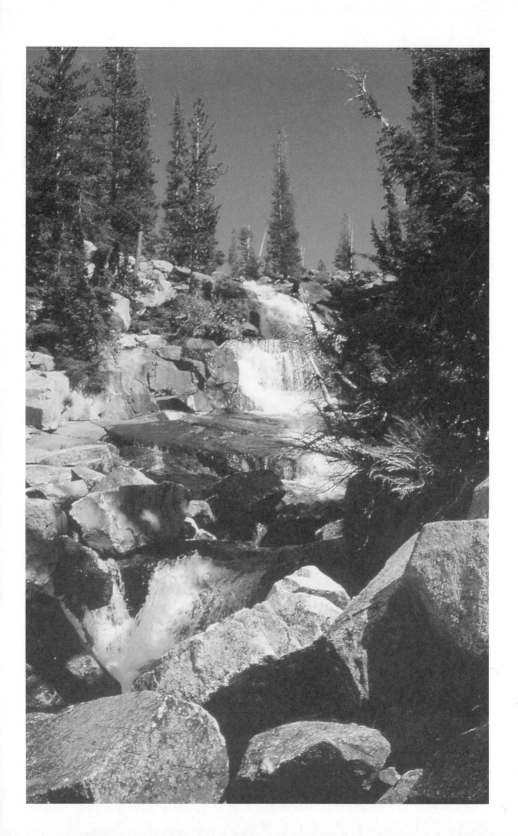

SIERRA NORTH

BACKCOUNTRY TRIPS IN
CALIFORNIA'S SIERRA NEVADA

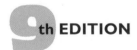th EDITION

**KATHY MOREY
& MIKE WHITE**

with **STACY CORLESS
& THOMAS WINNETT**

WILDERNESS PRESS · BERKELEY, CA

Sierra North: Backcountry Trips in California's Sierra Nevada

1st EDITION May 1967
2nd EDITION May 1971
3rd EDITION January 1976
4th EDITION May 1982
5th EDITION June 1985
6th EDITION May 1991
7th EDITION May 1997
8th EDITION June 2002
9th EDITION July 2005
  2nd printing February 2008

Front cover photo copyright © 2005 by Dan Patitucci/PatitucciPhoto
Interior photos, except where noted, by Kathy Morey
Maps: Bart Wright/Fineline Maps
Book & cover design: Larry B. Van Dyke
Book editor: Eva Dienel

ISBN: 978-0-89997-396-8
UPC: 7-19609-97396-6

Manufactured in China

Published by: **Wilderness Press**
               1200 5th Street
               Berkeley, CA 94710
               (800) 443-7227; FAX (510) 558-1696
               info@wildernesspress.com
               www.wildernesspress.com

Visit our website for a complete listing of our books and for ordering information.

Cover photo: Young Lakes camp at sunset
Frontispiece: Tilden Creek Falls (Trip 40)

SAFETY NOTICE: Although Wilderness Press and the author have made every attempt to
ensure that the information in this book is accurate at press time, they are not responsible for
any loss, damage, injury, or inconvenience that may occur to anyone while using this book. You
are responsible for your own safety and health while in the wilderness. The fact that a trail is
described in this book does not mean that it will be safe for you. Be aware that trail conditions
can change from day to day. Always check local conditions and know your own limitations.

ACKNOWLEDGMENTS

My thanks as always to my husband, Ed Schwartz, for his support. My thanks to Tom Winnett for inspiration, opportunity, and guidance. I'm grateful to my co-authors for their enthusiasm and support during this project. Thanks also to (in alphabetical order) J. Brian Anderson, Walt Lehmann, Steven K. Schuster, and Marshalle F. Wells for the fine photos they generously submitted. I would like also to acknowledge the forebearance of the long-suffering staff at Wilderness Press, particularly Eva Dienel and Roslyn Bullas. —KM

Working with Kathy Morey on this project proved to be quite enjoyable. As usual, thanks go to Eva Dienel and the staff at Wilderness Press for their stellar efforts. I greatly appreciated the company of Dan Palmer and Bob Redding on the trail. —MW

I would like to thank Kathy Morey for her hard work and for her guidance; my husband, Charlie Byrne; Debbie Clausen, for hiking; and Mark Clausen, for prompt Tuolumne pick-up. —SC

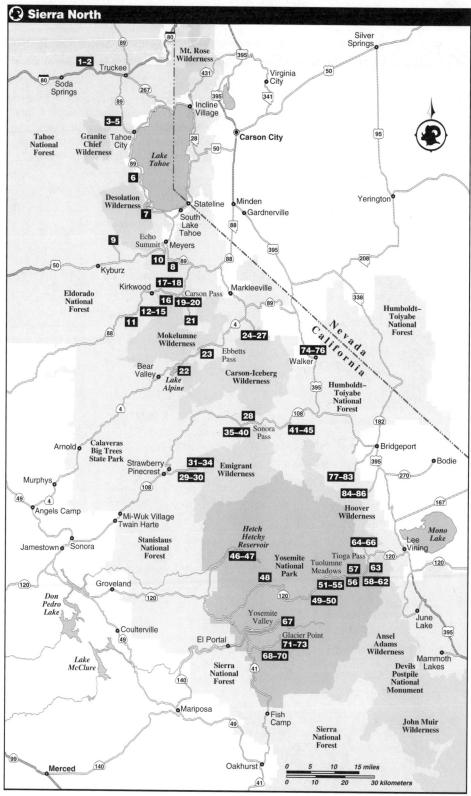

CONTENTS

State Highway 120 Trips   **165**

Western Yosemite Trips 231

US Highway 395 Trips 255

GOING HIGH TO GET HIGH
By Thomas Winnett, Wilderness Press Founder

As I write this, it is nearly 40 years since we at Wilderness Press held a celebration to promote the first edition of *Sierra North*, a one-of-a-kind book Karl Schwenke and I wrote to recommend 100 of the best backpacking trips into the northern Sierra.

It was the summer of 1967, and we celebrated in the backcountry with a high-altitude cocktail party. We invited everyone we thought would help get the word out about the book—people from the Sierra Club, outdoor writers, and friends. We held it in August, in Dusy Basin, in the eastern Sierra, 8 miles from the nearest car. The hike went over a 12,000-foot pass, so we were delighted when 15 people showed up. It was a real party. We used snow to make our martinis, ate hors d'oeuvres, and spent the night. In a mention of the event, *San Francisco Chronicle* columnist Herb Caen wondered, "How high can you get to get high?"

It was a spectacular occasion not only because we were launching the book, but because we were starting a new company. We founded Wilderness Press in 1965. Karl, a backpacking friend of mine, and I had been complaining about how hard it was to get accurate information about the out of doors. At the time, there were only one or two guidebooks to the Sierra—our favorite place—so we decided to write our own. We planned to create pre-packaged trips that specified which trails to take and where to stop each night. We would do a series of small books, each covering a 15-minute quadrangle, and they would be called the *Knapsacker/Packer Guide Series.*

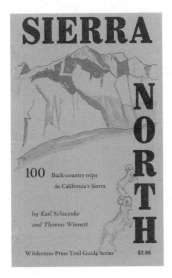

In the summer of 1966, we started doing the field research. Our approach was simple: We wanted to accurately describe where the trails lead and what was there. On my scouting trips, I carried more than your average backpacker. In addition to all the standard gear, I packed two cameras, two natural history books to help me indentify flowers and birds, and my Telmar tape recorder. The tape recorder ran about half the speed of the recording devices that are available today, and I'd walk along, dictating into the microphone everything I thought our customers would be interested in reading. So in addition to the basics—how to get to where you start walking, where to go, and the best campsites—we also described what we saw, the animals, flowers, birds, and trees.

By the end of the summer, we had enough material to cover most of the trails in the northern Sierra, so we published a book of 100 trails and called it *Sierra North*. We decided orange would be the official color of Wilderness Press, so we used an orange cover with some illustrations of bighorn sheep and mountains sketched by my wife, Lu.

That first edition sold like the proverbial hotcakes; we sold out our entire print run of 3000 books. Since then, this book has sold more than 150,000 copies, and it gives me great joy to see it in its ninth edition. As I think back to that high-altitude cocktail party in 1967, I wonder how many people have used this book to "go high to get high" in the Sierra. I have personally walked more than 2000 miles in this most beautiful of mountain ranges, and although I can't do that anymore, I am still hooked on the experience—the splendid isolation, the scenery that really lights up your eyeballs, the strength you feel climbing with the weight of your pack on your back, the myriad trout. I hope this guidebook hooks you, too.

TRIP CROSS-REFERENCE TABLE

TRIP NO.	TRIP TYPE				BEST SEASON			HIKING DAYS	MILEAGE	RECOMMENDED FOR BEGINNERS
	OUT & BACK	SHUTTLE	LOOP	SEMI-LOOP	EARLY	MID	LATE			
1	•					•	•	2	15.4	
2			•			•	•	3	16.4	
3	•					•	•	2	13.5	
4	•					•	•	4	27.5	
5		•	•			•	•	3	25/26.5	
6		•				•	•	4	30.2/27.5	
7				•		•	•	2	11.7	•
8		•				•	•	2	10.4	•
9			•			•	•	2	8	
10		•				•	•	2	13.4	•
11	•					•		2	18	
12	•					•		2	13	•
13	•					•		4	22	
14	•					•		6	33	
15		•				•		5	31.7	
16			•			•		2	5	•
17	•					•		2	10.2	•
18		•				•		2	13.4	•
19				•		•	•	2	14	
20		•				•		4	26.6	
21	•					•	•	2	12	
22		•				•	•	3	19.8	
23		•				•		3	8	•
24				•		•		2	20.5	
25		•				•		2	24	
26		•				•		3	30	
27				•		•		4	36.5	
28	•					•	•	4	22.6	
29	•					•	•	6	35.6	
30	•					•	•	2	10	•
31	•					•	•	4	24.8	
32		•				•	•	4	25.9	
33		•				•	•	5	33.3	
34		•				•	•	2	9.1	
35	•				•	•		2	13.6	
36	•					•	•	4	25.2	
37	•					•	•	4	26.8	
38				•		•	•	7	46	
39		•				•	•	7	43.1	
40		•				•	•	11	71.3	
41				•		•	•	2	19.5	
42	•					•	•	4	28	
43				•		•	•	4	34	

TRIP NO.	TRIP TYPE				BEST SEASON			HIKING DAYS	MILEAGE	RECOMMENDED FOR BEGINNERS
	OUT & BACK	SHUTTLE	LOOP	SEMI-LOOP	EARLY	MID	LATE			
44				•		•	•	5	40	
45				•	•	•		5	41.4	
46	•				•			2	13	•
47	•				•			4	18.6	
48			•		•	•	•	6	50	
49	•					•		2	11.4	•
50		•				•	•	2	17.3	
51	•					•	•	2	7.4	•
52	•					•	•	4	16.8	•
53		•	•			•	•	5	34/36.2	
54		•				•	•	4	25.4	
55		•				•	•	3	22.4	
56	•					•	•	2	11.8	
57				•		•	•	1	15.1	•
58	•				•	•	•	2	18	•
59	•					•	•	2	15.4	•
60				•		•	•	4	28.8	
61				•		•	•	6	40.3	
62				•		•	•	7	51.3	
63		•				•	•	3	20	
64			•			•	•	2	8.5	•
65	•					•	•	2	11/13.8	
66		•				•	•	3	20.2	
67	•				•		•	4	27.8	
68				•	•	•		5	27.9	
69		•			•	•		4	29.1	
70		•			•	•		4	32.7	
71	•				•			4	31.8	
72			•			•	•	10	71.5	
73		•				•	•	1	41.1	
74				•		•	•	2	14	
75			•			•		3	26.5	
76			•			•	•	5	41.5	
77	•					•	•	2	16	•
78		•				•	•	3	22.4	
79	•					•	•	2	16	•
80	•					•	•	4	23	
81				•		•	•	3	22	•
82	•					•	•	6	37.2	
83				•		•	•	8	49.6	
84	•				•	•	•	2	8	•
85		•				•	•	2	10.5	
86		•				•	•	4	26.7	

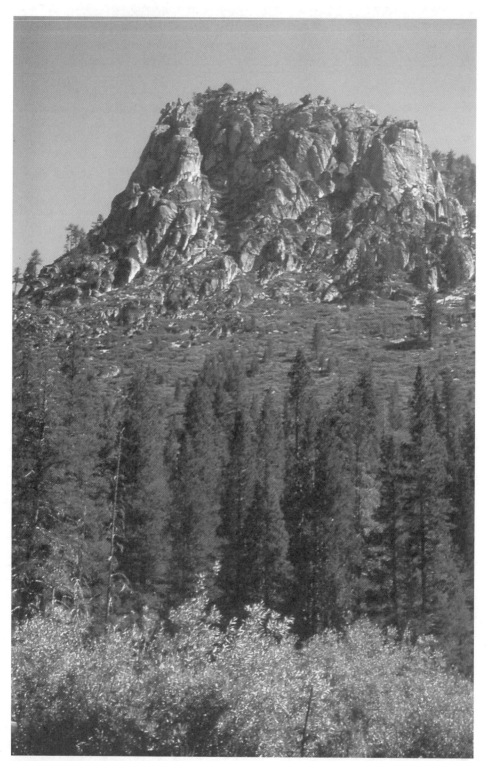

The Iceberg (Trip 34)

INTRODUCTION

Welcome to what we think is just about the most spectacular mountain range in the contiguous 48 states. The Sierra Nevada is a hiker's paradise filled with huge wilderness areas, hundreds of miles of trails, thousands of lakes, countless rugged peaks and canyons, vast forests, giant Sequoias, and terrain ranging from deep, forested river valleys to sublime, treeless alpine country.

Updates for the Ninth Edition

Welcome, too, to the ninth edition of Wilderness Press's flagship book, *Sierra North*. For this edition, we have some new co-authors as well as some exciting new elements that we think make this book better than ever before. Foremost among them is an expanded territory: *Sierra North* now spans existing and proposed wilderness areas from just north of I-80, south through Hwy. 120 and the rest of Yosemite National Park, and trailheads off Hwy. 395 between highways 108 and 120. (*Sierra South*, this book's companion, covers the Sierra south of Yosemite, including the Kern Plateau, Mt. Whitney, and the Great Western Divide.)

We have also reorganized this book, dividing it into major road sections so you can easily locate your favorite part of the northern Sierra. Each road section includes trailheads that serve as starting points for the many individual trips in the book. Additionally, each trailhead now includes a map showing every trip launching from that point, and each trip still includes an elevation profile. We've also incorporated Global Positioning System (GPS) data as UTM coordinates into our trips for GPS users.

Measuring distances in the backcountry is more an art than a science. We use decimal fractions for indicating distances, but don't imagine that we measured them to the tenths and hundredths of miles. The numbers represent our best estimates of distance based on techniques like the time it took us to get from point to point. You can't represent thirds accurately as decimal fractions, so we use 0.3 for one third and 0.6 for two thirds.

If you have used previous editions of *Sierra North*, you'll find many of your old favorite trips and, we hope, discover news ones as well. We have incorporated into this new edition an old favorite, the Tahoe-Yosemite Trail (TYT), 186 beautiful and adventurous miles from Lake Tahoe's Meeks Bay to Yosemite's Tuolumne Meadows. It's a worthy complement to, yet a very different experience from, the famed John Muir Trail (JMT) to the south. We treat the TYT in six legs (sections) from north to south.

It's our hope that this new edition will help you enjoy our magnificent northern Sierra as well as give you an incentive to work to preserve it.

We appreciate hearing from our readers. Many of the changes and updates for this edition are a direct result of readers' requests. Please let us know what did and didn't work for you in this new edition and about corrections you find. We're at 1200 5th St., Berkeley, CA 94710; mail@wildernesspress.com; 800-443-7227; 510-558-1666; fax 510-558-1696. Please visit us online at www.wildernesspress.com.

Care and Enjoyment of the Mountains

Be a Good Guest

The Sierra is home—the only home—to a spectacular array of plants and animals. We humans are merely guests—uninvited ones at that. Be a careful, considerate guest in this grandest of Nature's homes.

About a million people camp in the Sierra wilderness each year. The vast majority of us care about the wilderness and try to protect it, but it is threatened by some who still need to learn the art of living lightly on the land. The solution depends on each of us. We can minimize our impact. The saying "Take only memories (or photos), leave only foot-prints," sums it up.

Learn to Go Light

John Muir, traveling along the crest of the Sierra in the 1870s with little more that his overcoat and his pockets full of biscuits was the archetype.

Muir's example may be too extreme for many, but we think he might have appreciat-ed modern lightweight equipment and food as a great convenience. A lot of the stuff that goes into the mountains is burdensome, harmful to the wilderness, or just plain annoying to other people seeking peace and solitude. Please leave behind anything that is obtrusive or that can be used to modify the terrain: gas lanterns, radios, hatchets, gigantic tents, etc.

Carry Out Your Trash

You packed that foil and those cans and bags in when full; you can pack them out empty. Never litter or bury your trash. Anglers, take all your lures, bait, and monofilament out with you. Don't leave fishing line tangled over the trees, shrubs, and logs. We recom-mend you use biodegradable fishing line.

Sanitation

Eliminate body wastes at least 100 feet, and preferably 200 feet, from lakes, streams, trails, and campsites. Bury feces at least 6 inches deep wherever possible. Intestinal pathogens can survive for years in feces when they're buried, but burial reduces the chances that critters will come in contact with them and carry pathogens into the water. Where burial is not possible due to lack of enough soil or gravel, leave feces where they will receive maximum exposure to heat and sunlight to hasten the destruction of pathogens. Also help reduce the waste problem in the backcountry by packing out your used toilet paper, facial tissues, tampons, sanitary napkins, and diapers. It's easy to carry them out in a heavy-duty, self-sealing plastic bag.

Protect the Water

Just because something is "biodegradable," like some soaps, doesn't mean it's okay to put it in the water. In addition, the fragile sod of meadows, lakeshores, and streamsides is rapidly disappearing from the High Sierra. Pick "hard" campsites, sandy places that can stand the use. Camp at least 200 feet from water unless that's absolutely impossible; in no case camp closer that 25 feet. Don't make campsite "improvements" like rock walls, bough beds, new fireplaces, or tent ditches.

Avoid Campfires

Use a modern, lightweight backpacking stove. (If you use a gas-cartridge stove, be sure to pack your used cartridges out.) Campfires waste a precious resource: wood that would otherwise shelter animals and, upon falling and decaying, return vital nutrients to the soil. Campfires also run the risk of starting forest fires.

If your stove fails and you must cook over a campfire in order to survive, here are some guidelines: If possible, camp in an established site with an existing fireplace you can use. If you must build a fireplace, build with efficiency and restoration in mind: two to four medium-sized rocks set parallel along the sides of a narrow, shallow trench in a sandy place. Set the pot on the rocks and over the fire, which you can feed with small sticks and twigs (use only dead and downed wood). Never leave the fire unattended. Before you leave, thoroughly extinguish the fire and pour water over the ashes, stirring the ashes to be certain they're cold and wet, and then restore the site by scattering the rocks and filling the trench.

To use a stove or have a campfire where legal, you must have a California Campfire Permit. One such permit is good for the season. Your wilderness permit can double as your California Campfire Permit. If you're taking a trip that doesn't require a wilderness permit, you still need a California Campfire Permit, available at any ranger station.

Respect the Wildlife

Avoid trampling on nests, burrows, or other homes of animals. Observe all fishing limits and keep shorelines clean and clear of litter. If angling, use biodegradable line and never leave any of it behind. If you come across an animal, just quietly observe it. Above all, don't go near any nesting animals and their young. Get "close" with binoculars or telephoto lenses.

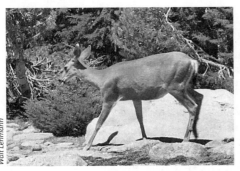
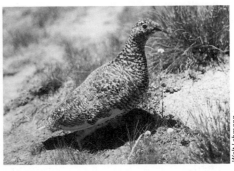

Deer   **Grouse**

Safety and Well Being

Hiking in the high country is far safer than driving to the mountains, and a few precautions can shield you from most of the discomforts and dangers that could threaten you.

Health Hazards

Altitude Sickness: If you normally live at sea level and come to the Sierra to hike, it may take your body several days to acclimate. Starved of your accustomed oxygen, for a few days you may experience shortness of breath even with minimal activity, severe headaches, or nausea. The best solutions are to spend time at altitude before you begin your hike and to plan a very easy first day. On your hike, light, frequent meals are best.

Giardia and Cryptosporidium: Giardiasis is a serious gastrointestinal disease caused by a waterborne protozoan, *Giardia lamblia*. Any mammal (which includes humans) can become infected. It will then excrete live giardia in its feces, from which the protozoan can get into even the most remote sources of water, such as a stream issuing from a glacier. Giardia can survive in snow through the winter and in cold water as a cyst resistant to the usual chemical treatments. Giardiasis can be contracted by drinking untreated water. Symptoms appear two to three weeks after exposure.

Cryptosporidium is another, smaller, very hardy pest that causes a disease similar to giardiasis. It's been found in the streams of the San Gabriel Mountains of Los Angeles, and is spreading throughout Southern California. Probably it will eventually infest Sierran waters.

At this time, boiling and filtering are the only sure backcountry defenses against giardia and cryptosporidium. Bring water to a rolling boil; this is easy to do while you're cooking and is now judged effective at any Sierra altitude. To be effective against both giardia and the much-smaller cryptosporidium, a filter must trap particles down to 0.4 micron.

Halogen treatments (iodine, chlorine) are ineffective against cryptosporidium and hard to use properly against giardia—but they are better than no treatment at all. Liquid chlorine-dioxide water-treatment kits and other devices are available for backpackers, but these treatments have not yet been proven effective by the FDA.

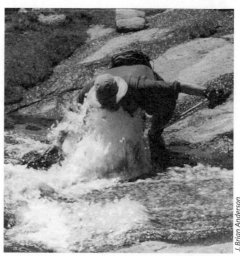

This may *feel* cool and refreshing, but it's advisable to filter or boil water before drinking it.

Hypothermia: Hypothermia refers to subnormal body temperature. More hikers die from hypothermia than from any other single cause. Caused by exposure to cold, often intensified by wet, wind, and weariness, the first symptoms of hypothermia are uncontrollable shivering and imperfect motor coordination. These are rapidly followed by loss of judgment, so that you yourself cannot make the decisions to protect your own life. Death by "exposure" is death by hypothermia.

To prevent hypothermia, stay warm: Carry wind- and rain-protective clothing, and put it on as soon as you feel chilly. Stay dry: Carry or wear wool or a suitable synthetic (not cotton), and bring raingear even for a short hike on an apparently sunny day. If weather conditions threaten and you are inadequately prepared, flee or hunker down.

Treat shivering at once: Get the victim out of the wind and wet, replace all wet clothes with dry ones, put him or her in a sleeping bag, and give him or her warm drinks. If the shivering is severe and accompanied by other symptoms, strip him or her and yourself (and a third party if possible), and warm him or her with your own bodies, tightly wrapped in a dry sleeping bag.

Lightning: Although the odds of being struck are small, almost everyone who goes to the mountains thinks about it. If a thunderstorm comes upon you, avoid exposed places—mountain peaks, mountain ridges, open fields, a boat on a lake—and avoid small caves and rock overhangs. The safest place is an opening or a clump of small trees in a forest.

The best body stance is one that minimizes the area where your body touches the ground. You should drop to your knees and put your hands on your knees. This is because the more area your body covers, the more chance that ground currents will pass through it. Also make sure to get all metal—such as frame packs, tent poles, etc.—away from you.

If you get struck by lightning, there isn't much you can do except pray that someone in your party is adept at CPR—or at least adept at artificial respiration if your breathing has stopped but not your heart. It may take hours for a victim to resume breathing on his or her own. If your companions are victims, attend first to those who are not moving. Those who are rolling around and moaning are at least breathing. Finally, a victim who lives should be evacuated to a hospital; other problems often develop in lightning victims.

Sunburn: Sierra altitudes demand strong sunblock (SPF 50 recommended).

Wildlife Hazards

Rattlesnakes: They appear at lower elevations (they are rarely seen above 7000 feet but have been seen up to 9000 feet) in a range of habitats, but most commonly near riverbeds and streams. Their bite is rarely fatal to an adult, but a bite that carries venom may still cause extensive tissue damage.

If you are bitten, get to a hospital as soon as possible. There is no substitute for proper medical treatment.

Some people carry a snakebite kit such as Sawyer's extractor when traveling in remote areas far from help and where snake encounters are more likely: below 6000 feet along a watercourse. This kit is somewhat effective if used properly within 30 minutes after the bite—but it's still no substitute for hospital care.

Better yet, don't get bitten: Watch where you place your hands and feet; listen for the rattle. If you hear a snake rattle, stand still long enough to determine where it is, then leave in the opposite direction.

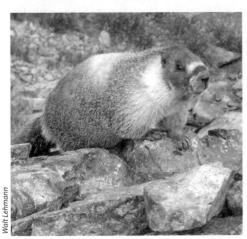

Marmot

Rodents and Birds: Marmots live from about 6000 feet to 11,500 feet. Because they are curious, always hungry, and like to sun themselves on rocks in full view, you are likely to see them. Marmots enjoy many foods you do, including cereal and candy (especially chocolate). They may eat through a pack or tent when other entry is difficult. Marmots cannot climb trees or ropes, so you can protect your food by hanging it (though this is illegal in some areas because of bears). Smaller, climbing rodents might get into hung food. We've heard reports of jays pecking their way into bags, too. Sealed bear canisters are excellent protection against all kinds of rodents, birds, and insects. (Please see pages 6–9 for information about bears.)

Mosquitoes: Insect repellent containing N, N diethylmeta-toluamide, known commercially as deet, will keep them off. Don't buy one without a minimum of about 30% deet. Studies show adults can use deet in moderation, but it is dangerous for children. To minimize the amount of deet on your skin, apply it to your clothes and/or hat instead—but test first to be sure that deet won't damage the garment.

Most non-deet and low-deet repellents work much more poorly than those with 30% deet or more, and electronic repellents are useless. Clothing may also act as a bar to mosquitoes—a good reason for wearing long pants and a long-sleeved shirt. If you are a favorite target for mosquitoes (they have their preferences), you might take a head net—a hat with netting suspended all around the brim and a snug neckband.

A tent with mosquito netting makes a world of difference during mosquito season (typically through late July). Planning your trip to avoid the height of the mosquito season is also a good preventive.

Terrain Hazards

Snow Bridges and Cornices: Stay off them.

Streams: In early season, when the snow is melting, crossing a river can be the most dangerous part of a backpack trip. Later, ordinary caution will see you across safely. If a river is running high, you should cross it only there is no safer alternative, you have found a suitable place to ford, and you use a rope—but don't tie into it; just hold onto it.

Here are some suggestions for stream-crossing:

- If a stream is dauntingly high or swift, forget it. Turn around and come back later, perhaps in late summer or early fall, when flows reach seasonal lows.

- Wear closed-toe shoes, which will protect your feet from injury and give them more secure placement.

- Cross in a stance in which you're angled upstream. If you face downstream, the water pushing against the back of your knees could cause them to buckle.

- Move one foot only when the other is firmly placed.

- Keep your legs apart for a more stable stance. You'll find a cross-footed stance unstable even in your own living room, much less in a Sierra torrent.

- One or two hiking sticks will help keep you stable while crossing. You can also use a stick to probe ahead for holes and other obstacles that may be difficult to see and judge under running water.

- One piece of advice used to be that you should unfasten your pack's hip belt in case you fell in and had to jettison the pack. However, modern quick-release buckles probably make this precaution unnecessary. Keeping the hip belt fastened will keep the pack more stable, and this will in turn help *your* stability. You may wish, however, to unfasten the sternum strap so that you have only one buckle to worry about.

The Bear Problem

The bears of the Sierra are American black bears; their coats range from black to light brown. Unless provoked, they're not usually aggressive, and their normal diet consists largely of plants. The suggestions in this section apply only to American black bears, not to the more aggressive grizzly bear, which is extinct in California.

American black bears run and climb faster than you ever will, they are immensely stronger, and they are very intelligent. Long ago they learned to associate humans with easy sources of food. Now, keeping your food away from the local bears is a problem. Remember, though, that they aren't interested in eating you. Don't let the possibility of meeting a bear keep you out of the Sierra. Respect these magnificent creatures. Learn what you can do to keep yourself and your food safe. Some suggestions follow.

Bears—Any Time, Anywhere: You may encounter bears anywhere in the areas this book covers. If they present special problems on that trip, we mention them in the "Heads Up!" paragraph of that trip. Bears are normally daytime creatures, but they've learned that our supplies are easier to raid when we're asleep, so they're working the night shift, too. Also, it used to be that you rarely saw bears above 8000 to 9000 feet. As campers moved into the higher elevations, the bears followed.

To avoid bears while hiking, some people make noise as they go, because most American black bears are shy and will scramble off to avoid meeting you. Others find noise-making intrusive, consider those who make noise rude, and accept the risk of meeting a bear. You will have to decide.

In camp, store your food properly and always scare bears away immediately. (See Food Storage, pages 7–8.)

Plan Ahead: Avoid taking smelly foods and fragrant toiletries; they attract bears—bears have a superb sense of smell. Ask rangers and other backpackers where there are bear problems, and avoid those areas; also ask them what measures they take to safeguard food and chase bears away.

Carry a bear canister (also see more below). If you need to counterbalance your food bags, practice the skill before you need it. After cooking, clean up food residue. Before going to sleep or leaving your camp, clean any food out of your gear and store it with the rest of your chow; otherwise, you could lose a pack to a bear who went for the granola bar you forgot in a side pocket. Don't take food into your tent or sleeping bag unless you want ursine company. Store your smelly toiletries and garbage just as carefully as you store your food. Set up and use your kitchen at a good distance from the rest of your camp. Also make sure your food, even in canisters, is stored a good distance from your campsite.

Food Storage: Backcountry management policies now hold campers responsible for keeping their food away from bears. You can even be fined for violating food-storage rules. If a bear gets your food, you're also responsible for cleaning up the mess once you're sure the bear won't be back for seconds. And you have an ethical responsibility to keep bears from becoming pests, which may mean that they have to be killed.

Here are some food-storage suggestions that will help you do this:

- **Bear Canisters:** The first ones were lengths of sturdy plastic pipe fitted with a bottom and a lid only a human can open. Today there are several more choices, including lighter-weight aluminum ones and still lighter ones of exotic aerospace materials. Using these canisters is the best method for protecting your food where bear boxes (below) aren't available.

  Canisters aren't perfect, but they work very well when used properly. Using a canister is much easier and more secure than counterbalance bearbagging. They make good in-camp seats, too.

  There's also an extremely lightweight Kevlar sack with an odor-barrier inner sack. It is less secure than a canister, is slightly more difficult to use properly (but much easier than counterbalancing), and may not be approved for use in areas that require you to use a canister, like Yosemite. One of us has had good luck with these sacks.

  The materials you receive with your permit will tell you whether canisters are required. If you don't own a canister, you can rent one from an outdoors store or perhaps from the agency that issues your permit.

- **Counterbalance Bearbagging:** If you don't have a bear canister or access to a bear box where you camp, counterbalance your food. Note that in areas with severe bear problems, like most of Yosemite National Park, counterbalance bearbagging is ineffective and probably against regulations.

  Assuming you're traveling in an area where bears aren't yet a severe problem, counterbalance bearbagging may protect your food not only from bears but from ground squirrels, marmots, and other creatures. It's best to get to camp early enough to get your food hung while there's light to do it. Counterbalancing is not completely secure, but it may slow the bear down and give you time to scare it away. When you get a permit, you may get a sheet on the counterbalance bearbagging technique. The technique is also well-covered in numerous how-to-backpack books. Practice it at home before you go.

  If a bear goes after your food, jump up and down, make a lot of noise, wave your arms—anything to make yourself seem huge, noisy, and scary. Have a stash of rocks to throw and throw them at trees and boulders to make more noise. Bang pots together. Blow whistles. The object is to scare the bear away. Never directly attack the bear itself. Note, however, that some human-habituated bears simply can't be scared off.

- **Bear Boxes (Food Storage Lockers):** Bear boxes are large steel lockers intended for storage of food only, and they will hold the food bags of several backpackers. Their latches, simple for humans, are inoperable by bears. Everyone shares the bear box; you may not put your own locks on one. Food in a properly fastened bear box is safe from bears;

however, some boxes have holes in the bottom through which, if the holes aren't plugged, mice will squeeze in to nibble on your goodies.

There are few bear boxes in the northern Sierra. In Yosemite National Park, there are bear boxes at each of the High Sierra camps and in two extremely popular backcountry camping areas, Little Yosemite Valley and Lake Eleanor.

The presence of a bear box attracts campers as well as bears, and these sites can become overused. However, it isn't necessary for everyone to cluster right around the box. A campsite a few hundred yards away may be more secluded and desirable; the stroll to and from the bear box is a pleasant way to start and end a meal.

Bear-box don'ts: Never use a bear box as a garbage can! Rotting food is smelly and very attractive to bears. Never use a bear box as a food drop; its capacity is needed for people actually camping in its vicinity. Never leave a bear box unlatched or open, even when people are around.

- **Above Timberline:** Above treeline, there are no trees to hang your food bags from. But there are still bears—as well as mice, marmots, and ground squirrels—anxious to share your chow. If you don't have a canister or Kevlar sack (the latter only where legal) but must hang your food, look for a tall rock with an overhanging edge from which you can dangle your food bags high off the ground and well away from the face of the rock. Unlike bears, marmots and other critters have not learned to get your food by eating through the rope suspending it.

  Another option is to bag your food and push it deep into a crack in the rocks too small and too deep for a bear to reach into—but be sure you can still retrieve it. One of us has had good luck with this technique; don't use it in Yosemite National Park, which discourages it, and use it only above timberline. You may lose a little food to mice or ground squirrels, but it won't be much.

  When dayhiking from a base camp where you can't put your food in a bear box or leave it in a canister, it's safer to take as much of it with you as you can.

If a Bear Gets Your Food: Never try to get your food back from a bear. It's the bear's food now, and the bear will defend it aggressively against puny you. You may hear that there are no recorded fatalities in bear-human encounters in recent Sierra history. Of course, this isn't true: Plenty of bears have been killed as a result of repeated encounters. Every time a bear gets some human food, that bear is a step closer to becoming a nuisance bear that has to be killed. And there have been very serious, though not fatal, injuries to humans in these encounters.

If, despite your best efforts, you lose your food to a bear, it may be the end of your trip but not of the world. You won't starve to death in the maximum three to four days it will take you to walk out from even the most remote Sierra spot. Your pack is now much lighter. And you can probably beg the occasional stick of jerky or handful of gorp from your fellow backpackers along the way. So cheer up, clean up the mess, get going, and plan how you can do it better on your next trip.

A Word About Cars, Theft, and Car Bears: Stealing from and vandalizing cars are becoming all too common at popular trailheads. You can't ensure that your car and its contents will be safe, but you can increase the odds. Make your car unattractive to thieves and vandals by disabling your engine (your mechanic can show you how), hiding everything you leave in the car, and closing all windows and locking all doors and compartments. Get and use a locking gas-tank cap. If you have more than one car, use the most modest one for driving to the trailhead.

Bearproof your car by not leaving any food in it and by hiding anything that looks like a picnic cooler or other food carrier—bears know what to look for. To a bear, a car with food in it is just an oversized can waiting to be opened. Some trailheads, especially in

Yosemite National Park, have bear boxes at trailheads. Leave any food and toiletries you're not taking into the backcountry in these bear boxes rather than in your car.

The Regulations: Call, write to, or get on the website of the agency in charge of the area you plan to visit in order to learn the latest regulations, especially those concerning bears and food storage. For each trailhead in this book, you'll find the agency's name, physical address, phone number, and web address (if there is one) under Information and Permits.

Maps and Profiles

Today's Sierra traveler is confronted by a bewildering array of maps, and it doesn't take much experience to learn that no single map fulfills all needs. There are topographic maps, base maps (US Forest Service), shaded relief maps (National Park Service), artistically drawn representational maps (California Department of Fish and Game), aerial-photograph maps, geologic maps, three-dimensional relief maps, soil-vegetation maps, and compact discs containing five levels of topographic maps already pieced together for you as well as software for drawing routes. Each map has different information to impart, and it's a good idea to use several of these maps in your planning.

For trip-planning purposes, the trailheads in this book include their own gray-scale map or maps, which show all trips and are based on the United States Geological Survey (USGS) topographic maps or USDA Forest Service wilderness maps. (More information about these maps is on page 14.) Each trip includes an elevation profile showing the ups and downs of that journey.

A useful map series for planning is the USDA Forest Service topographic series for most individual wilderness areas. (In this book, Granite Chief Wilderness seems to be the only wilderness that lacks such a map.) The scale of most maps of this series is 1:63,360 (1 inch = 1 mile), which is very close to that of the former USGS 15′ series (1:62,500), and each conveniently covers the entire wilderness area on one map. However, you may find these maps a bit bulky for the trail.

Most backpackers prefer to use a topographic (topo) map with finer detail than the above overview/planning maps. Hikers typically prefer the USGS 7.5′ series, where the elevation is usually shown in 40-foot contour intervals.

Wilderness Press still publishes and regularly updates a few 15′ topos for some areas covered by *Sierra North*. These Wilderness Press 15′ topos include indexes of the place names on them and are printed on waterproof, tear-resistant plastic. If any one or more of these maps covers all or part of a given trip, their titles appear in ***bold italics*** at the beginning of the trip under the section Topos. Unlike ordinary USGS topos, these maps show details of the adjacent national forest or park for your greater convenience in trip-planning. Wilderness Press still publishes the following 15′ quads that apply to *Sierra North: Hetch Hetchy Reservoir, Merced Peak,* and *Yosemite.*

Wilderness Press also publishes maps especially for Desolation Wilderness, Emigrant Wilderness, and Yosemite National Park. The *Desolation Wilderness* map is available separately and within Jeffrey P. Schaffer's *Desolation Wilderness and the South Lake Tahoe Basin.* The *Emigrant Wilderness* map is available separately and within Ben Schifrin's *Emigrant Wilderness and Northwestern Yosemite.* The *Yosemite National Park & Vicinity Recreation Map* is available separately and within Jeffrey P. Schaffer's *Yosemite National Park.* This map includes not only the park but also much of the adjacent Ansel Adams, Emigrant, and Hoover wildernesses.

You can also use commercially available software to print out your own topographic maps at your choice of scale and detail. Protect these printouts if the ink is prone to run.

How and Where to Get Your Maps

Order Wilderness Press 15' topos and other maps as well as books directly from Wilderness Press online at www.wildernesspress.com or by phone at 800-443-7227.

USGS topos for California as well as Wilderness Press maps and books are available by phone and email from the former Wilderness Press retail outlet, now independently owned: The Map Center at 510-658-3650 or Californiamaplady@netzero.net.

Also, backpacking stores and some bookstores—especially those near popular hiking areas—carry at least the topographic maps for hikes in their areas as well as the software required to print your own. USGS topographic maps and US Forest Service maps are available at many ranger stations and at stations that issue wilderness permits.

USGS's online store sells USGS maps at store.usgs.gov. Or contact the USGS Western Region office at 345 Middlefield Road, Menlo Park, CA 94025; 650-853-8300.

Maps for Ultralight Backpacking

We strongly recommend that you do not cut up your maps as some people recommend for ultralight backpacking. The weight saved is almost negligible, but the information lost is not: When you take a wrong turn and end up a mile or more off your planned route—and it will happen—you must have that information in order to get back on track.

How to Use This Book

Terms This Book Uses

Destination/UTM Coordinates: This new edition provides UTM coordinates for GPS users. For this edition, most of the UTM data are not from the field but are from software like National Geographic's TOPO! In the trip entries, we note which datum we obtained from the field by including "(field)" after the datum. Most of the UTM data in this edition are for trailheads and trip destinations. Because these data are all UTM data with the appropriate meters east (mE) and meters north (mN), we don't repeat those labels but show UTM data in this form: 10S 727068 4364426.

Trip Type: This book classifies a trip as one of four types. An **out-and-back** trip goes out to a destination and returns the way it came. A **loop** trip goes out by one route and returns by another with relatively little or no retracing of the same trail. A **semiloop** trip has an out-and-back part and a loop part; the loop part may occur anywhere along the way, and if it's in the middle, there are two out-and-back parts. A **shuttle** trip starts at one trailhead and ends at another; usually, the trailheads are too far apart for you to walk between them, so you will need to leave a car at the ending (take-out) trailhead, have someone pick you up there, or rely on California's scanty and ill-organized public transportation to get back to your starting (put-in) trailhead.

Best Season: Deciding when in the year is the best time for a particular trip is a difficult task because of yearly variations. Low early-season temperatures and mountain shadows often keep some of the higher passes closed until well into August. Early snows have been known to whiten alpine country in late July and August. Some of the trips described here are low-country ones, offered specifically for the itchy hiker who, stiff from a winter's inactivity, is searching for a warm-up excursion. These trips are labeled **early**, a period that extends roughly from late May to early July. **Mid** is from early July to the end of August, and **late** is from then to early October.

Pace: For each trip, we give the number of days you'd spend hiking at the trip's described pace as well as the number of layover days (below) you might want to take. Galen Clark, Yosemite's beloved "Old Man of the Valley," was once asked how he "got about" the park.

Clark scratched his beard and then replied, "Slowly!" And that is the philosophy we have adopted in this book. Since this book is written for the average backpacker, we chose to describe most trips on either a **leisurely** or a **moderate** basis, depending on where the best overnight camping places were along the route. We also call a few trips **strenuous**. A leisurely pace lets hikers absorb more of the sights, smells, and "feel" of the country they have come to see. Pace may not be everything, but Old Man Clark lived to the ripe old age of 96, and it behooves us to follow in his footsteps.

Layover Days: These are days when you'll want to remain camped at a particular site so you can dayhike to see other beautiful places around the area or enjoy some adventures like peak-bagging. The number of layover days you take and where are purely personal choices, to be balanced with how much time you have and how much food you can carry. Our trip descriptions will help you pick where and when you want to take layover days.

Total Mileage: The trips in this book range in length between about 5 miles and 73 miles, and many trips can be shortened or extended, based on your interest and time.

Campsites: Campsites are labeled poor, fair, good, or excellent. The criteria for assigning these labels were amount of use, immediate surroundings, general scenery, presence of vandalism, availability of water, kind of ground cover, and recreational potential—angling, side trips, swimming, etc. Camping is forbidden on meadows and other vegetated areas and within a certain distance of any stream or lake (we recommend 200 feet). You will be informed of these rules for your areas when you get your wilderness permit. "Packer campsite" indicates a semi-permanent camp (usually constructed by packers for the "comfort of their clients") characterized by things like nailed-plank table or benches, nails in the surrounding trees, and/or a large, rock fireplace.

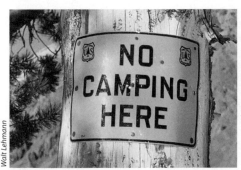
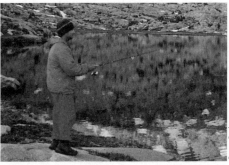

Be careful to oberve all camping and fishing regulations.

Fishing: Angling, for many, is a prime consideration when planning a trip, and many of the lakes in the Sierra are stocked. While we note the quality of fishing throughout the book, experienced anglers know that the size of their catch relates not only to quantity, type, and general size of the fishery, which are given, but also to water temperature, feed, angling skill, and that indefinable something known as "fisherman's luck." Generally speaking, the old "early and late" adage holds: Fishing is better early and late in the day, and early and late in the season.

Stream Crossings: Stream crossings vary greatly depending on snow-melt conditions. Often, June's raging torrent becomes September's placid creek. If a ford is described as "difficult in early season," fording that creek may be difficult because it is hard to walk through deep or fast water, and getting caught in the current would be dangerous. Whether you attempt such a crossing depends on the presence or absence of logs or other bridges, of downstream rapids or waterfalls, your ability and equipment, and your judgment. We mention manmade bridges and other manmade aids for you to cross on, but we usually don't mention chance aids like logs and rocks, because they can vary from year to year. (See pages 5–6 for tips for crossing streams more safely.)

Trail Type and Surface: Most of the trails described here are well maintained (the exceptions are noted) and are properly signed. If the trail becomes indistinct, look for blazes (peeled bark at eye level on trees) or ducks (two or more rocks piled one atop another). Trails may fade out in wet areas like meadows, and you may have to scout around to find where they resume. Continuing in the direction you were going when the trail faded out is often, but not always, a good bet.

Two other significant trail conditions have also been described in the text: the degree of openness (type and degree of forest cover, if any, or else "meadow," "brush," or whatever) and underfooting (talus, scree, pumice, sand, "duff"—a deep humus ground cover of rotting vegetation—or other material).

A "use trail" is an unmaintained, unofficial trail that is more or less easy to follow because it is well worn by use. For example, nearly every Sierra lakeshore has a use trail worn around it by anglers in search of their prey.

Landmarks: The text contains occasional references to points, peaks, and other landmarks. These places are shown on the appropriate topographic maps cited at the beginning of the trip. For example, "Point 9426" in the text would refer to a point designated simply "9426" on the map itself.

Fire Damage: The Forest Service and the Park Service have a policy of letting fires in the backcountry burn as long as they are not a threat to people or structures. One result has been some pretty poor-looking scenery on some trips in this book. However, most of the fire-damaged areas have begun to recover soon enough that we have chosen not to delete the affected trips from the book.

How This Book Is Organized

With one exception, the trips in this book are organized according to the highways that you must take to get to the trailheads in this book: US Interstate 80, State Hwy. 89, US Hwy. 50, State Hwy. 88, State Hwy. 4, State Hwy. 108, State Hwy. 120, and US Hwy. 395. One section, Western Yosemite Trips, is not organized around a highway. Within these major book sections are trailheads, from which the many trips begin.

TAHOE-YOSEMITE TRAIL

One trail, the 186-mile Tahoe-Yosemite Trail (TYT) is divided into six legs and extends throughout the book. We describe the TYT from north (Tahoe's Meeks Bay) to south (Yosemite's Tuolumne Meadows), but the trip can also be done from south to north by reversing those directions.

Trailhead and Trip Organization: As previously noted, each trip is located within trailhead sections in the book. These sections begin with a summary table, such as the fictitious one below, that uses the trailhead's name, destination, and UTM coordinates as its title:

Black Powder Trailhead

7654'; 10S 736921 4328622

DESTINATION/ UTM COORDINATES	TRIP TYPE	BEST SEASON	PACE (HIKING/ LAYOVER DAYS)	TOTAL MILEAGE
1 Bear Corral 10S 735694 4338773	Out & back	Early to mid	2/1 Moderate	18
2 Sunshine Lake 10S 733543 4347890	Out & back	Mid to late	4/1 Moderate, part cross-country	31

Following the table are details about information, permits, and driving directions to that trailhead.

Next comes the first trip from this trailhead. The trip data—UTM coordinates, total mileage, and hiking/layover days—are included with each trip entry. All trips include an elevation profile, a list of maps, and highlights. Some include *HEADS UP!*, or special considerations for that trip, and shuttle trips include directions to the take-out trailhead.

I Bear Corral

Trip Data: 10S 735694 4338773; 18 miles; 2/1 days

Topos: *Pickle Springs*

Highlights: Follow a pair of delightful streams to a secluded basin rimmed by granite cliffs on the eastern fringe of XYZ Wilderness.

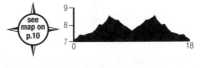

DAY 1 (Black Powder Trailhead to Bear Corral, 9 miles): From the trailhead, make a short climb northeast through a canopy of lodgepole, red fir, and white fir. Birds are abundant here, especially Steller's jays, white-crowned sparrows, juncos, and chickadees. Soon the route reaches a junction with the PCT. Turn right (east) here and….

…to the good camping at forested Bear Corral (7654'; 10S 735694 4338773).

DAY 2 (Bear Corral to Black Powder Trailhead, 9 miles): Retrace your steps.

After this comes the next trip, if any, from this same trailhead. Trips in the same general area, especially multiple trips from the same trailhead, often build upon each other. For example, the first trip from a trailhead is usually the shortest—one day out to a destination, the next day back to the trailhead. The second trip will build on—extend—the first trip by following the first trip's first day and then continuing on a second and subsequent days to more distant destinations. Rather than repeat the full, detailed description for the first trip's first day, we recapitulate it as briefly as possible with the essential trail instructions to get you to that day's destination. We also identify this as a recapitulation and give you a reference to the trip and day we're recapitulating, like this: *(Recap: Trip 1, Day 1.)*. If you wish, you can turn to that description to read everything we have to say about that day, which includes details about natural and human history—things that are fun to know but not essential for getting from the trailhead to the destination.

Trailhead Maps: Each trailhead section includes a map such as the one below. The legend that follows defines the symbols used in the maps in the book.

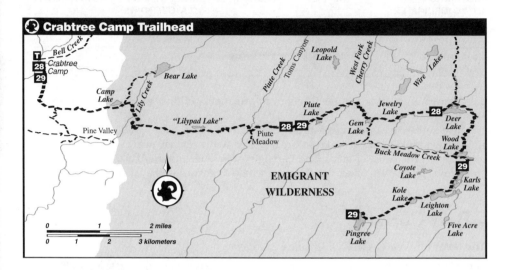

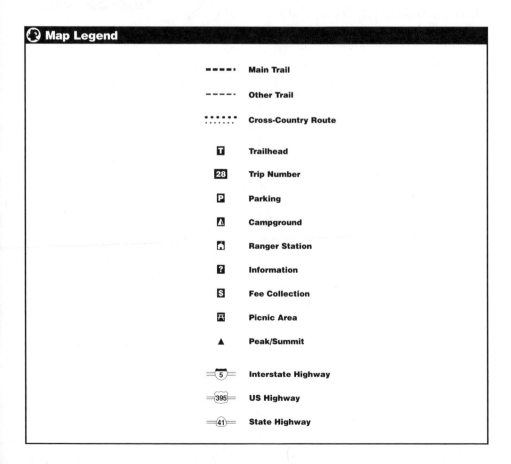

US INTERSTATE 80 TRIPS

The terrain around Donner Summit is a popular recreational playground for a host of northern Californian residents and visitors to the greater Lake Tahoe area. Despite this popularity, backpackers can find serenity at a trio of backcountry lakes cupped into granite cirques, part of the proposed Castle Peak Wilderness Area. The northbound PCT takes you from I-80 into this proposed wilderness. All trips from I-80 start from that northbound PCT trailhead.

TRAILHEAD: Castle Peak

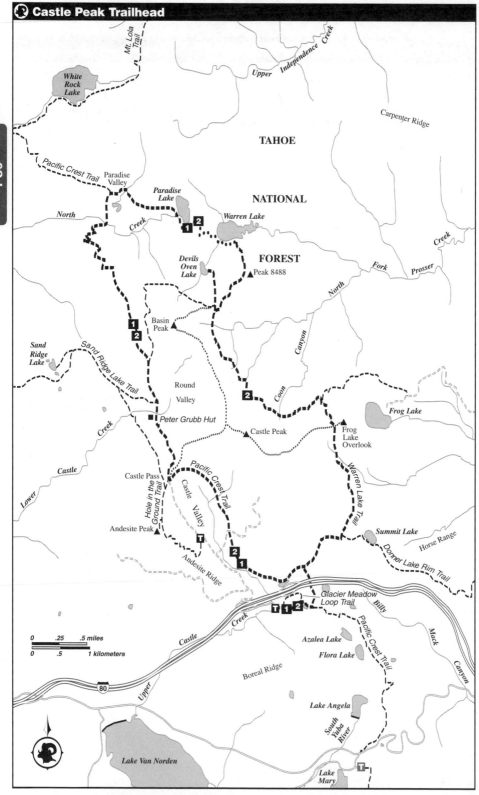

Castle Peak Trailhead

7200'; 10S 728986 4357808 (field)

DESTINATION/ UTM COORDINATES	TRIP TYPE	BEST SEASON	PACE (HIKING/ LAYOVER DAYS)	TOTAL MILEAGE
1 Paradise Lake 10S 727068 4364426	Out & Back	Mid to late	2/0 Moderate	15.4
2 Castle Peak Wilderness Loop 10S 728986 4357808	Loop	Mid to late	3/1 Moderate, part cross-country	16.4

Information and Permits: The proposed Castle Peak Wilderness is in Tahoe National Forest: 631 Coyote Street, Nevada City, CA 95959; 530-265-4531; www.fs.fed.us/r5/tahoe/. Specific information about Castle Peak Wilderness may not appear on the website until the area receives congressional wilderness designation. For now, you don't need a wilderness permit, but you do need a California Campfire Permit for campfires and stoves.

Driving Directions: West of Donner Summit, take the Castle Peak/Boreal Ridge Road exit from I-80, drive to the frontage road on the south side of the freeway, and then proceed east 0.3 mile to the PCT parking area. The large parking lot has trailer parking, pit toilets, and running water in season.

1 Paradise Lake

Trip Data: 10S 727068 4364426; 15.4 miles; 2/0 days

Topos: *Norden, Independence Lake*

see map on p.16

Highlights: The PCT combined with a 1-mile stretch of abandoned jeep road provides a well-graded route to island-dotted Paradise Lake, one of the most picturesque subalpine lakes in the greater Tahoe area. For those who aren't up to the more difficult trek of the full loop past Warren Lake, with a side trip to Devils Oven Lake on the way, an out-and-back trip to Paradise Lake is a great way to spend a couple of days or more.

DAY 1 (Castle Peak Trailhead to Paradise Lake, 7.7 miles): From the parking lot, follow a well-signed gravel path to a stone bridge over a seasonal stream and continue on dirt track through lodgepole pines, western white pines, and white firs. Soon you encounter a junction with the Glacier Meadow Loop and proceed ahead (east) toward the PCT. After a short distance you pass by a second junction with the Glacier Meadow Loop and continue ahead (east) toward the PCT. Head past a shallow pond, where mountain hemlocks join the mixed forest, and then make a short descent to the well-signed PCT junction near the edge of a grass-and-willow-filled meadow.

Turn left and head north on the PCT around the fringe of the meadow to a pair of large culverts underneath the eastbound and westbound lanes of I-80. Pass under I-80 and beyond the culverts, make a moderate climb to the crossing of a seasonal creek and then come to a well-signed junction, 1 mile from the trailhead.

At the junction, turn left (southwest) on the PCT, following signed directions to Castle Pass. The PCT rises and then drops to the north shore of a small pond and an unsigned path to the westbound Donner Summit Rest Area. Stay on the PCT here.

Beyond the unmarked junction, follow the gently graded PCT through mixed forest toward Castle Valley. The trail nears Castle Creek for a brief time and then travels just east of the verdant meadows of Castle Valley, where a pair of use trails branch away toward the creek and meadows. Cross a well-traveled dirt road and then continue upstream along the edge of Castle Valley, hopping over a number of lushly lined tributaries along the way.

Nearing the head of the valley, the PCT bends west, then south-southwest on an ascending traverse to a signed junction with a connecting trail from the Castle Valley Road. From there, make a short but stiff climb to Castle Pass and a junction with a trio of paths: northeast to the summit of Castle Peak, southeast to a connection with the trail to Andesite Peak, and north on the PCT toward Round Valley.

Take the middle fork north from Castle Pass, remaining on the PCT, on a traverse across a lightly forested slope. After about a half mile, begin a moderate, switchbacking descent toward Round Valley. Nearing the floor of the valley, pass a very short use trail on the left that leads to Peter Grubb Hut.

PETER GRUBB HUT

Following a ski trip to the Swiss Alps, Harold T. Bradley, university professor and former president of the Sierra Club, proposed a string of six alpine huts between Donner and Echo passes, similar to the ones he'd experienced in the Alps. Although only four of the six were eventually completed, the huts have provided warm shelter for many visitors since the late 1930s. Peter Grubb Hut is complete with a wood-burning stove and firewood, a gas stove and cooking utensils, a table and chairs, a loft with sleeping platforms, solar lights, and a detached outhouse. Interesting old photos and memorabilia cover the walls and provide a sample of the area's history. Except for emergency shelter, overnight use of Peter Grubb Hut is by reservation only. Contact the Sierra Club at Clair Tappaan Lodge, P.O. Box 36, Norden, CA 95724; 530-426-3632; www.sierraclub.org/outings/lodges/ctl/.

The PCT crosses Lower Castle Creek just north of the hut and then soon comes to a Y-junction with the Sand Ridge Trail, where you continue ahead, northbound.

Skirt the western fringe of Round Valley through light forest and then follow a moderate climb with occasional filtered views of the terrain to the west. Break out of the trees to sweeping views farther up the southwest shoulder of Basin Peak and ascend open slopes carpeted with willows and wildflowers.

BASIN PEAK

Peakbaggers can leave the trail anywhere near the high point and make a straightforward climb of flower-covered, volcanic slopes to the top of 9017-foot Basin Peak, which affords a wide-ranging vista of the northern Tahoe Sierra. A use trail along the crest of the ridge connecting the summits of Basin and Castle peaks offers climbers with some extra time the opportunity to double summit.

After cresting the shoulder of Basin Peak, the PCT follows a mellow descending traverse across flower-laden slopes before returning to light forest, where an extended, switchbacking descent heads toward the floor of Paradise Valley. At the bottom of the descent, stroll amid pines and firs with a lush understory of plants and flowers to a bridged crossing of lazy North Creek meandering through the tall grass. A gentle, winding climb from the bridge

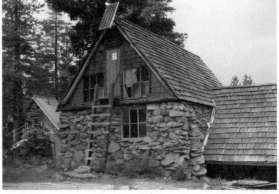

Mike White

Peter Grubb Hut

leads past a pond surrounded by the meadows of Paradise Valley to a signed junction with the track of an old jeep road traveling east toward Paradise Lake, 6.6 miles from the parking lot. Early season visitors to Paradise Valley will be alternately rewarded with a fine display of wildflowers and cursed with hordes of pesky mosquitoes.

Leaving the PCT, turn right (east) at the junction and follow the easy grade of the jeep road around the northern perimeter of Paradise Valley, a verdant clearing carpeted with a dense swath of plants and flowers. Leaving the clearing behind, the jeep road makes a moderate climb through scattered conifers and granite boulders. Eventually, the track of the old road falters, but a ducked route continues the climb toward the obvious location of the lake at the head of the cirque.

Several campsites are clustered around the west side of the picturesque lake (7728'; 10S 727068 4364426) in sandy pockets between the numerous granite slabs scattered around the shoreline. More secluded camping is available along the southwest shore and the saddle above the east shore, where the view down to Warren Lake is quite impressive

DAY 2 (Paradise Lake to Castle Peak Trailhead, 7.7 miles): Retrace your steps to return.

2 Castle Peak Wilderness Loop

Trip Data: 10S 728986 4357808 (field);
16.4 miles; 3/1 days

Topos: *Norden, Independence Lake*

Highlights: While the elevation gain and loss experienced along this route requires hikers to be in good physical condition, the rewards of incomparable views, picturesque lakes, vibrant wildflowers, and exquisite scenery more than make up for the extra effort. Additional cross-country routes to the summits of Basin or Castle peaks and plenty of connecting trails provide tantalizing ways to extend your visit to these lands.

HEADS UP! *Because of the potentially dangerous cross-country route between Paradise and Warren lakes and the indistinct trail to Devils Oven Lake, this trip is appropriate for experienced hikers only.*

DAY 1 (Castle Peak Trailhead to Paradise Lake, 7.7 miles): *(Recap: Trip 1, Day 1.)* From the Castle Peak Trailhead, take the gravel path over the stone bridge, and then follow dirt track eastward, going ahead (east) at both junctions with the Glacier Meadow Loop. Where you meet the PCT, turn left (north) and pass under I-80 to a seasonal stream and a signed junction where you turn left (southwest) to stay on the PCT, heading for Castle Pass. The trail presently curves northwest to an unsigned junction where you go ahead (north) to stay on the PCT along Castle Valley, passing by use trails into it. Cross a dirt road and continue on the PCT as it bends west and then southwest to a junction with a trail to Castle Valley Road. Stay on the PCT here, climbing southwest to Castle Pass and a junction with three trails. Take the middle fork, the PCT, north toward Round Valley, passing the use trail to the Peter Grubb Hut. Skirt Round Valley, ascend the shoulder of Basin Peak, and descend into Paradise Valley. At the junction with the old road to Paradise Lake, turn left (east) to leave the PCT and follow first the road and then ducks to the lake (7728'; 10S 727068 4364426).

DAY 2 (Paradise Lake to Devils Oven Lake, 2 miles, part cross-country): A short climb up and over some bedrock cliffs at the south end of Paradise Lake is necessary in order to reach the saddle and the continuation of the loop trip via the cross-country route down to Warren Lake.

From the saddle above the east shore of Paradise Lake, look for a large cairn at the head of a rock slot that signifies the beginning of the ducked cross-country route down to

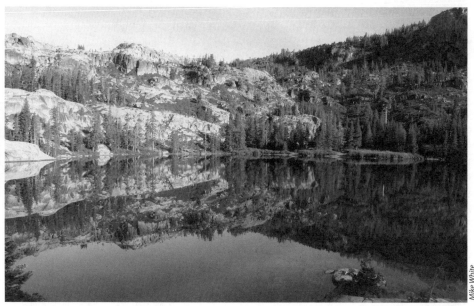

Mike White

Warren Lake

Warren Lake. Head south from the saddle on an angling descent across the headwall of Warren Lake's cirque to a slightly rising traverse below the base of some steep cliffs. Drop down some steep rocks and then follow a rocky swale through shrubs to easier terrain below, where the route bends left to avoid some talus. Continue the descent over rock slabs interspersed with sandy patches through waist-high shrubs toward the tree-lined southwest shore. Nearing the lake, very briefly follow an alder-lined stream to a secluded campsite and proceed a very short distance to the use trail that hugs the shoreline. Head right (east) on the use trail and stroll past several campsites and over a couple of tiny streams to the midpoint of Warren Lake's south shore (7210'; 10S 727068 364426), where a maintained trail resumes in an attack of the steep, 1000-foot slope above.

Leaving the south shore of Warren Lake, one of the steepest miles of trail in the greater Lake Tahoe region winds tightly up a bedrock gully toward a high saddle in the ridge directly southwest of Peak 8488. Complicating matters somewhat, the trail is quite rocky in places, providing laboring hikers with poor footing for a steep ascent. By getting an early start, at least the seemingly interminable climb can be done under shade and the relatively cool temperatures of morning. After cresting the lip of the basin, a more moderate climb over the last 150 vertical feet leads across drier slopes with widely scattered mountain hemlocks and western white pines. Persistence is finally rewarded at the saddle with an impressive view to the south of North Fork Prosser Creek's sweeping basin arcing past Basin Peak and the impressive battlements of Castle Peak to Frog Lake Overlook, and also westward down the creek's verdant canyon to Carpenter Valley. At the saddle a use trail veers left, petering out before reaching an exposed overlook of the canyon below, including an inviting-looking pond surrounded by lush greenery.

Turn right (west) at the saddle and follow a more reasonably graded trail to the crest of a ridge and across an open, flower-filled slope to a junction with the trail to Devils Oven Lake. A sign at the junction provides this ominous warning for those bound for the lake: ROUGH TRAIL.

To reach Devils Oven Lake, turn sharply right (north), away from the Warren Lake Trail, and follow the Devils Oven Lake Trail on a climb to a level area on the crest of a ridge. Close attention must be paid here, as the more obvious route on the ground leads not to the lake but on an arcing traverse on abandoned roads around the north and east sides of Basin Peak to a connection with the PCT southwest of the summit (a route that seems to be increasingly popular with the equestrian crowd). The deteriorating route to Devils Oven Lake heads north from the level area on a curving descent that bends northwest before arriving at the southeast shore (7874'; 10S 727629 4363411). Campsites appear to be more limited here than at the neighboring lakes, a testament to the fact that most backpackers are unwilling to make the steep climbs out of both Devils Oven and Warren lakes.

DAY 3 (Devils Oven Lake to Castle Peak Trailhead, 6.7 miles): Return to the junction between the Devils Oven Lake and Warren Lake trails. From the junction, turn right (south) to begin an undulating 2.5-mile traverse of the head of North Fork Prosser Creek's upper basin, across flower-filled slopes and several willow-and-flower-lined streams. Over the course of this traverse between the junction and the saddle below Frog Lake Overlook, the trail gradually curves east as it gains and loses a considerable amount of elevation due to the uneven terrain of the upper basin. After crossing the last stream in Coon Canyon, the trail begins a final, stiff climb toward the saddle. You reach a junction at a small flat on the top of a ridge midway through this climb, where an old, seldom-used trail heads left (east) to the privately owned environs around Frog Lake. You go right (south). After the brief respite, the gently rising trail leads across a stream before a steep, winding climb to a junction on the saddle below Frog Lake Overlook. The short path on the left (east) to the overlook shouldn't be missed, as the view straight down Frog Lake Cliff to the lake is a dramatic sight.

Return to the main trail and turn left (south) back onto the Warren Lake Trail. After the previous undulating route across North Fork Prosser Creek's basin, you're grateful to find that the trail from the saddle is all downhill back to the parking lot. Initially, the trail follows a gentle-to-moderate descent across a slope covered with acres and acres of mule ears—a beautiful sight at peak bloom—before a steeper descent leads back into the cover of mixed forest. Amid the trees, the trail crosses several trickling, flower-lined little streams on the way to an extensive clearing covered with wildflowers and shrubs that grants one

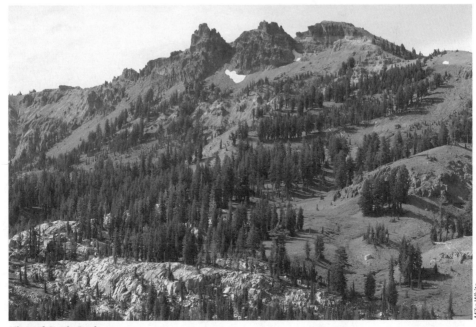

View of Castle Peak

Mike White

last expansive vista—this one of the Carson Range to the east and the Donner Pass peaks to the south. Returning to a shady forest, the trail makes a winding descent down to a junction on the left with the short lateral heading eastward to tree-rimmed Summit Lake. Backpackers reluctant to end their journey may find reasonable campsites at this popular lake.

Go right (west) from the Summit Lake junction and continue through the forest cover, broken momentarily by a substantial, open meadow thick with flowers and willows. The forest thins for a while again where the trail passes through an area sprinkled with granite boulders and slabs as the trail makes its way to closing the loop at the junction with the PCT. From there, turn right (south-southeast) to retrace your steps 1 mile to the parking lot.

I-80

STATE HIGHWAY 89 TRIPS

Trips in this section start from four trailheads (from north to south): the Powderhorn Trailhead into Granite Chief Wilderness; into Desolation Wilderness, Lake Tahoe's Meeks Bay Trailhead, start of Section 1 of the TYT, and Lake Tahoe's Bayview Trailhead; and the Big Meadow Trailhead into Meiss Country.

Although set within the popular Tahoe Basin, Granite Chief Wilderness is extremely lightly used in comparison to other areas around the lake, particularly the ever-popular Desolation Wilderness. Instead of permits and quotas, backpackers will experience deep forests, rushing streams, seasonal wildflowers, excellent views, and fewer people.

Above the southwest shore of Lake Tahoe, Desolation Wilderness encompasses 63,690 acres of federally protected backcountry. The terrain resembles a miniature High Sierra, albeit at a lower elevation, with deep blue lakes, craggy summits, and granite peaks and basins showing extensive signs of glaciation from the last Ice Age. The Meeks Bay Trailhead also features the beginning of the TYT, which stretches almost 186 miles from Lake Tahoe's Meeks Bay to Yosemite's Tuolumne Meadows and traverses some of the northern Sierra's loveliest territory. It's a fine complement to the JMT and is even more of an adventure.

South of Lake Tahoe, bounded on the east by Hwy. 89, and in between Hwy. 50 and Hwy. 88 lies Meiss Country, a proposed wilderness area of deep forests, scenic lakes, and expansive meadows that saw far fewer visitors before the fairly recent creation of the Tahoe Rim Trail. Despite this increased popularity, the area still affords backpackers a reasonable dose of serenity along with the stunning scenery.

TRAILHEADS: Powderhorn
Meeks Bay
Bayview
Big Meadow

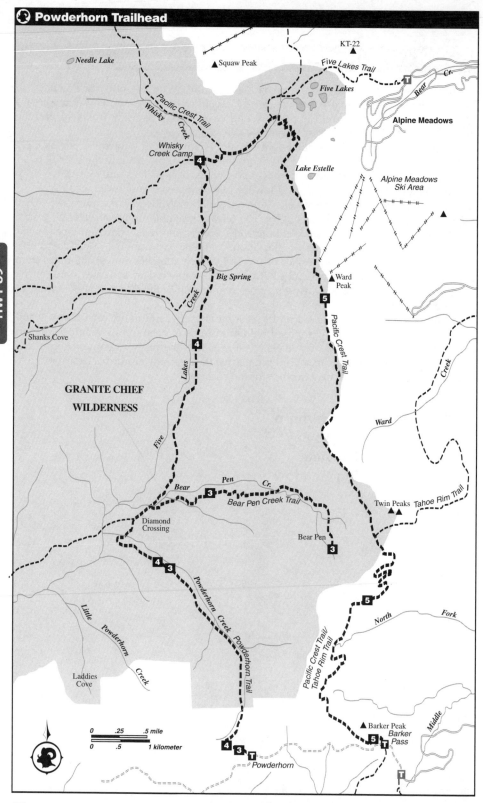

HWY 89

Needle Lake

▲ Squaw Peak

KT-22 ▲

Five Lakes Trail

Five Lakes

1

Bear Cr.

Alpine Meadows

Pacific Crest Trail

Whisky Creek

Whisky Creek Camp

4

Lake Estelle

Alpine Meadows Ski Area

▲

Big Spring

Creek

5

▲ Ward Peak

Pacific Crest Trail

Shanks Cove

4

GRANITE CHIEF WILDERNESS

Five Lakes

Creek

Ward

Creek

Bear Pen *Cr.*

3

Bear Pen Creek Trail

Twin Peaks ▲▲

Tahoe Rim Trail

Diamond Crossing

Bear Pen

3

4 **3**

5

Powderhorn Creek

North Fork

Little Powderhorn Creek

Powderhorn Trail

Pacific Crest Trail/ Tahoe Rim Trail

Laddies Cove

0   .25   .5 mile
0   .5   1 kilometer

▲ Barker Peak

5 *Barker Pass*

1

4 **3** **1**

Powderhorn

Middle

1

Powderhorn Trailhead

7640'; 10S 736921 4328622 (field)

DESTINATION/ UTM COORDINATES	TRIP TYPE	BEST SEASON	PACE (HIKING/ LAYOVER DAYS)	TOTAL MILEAGE
3 Bear Pen 10S 738116 4332843	Out & back	Mid to late	2/1 Moderate	13.5
4 Whisky Creek Camp 10S 735694 4338773	Out & back	Mid to late	4/1 Moderate	27.5
5 Barker Pass 10S 739116 4328964 for loop (field) 10S 736921 432862 for shuttle (field)	Shuttle or loop	Mid to late	3/1 Strenuous	25 (shuttle) or 26.5 (loop)

Information and Permits: Granite Chief Wilderness is in the Tahoe National Forest: 631 Coyote Street, Nevada City, CA 95959; 530-265-4531; www.fs.fed.us/r5/tahoe/recreation/gchief/. You don't need a wilderness permit for overnight travel, but you do need a California Campfire Permit for campfires and stoves. Currently, dogs are banned from fawning areas from May 15 to July 15; check with Tahoe National Forest for details.

Driving Directions: From Hwy. 89, about 4 miles south of its junction with Hwy. 28 in Tahoe City, turn west onto Barker Pass Road (FS Road 03), marked SNO-PARK and KASPIAN CAMPGROUND. Follow FS Road 03 along the north side of the valley, bend left to cross Blackwood Creek near the 2-mile mark, and then continue up the south side of Blackwood Canyon to the PCT trailhead parking area near Barker Pass (7644'; 10S 739116 4328964), 7 miles from Hwy. 89. To get to the Powderhorn Trailhead, continue downhill from Barker Pass another 1.5 miles to the signed Powderhorn Trailhead (7640'; 10S 736921 4328622), where limited parking is available for two or three vehicles.

3 Bear Pen

Trip Data: 10S 738116 4332843; 13.5 miles; 2/1 days

Topos: *Wentworth Springs*

Highlights: Follow a pair of delightful streams to a secluded basin rimmed by granite cliffs on the eastern fringe of Granite Chief Wilderness.

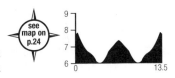

DAY 1 (Powderhorn Trailhead to Bear Pen, 6.75 miles): From the trailhead, make a short climb through selectively logged fir forest to a dirt road and follow that road to a bend, where the marked route continues ahead. Descend the old roadbed to a sharp curve, where a trail marker directs hikers to veer left (generally north) onto single-track trail. This section of trail makes a steep, winding descent across a flower-lined seasonal stream to another dirt road, which you briefly follow until the single-track trail resumes.

Continue the descent past the signed Granite Chief Wilderness boundary down Powderhorn Creek's canyon. Along the descent, avalanche swaths have thinned the forest enough in spots to allow a profusion of wildflowers, plants, and shrubs to flourish. Amid a thickening forest, cross a narrow stream flowing through a tangle of alders and colorful wildflowers and proceed on a gentle to moderate descent down the canyon. The grade eventually eases where the trail crosses a wildflower-carpeted meadow and then encounters a boulder-hop ford of Powderhorn Creek (may be difficult in early season). There's a marginal campsite near the crossing.

Heading northeast, the trail proceeds through the trees for about 300 yards to the open meadow known as Diamond Crossing. Pass by a marked junction in this meadow, where a very faint trail (the old Hell Hole Trail) heads southwest toward a trailhead near Hell Hole Reservoir. Bear right (northwest) at this junction to continue through the meadow, and then reenter forest on the way to a second junction, this one with a slightly more distinct trail heading up the canyon of Bear Pen Creek.

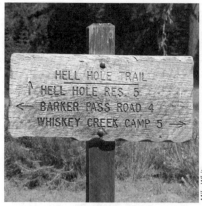

Turn right and head east on the Bear Pen Creek Trail on a moderate climb up a canyon filled with thick forest. The trail to Bear Pen is infrequently used and the tread tends to falter where it crosses a small meadow. After 2.75 miles from the last junction of the mostly forested trail, reach a willow-and-grass-filled meadow known as Bear Pen (7436'; 10S 738116 4332843), an opening in the thick forest backdropped by a dramatic

Trail sign for the old Hell Hole Trail

amphitheater of cliffs. Little-used, hemlock-shaded campsites around the meadow's perimeter offer secluded camping to solitude seekers. With a little luck, visitors may also see a namesake critter or two.

DAY 2 (Bear Pen to Powderhorn Trailhead, 6.75 miles): Retrace your steps.

4 Whisky Creek Camp

Trip Data: 10S 735694 4338773;
27.5 miles; 4/1 days

see map on p.24

Topos: *Wentworth Springs,*
Granite Chief

Highlights: Increase your enjoyment of
peaceful Granite Chief Wilderness by extending your trip to Whisky Creek Camp, where you can spend the night in the company of historic structures.

DAY 1 (Powderhorn Trailhead to Bear Pen, 6.75 miles): *(Recap: Trip 3, Day 1.)* From the Powderhorn Trailhead, climb on trail to a dirt road and follow that road to a bend where the marked route continues ahead. Descend the old roadbed to a sharp curve, where a trail marker directs hikers to veer left (generally north) onto single-track trail. Make a steep, winding descent to another dirt road, which you briefly follow until the single-track trail resumes. Continue on this trail to the wilderness boundary and then down Powderhorn Creek's canyon to the junction with the Bear Pen Creek Trail. Turn right and take this trail 2.75 miles to Bear Pen (7436'; 10S 738116 4332843).

DAY 2 (Bear Pen to Whisky Creek Camp, 7 miles): Retrace your steps 2.75 miles to the junction of the Bear Pen Creek and Five Lakes Creek trails. From the junction, turn right and head north on the Five Lakes Creek Trail through a mixed forest of incense cedar, Jeffrey pine, and red and white firs, immediately encountering the crossing of Bear Pen Creek. Beyond the crossing, briefly follow alongside the alder-lined course of Bear Pen Creek until it bends eastward, and then proceed up the trail on a gentle ascent of forested Five Lakes Creek's canyon. About a mile from the junction, damp soils allow a sprinkling of aspens to join the forest, a few specimens with trunks as massive as 2 feet in diameter. A half mile farther on, the trail crosses the rocky channel of the seasonal outlet from Grouse Canyon and then continues another quarter mile to a trickling, spring-fed rivulet lined with grasses and wildflowers.

Another half mile of gently graded trail from the spring-fed rivulet leads to a signed junction just before a good-size meadow. Despite directions on a sign for Whisky Creek Camp to the left, any indication of a trail on the ground has almost completely disappeared, and it is virtually impossible to follow. Therefore, continue straight ahead (north), following signed directions for Big Spring.

Crossing the meadow north of the junction, the tread may be difficult to follow through the tall grasses, but a distinct path reappears where the trail reenters the forest. From the meadow, a shady half mile of easy walking leads to Big Spring, a gurgling eruption of water surrounded by alders at the south end of a large meadow, where a nearby grove of conifers harbors a couple of decent campsites. Although defined trail disappears in the meadow grass beyond the spring and the campsites, find where the trail resumes at the west edge of the meadow, about midway through the clearing. This path leads shortly down to a ford of Five Lakes Creek and just as shortly up to a junction (10S 735706 4336951) with a faint trail heading south toward Shanks Cove and more pronounced tread heading north toward Whisky Creek Camp.

Turn right (north) at the junction and follow a gently graded trail on the west side of alder-lined Five Lakes Creek for 0.3 mile to the crossing of a side stream. Beyond this stream, the grade of the ascent increases to moderate until you experience a momentary respite upon reaching the forested flat that harbors Whisky Creek Camp (6925'; 10S 735694 4338773). A log cabin with metal roof, a smaller shed, and a cooking fireplace are the three historic structures that occupy the south side of the flat. (Camping is not allowed inside the cabin or within 250 feet of the structures). Nearby is a three-way junction with a trail headed west toward the Greyhorse Valley Trailhead. Overnighters will find a couple of shady campsites on the north side of the flat. Nearby Five Lakes Creek supplies water.

DAYS 3–4 (Whisky Creek Camp to Powderhorn Trailhead, 13.75 miles): Retrace your steps.

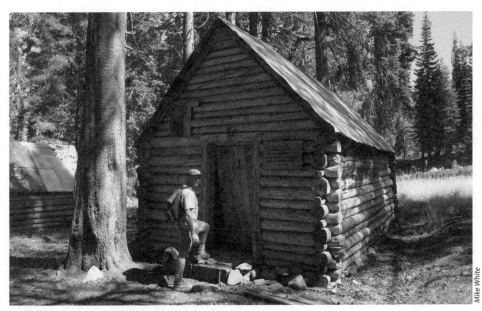

Mike White

Historic structures at Whisky Creek Camp

5 Barker Pass

Trip Data: 10S 739116 4328964 (field);
25 miles (shuttle) or 26.5 miles (loop);
3/1 days

Topos: *Wentworth Springs, Granite Chief,*
Tahoe City, Homewood

Highlights: On the first part of this journey, backpackers are treated to a shady, old-growth forest that escaped the axes of the lumbermen who denuded the Tahoe Basin of most of its timber during the Comstock Lode frenzy in the 19th century. Secluded camping, colorful wildflowers, and dancing streams are delightful attractions. The second part of the trip follows a section of the PCT on a ridge route that offers sweeping vistas. To do this trip as a loop, see the loop directions on page 30.

HEADS UP! *The heart of Granite Chief Wilderness is a lonely parcel of land where little-used trails can disappear in grassy meadows—make sure you carry a map and compass.*

Shuttle Directions: If taking the shuttle trip between the Powderhorn Trailhead and the Barker Pass Trailhead, leave your first car at the Barker Pass Trailhead (7644'; 10S 739116 4328964 (field)) and your second at the Powderhorn Trailhead (7640'; 10S 736921 4328622 (field)), 1.5 miles farther west down Barker Pass Road.

DAY 1 (Powderhorn Trailhead to Bear Pen, 6.75 miles): *(Recap: Trip 3, Day 1.)* From the Powderhorn Trailhead, climb on trail to a dirt road and follow that road to a bend where the marked route continues ahead. Descend the old roadbed to a sharp curve, where a trail marker directs hikers to veer left (generally north) onto single-track trail. Make a steep, winding descent to another dirt road, which you briefly follow until the single-track trail resumes. Continue on this trail to the wilderness boundary and then down Powderhorn Creek's canyon to the junction with the Bear Pen Creek Trail. Turn right and take this trail 2.75 miles to Bear Pen (7436'; 10S 738116 4332843).

DAY 2 (Bear Pen to Whisky Creek Camp, 7 miles): *(Recap: Trip 4, Day 2.)* Retrace your steps 2.75 miles to the junction of the Bear Pen Creek and Five Lakes Creek trails. From the junction, turn right and head north on the Five Lakes Creek Trail, immediately encountering the crossing of Bear Pen Creek. Beyond the crossing, briefly follow alongside the alder-lined course of Bear Pen Creek until it bends eastward, and then proceed up the trail in forested Five Lakes Creek canyon. Cross the rocky channel of the seasonal outlet from Grouse Canyon and then continue another quarter mile to a rivulet.

Another half mile from the rivulet leads to a signed junction just before a good-size meadow. The signed trail to Whisky Creek Camp is virtually impossible to follow. Therefore, continue straight ahead (north), following signed directions for Big Spring.

Crossing the meadow north of the junction, the tread may be difficult to follow through the tall grasses, but a distinct path reappears where the trail reenters the forest. From the meadow, an easy half mile leads to Big Spring at the south end of a large meadow; nearby conifers harbor campsites. Although defined trail disappears in the meadow grass beyond the spring and the campsites, the trail resumes at the west edge of the meadow, about midway through the clearing and shortly to a ford of Five Lakes Creek and then to a junction (10S 735706, 4336951).

Turn right (north) at the junction and follow the west side of alder-lined Five Lakes Creek for 0.3 mile and then cross a side stream. Beyond this stream, climb moderately to the forested flat that harbors Whisky Creek Camp (6925'; 10S 735694, 4338773). Observe posted regulations here.

DAY 3 (Whisky Creek Camp to Barker Pass, 11.25 miles, or to Powderhorn Trailhead, 12.75 miles): From Whisky Creek Camp, head east a short distance to the crossing of Five Lakes Creek, and then make a 0.3-mile switchbacking climb through the trees to a T-junction with the PCT. Turn right at the junction, following signed directions for the Alpine Meadows Trailhead, and proceed on the PCT on a moderate climb through a gradually lightening forest, where shrubs and wildflowers become more and more prominent. Follow occasional switchbacks up the left-hand side of Five Lakes Creek canyon across initially dry slopes, followed by a hillside of flourishing wildflowers and willows. Beyond this incredibly verdant hillside, where conifers start to reappear, is a signed junction with a lateral to Five Lakes. (Backpackers seeking campsites must find one at least 600 feet away from any of the lakes in the Five Lakes basin.)

From the junction with the Five Lakes lateral, veer right (east), remaining on the PCT, and follow the gently graded trail across a meadow sprinkled with lodgepole pines and firs to a boulder-hop of Five Lakes Creek. From the crossing, climb an open hillside carpeted with patches of alder and willows and interspersed with a fine assortment of wildflowers, including delphinium, yarrow, paintbrush, aster, corn lily, and daisy. Beyond this colorful area, many long switchbacks zigzag up a forested hillside towards the crest of the ridge above. Before the end of these switchbacks, thinning trees allow the first of many sweeping views to come: Squaw Peak is the prominent mountain to the northwest, and below to the west is the heart of Granite Chief Wilderness; farther on, where the switchbacks end and the trail approaches the crest, views expand to the south of peaks in Desolation Wilderness, along with a varied assortment of communications equipment and ski-lift machinery littering the summit of Ward Peak directly ahead. When the trail reaches a small saddle, the views include Lake Tahoe and Alpine Meadows to the east. Reaching a small saddle, the trail offers views to the east of Lake Tahoe and Alpine Meadows.

With the stiff climbing behind you, traverse around Peak 8474 to a second saddle, pass by a snow fence built to minimize cornices overhanging the ski slopes of Alpine Meadows, and continue through low-growing flowers and shrubs across the west side of Ward Peak, enjoying continuous views of the surrounding terrain along the way. Beyond Ward Peak, the PCT reaches two more saddles before dipping below impressive-looking volcanic cliffs on the west side of Peak 8522.

Briefly enter a grove of western white pines, firs, and hemlocks, the first significant pocket of forest since the switchbacks above the crossing of Five Lakes Creek. Leave the trees for a while to regain the crest and enjoy fine views of Ward Canyon and Lake Tahoe to the east and ahead to Twin Peaks. Then head back into the trees, where a subsidiary ridge abuts the main crest, and follow a pair of short switchbacks on a brief climb back to the top of the shrub-covered ridge.

Continue along the ridge, where waist-high tobacco brush threatens to overgrow the path in places and where proclaiming the expansive views along this part of the journey becomes redundant. Eventually, the views diminish as the trail follows a gentle grade through mixed forest to a junction with the TRT just southwest of Twin Peaks.

CLIMBING TWIN PEAKS

Peakbaggers can easily add a notch to their belts by heading east from the junction on the TRT to a use trail that ascends the east ridge of the easternmost of Twin Peaks' summits. The route climbs steeply up the ridge, offering excellent views of Lake Tahoe, the summits of Desolation Wilderness, and the surrounding canyons along the way, culminating in an even more impressive 360-degree view from the top.

From the junction, the PCT and TRT share a similar course for many miles, almost to Carson Pass. Initially the trail continues through the trees, but eventually it emerges into the open again with excellent views of Twin Peaks and Blackwood Canyon. In order to avoid a knife-edged ridge, the trail next makes several long switchbacks down into the canyon of North Fork Blackwood Creek. The switchbacking trail loses 600 feet of elevation before ultimately climbing back out of the canyon. The trail crosses a few lushly lined streams and seeps along the way, all tributaries of North Fork Blackwood Creek, where a limited number of nearby campsites serve overnighters.

A short but stiff climb from the campsites leads to the top of a ridge directly west of Peak 8355. An extremely short use trail leads to a scramble of this volcanic pinnacle, where hikers can enjoy fine views of the surrounding terrain.

Away from the ridge, the trail traverses the head of a canyon of a subsidiary steam of Middle Fork Blackwood Creek, passing in and out of a light fir forest. Good views of Lake Tahoe, Barker Peak, and Ellis Peak are available along the way through gaps in the forest. A final, moderate descent across the south slopes of Barker Peak leads to the Barker Pass Trailhead (7644'; 10S 739116 4328964 (field)), where your shuttle ride is waiting.

If you are doing the loop option, add 1.5 miles to your day and close the loop by turning right and descending generally west on Barker Pass Road to the Powderhorn Trailhead (7640'; 10S 736921 4328622 (field)).

Meeks Bay Trailhead

6231'; 10S 748752 4324856 (field)

DESTINATION/ UTM COORDINATES	TRIP TYPE	BEST SEASON	PACE (HIKING/ LAYOVER DAYS)	TOTAL MILEAGE
6 Tahoe-Yosemite Trail Section 1: To Echo Summit 10S 757559 4300186 (field)	Shuttle	Mid to late	4/1 Moderate	30.2 or 27.5

Information and Permits: All backpackers must secure and pay for a wilderness permit for entry into Desolation Wilderness. The region is heavily used, and strict quotas are in place for the number of overnighters departing from every trailhead that enters the wilderness. A majority of permits are available by reservation, with the remainder handed out on a first-come, first-served basis. Reserved permits are currently mailed out. For east-side entry, contact Eldorado National Forest: 100 Forni Road, Placerville, CA 95667; 530-622-5061; www.fs.fed.us/r5/eldorado/wild/moke/index.html. During the summer only, stop by the Lake Tahoe Visitor's Center located 3 miles north of the Hwy. 50/Hwy. 89 junction at South Lake Tahoe, on Hwy. 89. Call for hours: 530-543-2674. See also www.fs.fed.us/r5/eldorado/deso/.

Driving Directions: Follow Hwy. 89 on the west shore of Lake Tahoe to Meeks Bay and locate the trailhead near a closed gate on the west side of the highway, 0.1 mile north of the entrance into Meeks Bay Campground. The trailhead is approximately 16.5 miles north of the junction of highways 89 and 50 in South Lake Tahoe or 11 miles south of the junction of highways 89 and 28 in Tahoe City.

6 Tahoe-Yosemite Trail Section 1: To Echo Summit

Trip Data: 10S 757559 4300186; 30.2 or 27.5 miles; 4/1 days

see map on p.32

Topos: *Homewood, Rockbound Valley, Pyramid Peak, Echo Lake*

Highlights: This first section of the TYT, from Meeks Bay to a Sno-Park just west and south of Hwy. 50's Echo Summit, lies almost entirely within one of California's best-known wilderness areas, Desolation. The section is never far from a road, and frequent glimpses of Lake Tahoe may call forth images of noisy casinos and crowded beaches. Yet near the trail you may find many campsites that possess a feeling of utter remoteness.

HEADS UP! *Extensive sections of the trail are strewn with sharp, angular rock—be sure to wear sturdy footwear. Wood fires are banned within the wilderness, so plan on using a stove for cooking.*

Shuttle Directions: Follow Hwy. 50 to Echo Summit, and from there go west to a paved access road on the south side of the highway, 0.2 mile west of Echo Summit. A sign reading SNO-PARK marks the turnoff. Proceed 0.2 mile to the large PCT parking lot just before the Sno-Park.

DAY 1 (Meeks Bay Trailhead to Rubicon Lake, 8 miles): The "trail" begins as a dirt road beyond a locked gate near Hwy. 89. The gate bars access to the general public, but vehicles may still be infrequently encountered along the road. Beyond the gate, head generally southwest through mixed forest of incense cedars, white firs, lodgepole pines, and sugar pines on the right, and verdant meadows along Meeks Creek on the left. Continue along the dusty road to a junction about 1.5 miles from the trailhead.

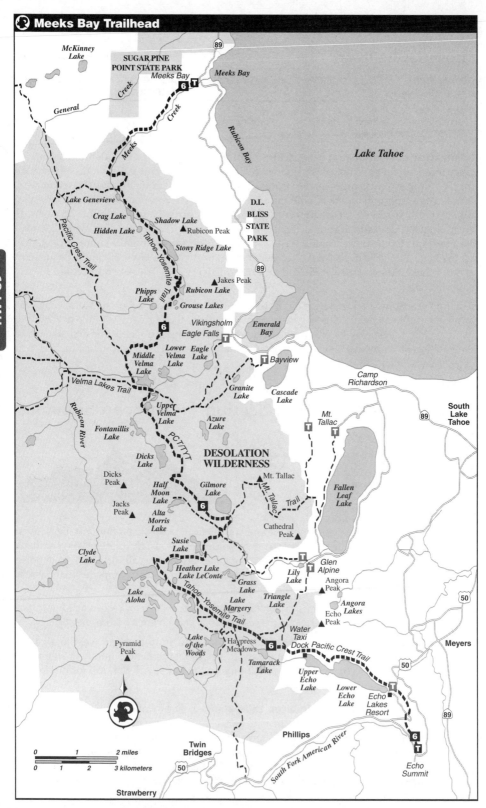

89

McKinney
Lake

SUGAR PINE
POINT STATE PARK
Meeks Bay
6 T   Meeks Bay

Creek

General

Meeks Creek

Lake Tahoe

Rubicon Bay

Pacific Crest Trail

Lake Genevieve

Crag Lake

Shadow Lake

Hidden Lake   ▲ Rubicon Peak

Stony Ridge Lake

Tahoe-Yosemite Trail

D.L.
BLISS
STATE
PARK

89

Phipps
Lake

Rubicon Lake   ▲ Jakes Peak

Grouse Lakes

6   Vikingsholm
Eagle Falls
T

Emerald
Bay

Lower   Eagle
Velma   Lake
Lake

T Bayview

Middle
Velma
Lake

Camp
Richardson

Velma Lakes Trail

Upper Velma
Lake

Granite
Lake

Cascade
Lake

South
Lake
Tahoe

89

Rubicon River

Fontanillis
Lake

Azure
Lake

Mt.
Tallac
T

PCT/TYT

DESOLATION
WILDERNESS

Dicks
Lake

Dicks
Peak ▲

Half
Moon
Lake

Gilmore
Lake

6

Mt. Tallac ▲

Mt. Tallac Trail

Fallen
Leaf
Lake

50

Jacks
Peak ▲

Alta
Morris
Lake

Cathedral
Peak ▲

Clyde
Lake

Susie
Lake

Heather Lake
Lake LeConte

Glen
Alpine
T

Grass
Lake

Lily
Lake

T

Angora
Peak ▲

Angora
Lakes

50

Lake
Aloha

Tahoe-Yosemite Trail

Lake
Margery

Triangle
Lake

Echo
Peak ▲

Meyers

Pyramid
Peak ▲

Lake
of the
Woods

Haypress
Meadows

6

Water
Taxi
Dock   Pacific Crest Trail

50

Tamarack
Lake

Upper
Echo
Lake

Lower
Echo
Lake

Echo
Lakes
Resort

T

89

Phillips

South Fork American River

6
T

0   1   2 miles
0   1   2   3 kilometers

Twin
Bridges

50

Echo
Summit

Strawberry

HWY 89

Obeying signed directions for the TYT, turn right (southwest) and leave the road behind to follow a climbing single-track trail past luxuriant foliage bordering a seeping spring to the signed Desolation Wilderness boundary, 2.5 miles from the trailhead.

A moderate ascent on rocky trail continues and leads past a spring surrounded by thriving currant bushes and corn lilies. Above the spring, purple lupine and red paintbrush carpet the slope. Beyond the spring, the grade eases, and mountain junipers start to line the path.

MOUNTAIN JUNIPERS

These rugged trees with thick, sienna-barked trunks are members of the cypress family, very unlike the more common needle-bearing conifers of the High Sierra. Botanists consider junipers to be more closely related to the incense-cedars, also members of the cypress family. The twigs of junipers, incense-cedars, and giant sequoias (not in the cypress family) are covered with overlapping scale-like leaves rather than having needle-like leaves that extend from the twig as do the pines, firs, and spruces.

Nearing Meeks Creek, the sound of the gurgling stream delights passersby. Along the banks of a seep beside the creek, paintbrush, monkey flower, columbine, and tiger lily blossom in early summer. Veering away from the stream, the sandy, now-level tread passes through a meadow and then a forested, meadowy glade of ferns before encountering another meadow holding a forest of drowned trees, bare and silvery in death. The large yellow flowers from a garden of mule ears soften the bleak ambiance created by the dead trees. A gentle-to-moderate ascent under sparse, mixed forest cover gives way to a short, moderate to steep climb on rocky trail, where red fir joins the other conifers.

RED FIRS

Sometimes referred to as silvertips, red firs are found between 5000 and 9000 feet in California, although they are most common around 7000 and 8000 feet. In fully developed stands, very little groundcover is found due to the lack of sunlight reaching the forest floor. Saprophytes—plants that don't perform photosynthesis, such as snow plant and pine drops—may be found randomly thrusting out of the shady soil.

Near a sturdy log-and-timber bridge over Meeks Creek is an attractive campsite—unfortunately, its close proximity to the creek makes the site illegal for camping. However, across the bridge and 80 yards upstream is a shady campsite that's suitable for overnight stays. Nearby, pan-size brook and brown trout lie in small holes shaded by thickets of dogwood, alder, willow, and mountain ash.

The sandy trail steadily ascends the east wall of the canyon, looping away from the creek to gain the height of a steep cascade, as the gracefully curved tips of mountain hemlocks herald your arrival in the higher elevations. Just beyond a waterfall, the trail leads to a junction with the seldom-used Lake Genevieve Trail and then soon reaches the shore of Lake Genevieve, a shallow, warm, pine-rimmed, green lake. A few fair campsites at the north end and along the east side provide views across the water of photogenic Peak 9054, a beautiful sight in early morning with sunrise light crowning a mantle of blue shadows. Campsites at Genevieve and the upcoming lakes are limited and are generally fair to poor in quality. With the canyon's floor shoehorned between steep ridges, the campsites are sandwiched tightly between the trail and the shorelines.

From Lake Genevieve the trail makes a short, gentle ascent under red fir, western white pine, and Jeffrey pine to Crag Lake, where fair campsites on the glacial moraine forming the east side of the lake's basin may tempt overnighters.

DAMS

The flow-maintenance dam across Crag Lake's outlet is one of many such dams in the high country built by the state's Department of Fish and Game (DF&G), US Forest Service, or private sportsmen's groups. DF&G biologists and wardens making adjustments of the outlet valve during the summer insure adequate flow continues into Meeks Creek.

The route now ascends moderately on rocky tread to a ford of Meeks Creek. Just beyond the ford is a junction with a path right (south) and down to Hidden Lake, which appears through gaps in the forest a short distance farther up the trail. Despite increasing use, Hidden Lake seems to maintain a healthy population of brook trout.

Go ahead (southeast) here, veering away from the creek, to make a gentle ascent through dense pine forest that passes above meadow-bordered and lily-dotted Shadow Lake. Make a steady diagonal ascent up a curving moraine, beside rapids and cataracts, to Stony Ridge Lake, the largest of the six Tallant Lakes occupying this valley, 6.3 miles from the trailhead. Backpackers will find fair campsites near the outlet, as well as a few along the west shore. Anglers can test their skills on both rainbow and brown trout. A forest primarily of lodgepole pines rims the lake except along the eastern shore. A short distance up the rocky western slope, gray-green sagebrush calls into question the notion that sagebrush defines desert.

At the head of Stony Ridge Lake, make a slight ascent overlooking a pond and a green, marshy meadow above the lake. For the next half mile, the trail is mostly level across a wet hillside carpeted by the best flower gardens seen so far on the TYT. After a 300-foot elevation gain via a series of switchbacks, the trail turns south, paralleling the east side of a small, north-facing glacial cirque. Black, lichen-streaked cliffs stand 200 feet high above a talus-block fan. In early season, the wide, sweeping snowbank in this cirque, stained red by millions of minute algae, is a small reminder of the glacier that sculpted the curving headwall.

Eight miles from the trailhead you find Rubicon Lake (8309'; 10S 748203 4316991), the crown jewel of the Tallant Lakes. Encircled by lodgepole pines and mountain hemlocks, the lake offers a number of fair-to-good campsites scattered around the shoreline of the green-tinted lake.

DAY 2 (Rubicon Lake to Dicks Lake, 7.1 miles): About 100 yards up the cool, shaded trail from Rubicon Lake is a lateral on the left to Grouse Lakes. The TYT goes right (ahead, south) here, and, after a couple of switchbacks, the snow-covered north slope of Mt. Tallac springs into view above the gray-green valley of Eagle Creek.

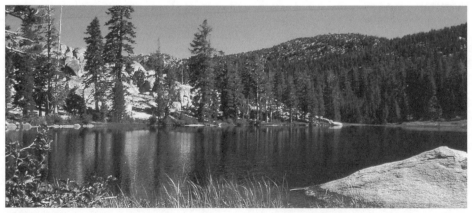

Rubicon Lake

On rocky trail, ascend moderately until the grade eases on a traverse of the far side of a ridge overlooking Grouse Lakes and the Eagle Creek drainage, along which Cascade and Fallen Leaf lakes are visible to the southeast. Where the route to Phipps Lake departs to the right (west), the TYT continues ahead (south-southwest) as the traverse is interrupted by a set of steps of milled lumber held in place by steel pegs. For some unclear reason, the next section of trail contours around the south side of Phipps Peak until it heads almost due north, at which point hikers might begin to worry, knowing that they should be heading south toward the Velma Lakes. Ultimately, they will.

Dicks Peak comes into view near Phipps Pass, and some of the mountains of the Crystal Range appear over its right shoulder. You've been traveling through gray granite country since the beginning of the journey; now, the reddish-brown metasedimentary rocks of Dicks Peak and its outliers are quite striking. Leaving the pass, the trail descends briefly but over the next half mile seems to climb more often than drop.

Soon, all three Velma Lakes come into view at once. Named for a daughter of Nevada mining king Harry Comstock, the lakes lie close together in a single basin—but Upper and Lower Velma lakes drain into Lake Tahoe and ultimately Nevada's Pyramid Lake, while Middle Velma Lake drains into the Rubicon River and ultimately the Pacific Ocean. From this vantage point, experienced cross-country enthusiasts may elect to head straight for Middle Velma Lake, as the TYT route is quite indirect.

Veering west onto Phipps Peak's dry and exposed west flank, the TYT provides excellent views of the north part of the Crystal Range, including Rockbound Pass—the deepest notch visible—and the basins of lakes Lois and Schmidell, landmarks that remain visible for a mile or more as the trail arcs around Phipps Peak. Finally, at a hairpin turn, the trail heads back toward Velma Lakes. A few yards northwest of this turn, a viewpoint overlooks much of Rockbound Valley, including the namesake lake, which sits near the wilderness's northwest corner. Beyond this vista point, a steady, sandy descent incorporating three long switchbacks passes through moderate-to-dense forest cover to a junction with the 2600-mile PCT, 4 miles from Rubicon Lake.

Turn left (south-southeast) onto the southbound PCT. From the PCT junction to Middle Velma Lake, the route wanders more than seems necessary, eventually crossing a sluggish creek to reach the first of two junctions with the Velma Lakes Trail, which here heads right (generally west) to Camper Flat on the Rubicon River. The PCT/TYT, briefly joined by the Velma Lakes Trail, goes left (generally east) at this junction. At the southwest end of forested Middle Velma Lake, the PCT/TYT skirts a cove and rises above the lake into red fir forest.

MORE ON RED FIRS

Red fir is more vulnerable to breakage than any other Sierra conifer, as evidenced by the numerous downed trees and tree parts scattered about the forest floor by winter storms. Also strewn across the ground are the ragged cores of fir cones that remain following a chickaree's meal of cone seeds. The Sierra chickaree, a kind of squirrel, climbs the fir in autumn to cut the green cones and caches them for later use, the cool seasonal temperatures keeping the cones fresh until needed. Fir cones, unlike pinecones, disintegrate while on the tree. You usually won't find a fir cone on the ground unless a chickaree has nibbled it off and then lost it.

The shady duff tread of the PCT/TYT soon leads to the second junction with the Velma Lakes Trail, which here goes left (east) while the PCT/TYT goes right (generally south). (To visit Upper Velma Lake, make a 200-yard stroll up this trail to a junction marked by a post and turn south, reaching the southwest shore of the lake after another half a mile. Backpackers will find fair campsites near the inlet.)

POCKET GOPHER TUNNELS

In a meadow of sedge and corn lilies, where the trail first nears Upper Velma Lake, "ropes" of soil are the telltale signs of the pocket gopher. During the winter, the rodent tunnels in the snow to eat the aboveground parts of plants. Later, the gopher tunnels in the earth, filling the snow tunnels with the extracted dirt. Following snowmelt, these casts of dirt that once filled snow tunnels descend to the ground, where you see them.

From the second Velma Lakes Trail junction, the PCT/TYT ascends south on a moderate grade while overlooking Upper Velma Lake. As the slope eases to gentle, Dicks Pass, Lake Tahoe, and then Fontanillis Lake come into view. After a short, gentle descent, cross the outlet and reach Fontanillis Lake, cradled in a rocky basin and towered over by Dicks Peak. Fair campsites are shaded by stands of lodgepole pines and mountain hemlocks. On the east shore, a lavish display of red and sienna rocks complement the familiar gray granite—scramble up the slope to find them.

Leaving Fontanillis Lake, the sandy trail ascends a boulder-covered granite hillside with several meltwater tarns that could offer a refreshing swim at just the right time of the season. At the top of this rise, there's a junction where a short lateral heads right (south) to Dicks Lake (8422'; 10S 747505 4311188). This cirque lake below Dicks Peak offers several fair campsites and one good one on the timbered east shore. Anglers will appreciate a self-sustaining population of brook trout.

DAY 3 (Dicks Lake to Tarn Above Heather Lake, 7.4 miles): At the junction of the PCT/TYT and the Dicks Lake lateral, the PCT/TYT turns north (left if you've not gone down to Dicks Lake, right if you are coming from the lake) and proceeds a short distance to another junction in a saddle overlooking the drainage of Eagle Creek to the east. Turn right (southeast) here as the rocky trail ascends steadily on a granite slope sparsely dotted with lodgepole pines. Far below, a large area of downed timber on the southwest slope of the Dicks Lake cirque provides graphic evidence of a former avalanche.

The grade increases as more than a dozen switchbacks assault the northwest slope of Peak 9579, which often remains snow covered into July. The ascent concludes at Dicks Pass (9380'), which is somewhat east of the actual low point of the divide. Standing at the pass with pack off and shoulders recuperating, the backpacker surveys a considerable part of California, from Sierra Buttes beyond Yuba Pass in the north to Round Top beyond Carson Pass in the south. Nearer to the south, Pyramid Peak rises majestically above island-dotted Lake Aloha, and from just beyond the pass, Susie and Grass lakes are clearly seen in the wooded basin of Glen Alpine Creek. The trail sign at the pass stands at the center of several almost flat acres, strewn with the rocky products of erosion, technically referred to as "erosion pavement." The surrounding trees are all whitebark pines, the highest-dwelling conifer encountered along the TYT. When snowmelt provides a reliable source of water, good campsites provide an overnight haven east of the pass.

Descending from the pass to the actual saddle, Susie, Gilmore, and Half Moon lakes and Lake Aloha can be seen ahead, while Fontanillis and Dicks lakes are visible to the rear. The trail descends the warm, south-facing slope, and when there is still much snow on the north side, the south side offers a springtime display of vibrant wildflowers, including paintbrush, sulfur flower, white heather, western wallflower, white and lavender phlox, and elderberry. At the saddle on this divide, a use trail provides access westward to the summit of Dicks Peak.

Go left (southeast) here to stay on the PCT/TYT as it traverses gently down the side of a ridge toward Gilmore Lake. Along this traverse, the variety of wildflowers seems to multiply with each step. At the peak of the blossoming season, delphinium, deerbrush, spiraea, creamberry, red heather, buckwheat, groundsel, serviceberry, corn lily, penstemon, white heather, pussypaws, and buttercups will delight passersby. Near the first sign of red firs, a lateral heads left (northeast) a short way to Gilmore Lake, where backpackers will find good campsites and anglers can test their skill on three species of trout. For peakbaggers, the trail to Gilmore Lake continues toward the 9735-foot, view-packed summit of Mt. Tallac.

The PCT/TYT goes right (ahead, east) at the junction to begin a switchbacking descent through mixed forest to a junction where a trail on the right heads north to Half Moon Lake and a trail to the left goes east-southeast to Glen Alpine. You go ahead (southwest) on the PCT/TYT down rocky trail toward Susie Lake for a half mile to a swampy, flower-filled meadow and a junction with another trail left (south) to Glen Alpine and Fallen Leaf Lake. Go right (west-southwest) and make a short, moderate, winding ascent that culminates at a rise overlooking Susie Lake, one of the most popular lakes in Desolation Wilderness, despite the poor-to-fair campsites. After crossing the outlet, a difficult ford in early season, the PCT/TYT meets a use trail heading down the canyon to large, forested campsites.

Staying on the PCT/TYT, curve right (southwest) to continue around the shore of Susie Lake and then climb steadily up to the V at the outlet of the Heather Lake basin, formed by the slopes of Jacks Peak on the north and Cracked Crag on the south. (In early season there is always snow here.) Notice the clear line of division on Jacks Peak that separates the metasedimentary rock of the "Mt. Tallac pendant" and the gray granite to the south. Follow a rocky course well above Heather Lake over a small ridge and then just above a placid tarn. Although Heather Lake offers no decent, legal places to camp, good campsites can be found beside a tarn (8065'; 10S 747672 4307047) that lies just below the headwall of the lake's cirque. This is the better place to stop, as upcoming Lake Aloha is extremely windy and has almost no decent, legal campsites. Heather Lake has rainbow, brook, and brown trout.

DAY 4 (Tarn Above Heather Lake to Echo Summit, 7.7 miles or 5 miles via water taxi): A short, rocky climb leads to the crest of the divide that separates the Heather Lake basin and Desolation Valley. This high point offers a magnificent, close-up view of the Crystal Range.

CRYSTAL RANGE

Rising above the far shore of shallow, island-dotted Lake Aloha, this classic range is a superb glacial ridge left standing high after moving ice on both sides plucked immense quantities of rock from its flanks and carried them downslope. Parts of the ridge are knife-edged—which geologists call an arête—and the snowfields at the base of the knife blade look like little glaciers. As the rivers of ice retreated, forests and meadows advanced to clot the moraines, rock-rimmed basins, and rugged cliffs. Along with the plants came animals—mammals, birds, reptiles, amphibians, and insects.

Foregrounding Mt. Price, Pyramid Peak, and the peaks between is a blue sheet of water, Lake Aloha, which is more than 2 miles long and is dotted with a thousand tiny granite islands, some of which harbor a single weather-beaten lodgepole snag. Campsites at Lake Aloha are very few, very poor, and very windy. However, some will find camping near the lake worthwhile for the sight of the morning sun turning the Crystal Range from blue-gray to gold.

Nearing the northeast edge of Lake Aloha, the trail to Mosquito Pass and Rockbound Valley heads right (west), but the PCT/TYT veers left (southeast) to follow the shore of the lake, composed of glacier-polished, barren granite. After a half mile the trail turns and immediately comes to a flat, where an unsigned and little-used spur darts left (north) to Lake Le Conte. This lake has several small, fair campsites on the east side. The PCT/TYT goes right and continues southeast around Lake Aloha's shore.

Approaching sparse forest cover, as stands of lodgepole pine alternate with meadows, the PCT/TYT goes left (southeast) at a junction with a trail straight ahead (south) to Lake

DESOLATION VALLEY

Even in this "desolation valley," formerly called Devils Basin, life is plentiful. Coyotes are often heard and sometimes seen, and yellow-bellied marmots virtually infest the talus slopes of Cracked Crag. Water snakes and skinks fill their ecological niches. Lake Aloha itself has thousands of brook and rainbow trout. The bountiful crop of wildflowers includes white heather, Douglas phlox, buckwheat, groundsel, paintbrush, mountain penstemon, stonecrop, streptanthus, pennyroyal, and buttercup. Besides lodgepole pine, conifers include mountain hemlock, western white pine, red fir, and junipers.

of the Woods. After a short ascent, the trail enters a highly scenic area, where, in early to mid-season, numerous tarns reflect the green pines and hemlocks and the house-size gray boulders dumped here by the glacier. Near the westernmost tarn, a trail to lakes Margery and Lucille leads off left (east) to good campsites around both lakes and to bearably warm swimming. The PCT/TYT goes right (southeast).

In a short quarter mile, a well-used spur trail from Lake Aloha merges with the TYT from the right, and 0.3 mile farther, the southern trail to Lake Lucille goes left (north). The excavated, level patch of ground next to the junction once held a log cabin used by trail crews and others needing emergency shelter. Go right (east-southeast) here to stay on the PCT/TYT.

The PCT/TYT next meets a pair of laterals that go right to Lake of the Woods, one in about 200 yards from the last junction and the other 350 yards farther on. Continue ahead (east-southeast) on the PCT/TYT at both junctions as the wide, sandy trail skirts above Haypress Meadows, site of one of the largest expanses of grass on the TYT. The grass was once harvested for sale to wagon trains crossing Echo Summit. Raised walkways help protect the fragile meadows from being trampled. As the PCT/TYT passes an abandoned trail, Echo Lakes come into view down the valley of Echo Creek, and the trail becomes steep and rocky. Where a trail veers left (east) up the hill toward Lily and Fallen Leaf lakes, the PCT/TYT continues ahead (east-southeast) toward Echo Lakes. At the last switchback in a series, rocks to sit on, water, and shade provide a fine place for a rest stop.

Watch your footing on the next section, a long traverse down a moderately graded tread filled with loose granite rocks. Even though many dayhikers and equestrians routinely travel this far from Echo Lakes, it's hard to justify the extensive blasting and grading of this section of trail that many refer to as a freeway.

Go left (briefly northeast) at a junction with a lateral right (southwest) to Tamarack Lake (camping prohibited) and reenter forest: a heavy cover of lodgepole, later thinning somewhat and showing inclusions of Jeffrey pine. Beyond the forest, another unsigned trail to the Fallen Leaf Lake area goes left (north) up the hill as the PCT/TYT continues ahead (generally southeast). Exit Desolation Wilderness in 300 more yards and soon encounter the signed lateral going right to the water taxi landing at the north shore of Upper Echo Lake.

WATER TAXI

The Echo Lake Chalet offers water-taxi service from the resort's upper dock at the south end of Lower Echo Lake to the public dock at the far end of Upper Echo Lake, reducing the hiking distance by 2.5 miles. The normal season runs from the Fourth of July through Labor Day weekend, although service is usually extended through September, depending on weather conditions and lake levels. The fee in 2004 was $7 per person one way with a two-person minimum for service. A direct-line phone to the Chalet at the upper dock can be used to arrange for pickup. (Call 530-659-7207, 8 A.M. to 6 P.M. during summer, for more information.)

HWY 89

Beyond the water-taxi lateral, the trail skirts the north side of Upper and Lower Echo lakes. The 2.5-mile walk is unremarkable on a wide and well-trod trail that travels discouragingly high above the lakes. The final section is on a dusty, exposed, south-facing slope, making the trip uncomfortably warm in the afternoon sun.

After a milkshake or other morale-booster at Echo Lake Resort, take a very steep trail from the back of the public restrooms next to the resort up to the large parking lots, and on the west edge of the paved lot, find a segment of PCT/TYT built in 1978. This segment first makes a long switchback leg west before turning east to climb gently through red firs above the many summer-home cabins. The trail veers south and then southwest and just past a rusty tank on the left, meets a junction: Ahead is a 4WD road; turn left (southeast) to continue on the signed PCT/TYT. Immediately dip across a small seasonal stream and follow the trail on a gradual curve through white fir and lodgepole pine to meet paved Johnson Pass Road at a ditch so abrupt you may wish to cut left, almost to a driveway, to avoid the ditch.

From the ditch intersection, angle right across the road toward PCT signs and continue gently winding down to meet Hwy. 50 about 100 yards east (uphill) of the defunct Little Norway Resort. Cross the highway and on the south side find the next section of trail, which crosses another ditch and turns left (south-southeast) to climb as it parallels the highway toward Echo Summit. After a mile, this section meets a paved road coming south from Hwy. 50. Turn right (south) onto the paved road and end Section 1 of the TYT at a paved PCT trailhead parking lot (7389'; 10S 757559 4300186 (field)), south of which is an area that doubles as a California Sno-Park in winter.

See Hwy. 50, Echo Summit Trailhead, for Section 2 of the TYT.

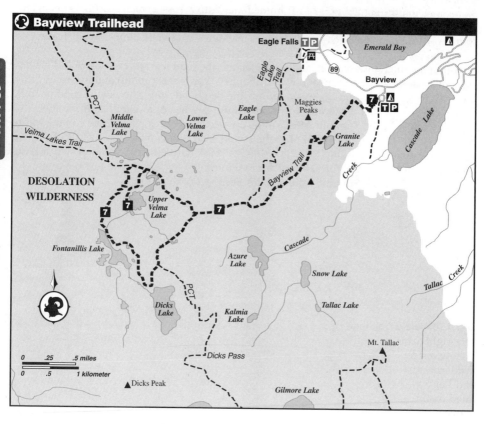

HWY 89

Bayview Trailhead

Eagle Falls

Emerald Bay

Bayview

Eagle Lake Trail

Eagle Lake

Maggies Peaks

Middle Velma Lake

Lower Velma Lake

Granite Lake

Cascade Lake

Velma Lakes Trail

Bayview Trail

Creek

DESOLATION WILDERNESS

Upper Velma Lake

Fontanillis Lake

Cascade

Azure Lake

Snow Lake

Tallac Creek

Dicks Lake

PCT

Kalmia Lake

Tallac Lake

Mt. Tallac

0   .25   .5 miles

0   .5   1 kilometer

Dicks Pass

Dicks Peak

Gilmore Lake

Bayview Trailhead

6878'; 10S 751336 4314584 (field)

DESTINATION/ UTM COORDINATES	TRIP TYPE	BEST SEASON	PACE (HIKING/ LAYOVER DAYS)	TOTAL MILEAGE
7 Upper Velma Lake 10S 747035 4312518	Semiloop	Mid to late	2/1 Moderate	11.7

Information and Permits: All backpackers must secure and pay for a wilderness permit for entry into Desolation Wilderness. The region is heavily used, and strict quotas are in place for the number of overnighters departing from every trailhead that enters the wilderness. A majority of permits are available by reservation, with the remainder handed out on a first-come, first-served basis. Reserved permits are currently mailed out. For east-side entry, contact Eldorado National Forest: 100 Forni Road, Placerville, CA 95667; 530-622-5061; www.fs.fed.us/r5/eldorado/wild/moke/index.html. During the summer only, stop by the Lake Tahoe Visitor's Center located 3 miles north of the Hwy. 50/Hwy. 89 junction at South Lake Tahoe, on Hwy. 89. Call for hours: 530-543-2674. See also www.fs.fed.us/r5/eldorado/deso/.

Driving Directions: Follow Hwy. 89 to Emerald Bay and find the turnoff for the Bayview Campground and Trailhead on the south side of the highway, approximately 7.5 miles from the junction of Hwy. 50 in South Lake Tahoe, or 19.5 miles south from the junction of Hwy. 28 in Tahoe City. The trailhead is at the south end of Bayview Campground.

7 Upper Velma Lake

Trip Data: 10S 747035 431251; 11.7 miles; 2/1 days

Topos: *Emerald Bay, Rockbound Valley*

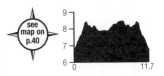

see map on p.40

Highlights: This hike through the heart of Desolation Wilderness visits several cirque-bound lakes surrounded by the characteristic granite terrain for which the area is renowned.

DAY 1 (Bayview Trailhead to Upper Velma Lake, 4.6 miles): Soon after leaving the trailhead, turn right to go generally southwest at a junction with the trail on the left to Cascade Lake. Follow a steep, switchbacking climb through mixed forest. After crossing the Desolation Wilderness boundary, follow the crest of a ridge, from where good views of Emerald Bay and Lake Tahoe appear through gaps in the forest. Leave the ridge and follow the alder-lined outlet of Granite Lake on a gentle ascent through lush foliage, reaching the hillside above Granite Lake. To visit the lake, drop down to the shoreline via one of the use trails on the northwest side.

Well above the far end of the lake, the Bayview Trail begins a steep, switchbacking climb across the south-facing slope below Maggies Peaks. Exiting Granite Lake's basin, the grade mercifully eases to a gentle stroll along the back side of South Maggies Peak, followed by a gentle descent along the forested southwest ridge. You reach a junction with the Eagle Lake Trail at a saddle, 2.7 miles from the trailhead (10S 749062 431274).

Turn right (generally west) at the junction and follow sandy tread on a gently undulating route through scattered conifers and around granite boulders and slabs for 0.6 mile to a junction with the Velma Lakes Trail (10S 749288 4312702).

Bear right (north-northwest) here and descend, with occasional glimpses through scattered pines of the unnamed pond directly north of Upper Velma Lake. Reach the floor of the basin and follow the north shore of the pond to a ford of the outlet and to a junction just beyond, 4.1 miles from the trailhead. Turn left (south) and proceed 0.6 mile to campsites near the inlet on the southwest shore of Upper Velma Lake (7960'; 10S 747035 4312518).

DAY 2 (Upper Velma Lake to Bayview Trailhead, 7.1 miles): Retrace your steps 0.6 mile to the last junction and turn left (west) to make a short climb to a junction with the PCT (10S 747133 4313270). (To see Middle Velma Lake, continue west on the PCT a short distance to a fine viewpoint. A number of pleasant and popular campsites on the south shore are easily reached cross-country from the PCT.)

To continue the loop part of this trip, follow the PCT south-southwest on a moderate, winding climb along a forested ridge above the west shore of Upper Velma Lake. Eventually, Dicks Pass and Fontanillis Lake pop into view as the trees thin and the grade eases. A short drop leads to the crossing of Fontanillis Lake's outlet, followed by a traverse across the east side of the lake's multihued rock basin, which lies in the shadow of towering Dicks Peak. Legal campsites are absent on the trail side of the lake, but open benches above the west shore provide a number of excellent opportunities for overnight accommodations.

Leaving Fontanillis Lake, a brief ascent across boulder-covered slopes leads to the top of a rise and a junction with a 100-yard lateral right (south) to Dicks Lake. Backpackers will find excellent, although popular, campsites on the north shore and east peninsula of Dicks Lake.

Assuming you don't take the lateral, the PCT heads left (generally north), away from Dicks Lake, on an easy ascent to a junction where the PCT and the TYT turn right (southeast) toward Dicks Pass. You go ahead here (north) to descend moderate switchbacks to the floor of a pond-dotted basin, and then traverse the basin northeastward to the junction of the Eagle Lake and Velma Lakes trails, closing the loop part of this trip.

From there, turn right (east) and retrace your steps 2.7 miles past Granite Lake to the Bayview Trailhead.

HWY 89

Big Meadow Trailhead

7260'; 10S 760498 4297599 (field)

DESTINATION/ UTM COORDINATES	TRIP TYPE	BEST SEASON	PACE (HIKING/ LAYOVER DAYS)	TOTAL MILEAGE
8 Carson Pass West 11S 239819 4287379 (field)	Shuttle	Mid to late	2/0 Moderate	10.4

Information and Permits: Meiss Country is administered by the Lake Tahoe Basin Management Unit: USDA Forest Service, Lake Tahoe Basin Management Unit, 35 College Drive, South Lake Tahoe, CA 96150; 530-543-2600; www.fs.fed.us/r5/ltbmu/. No wilderness permits are required, but you must have a California Campfire Permit to have a campfire or use a stove.

Driving Directions: Drive on Hwy. 89 to the well-signed Big Meadow/Tahoe Rim Trail parking lot, 6 miles from the Hwy. 88 junction in Hope Valley, and 5 miles from the Hwy. 50 junction near Myers.

8 Carson Pass West

Trip Data: 11S 239819 4287379; 10.4 miles; 2/0 days

Topos: *Caples Lake, Carson Pass*

see map on p.44

Highlights: This trip travels through the heart of the proposed 31,100-acre Meiss Meadows Wilderness. Following sections of the TRT, the TYT, and the PCT, recreationists can travel from Hwy. 89 to Hwy. 88, visiting Big Meadow, Dardanelles Lake, Round Lake, and Meiss Meadows along the way.

Shuttle Directions: To get to the Carson Pass West Trailhead, follow Hwy. 88 0.3 mile west of Carson Pass. There's a daily fee to park, and the drive between the trailheads is approximately 16 miles.

DAY 1 (Big Meadow Trailhead to Dardanelles Lake, 3.5 miles): Leave the parking area and follow the single-track TRT a short distance south to a crossing of Hwy. 89. Once across the highway, pick up the TRT and start a winding, moderate, southward climb through a forest of Jeffrey pines, lodgepole pines, and red firs. At a switchback, you have a fine view of the aspen-lined, rocky channel of Big Meadow Creek, which is vibrantly alive with snowmelt in early July and golden color in autumn. Following more switchbacks, the grade eases just before reaching a junction a half mile from the trailhead, where a trail to Scott Lake branches left (southeast).

Go right (south) at the junction and quickly leave the trees behind, emerging into grassy, flower-covered Big Meadow. Follow the trail through the meadow to a wood-plank bridge that spans the gurgling creek and proceed to the far edge, where a lightly forested ascent resumes. Sagebrush, currant, and drought-tolerant wildflowers, principally mule ears, line the path. Farther up the trail, wood-beam-reinforced steps help you over the steeper sections of trail that follows a diminishing tributary of Big Meadow Creek, a sprightly watercourse lined with luxuriant foliage.

Continue climbing to a densely forested saddle and then follow a switchbacking descent into the next canyon, through which flows an Upper Truckee River tributary. Reach the floor of the canyon and a junction marked by a post, where you meet the Meiss Meadows Trail, 2.2 miles from the trailhead.

From the Meiss Meadows Trail junction, turn right and head northwest for 0.2 mile to another junction, this one with the Dardanelles Lake Trail. Turn left (west), make a very brief descent to ford an Upper Truckee River tributary, and soon ford a wider stretch of the

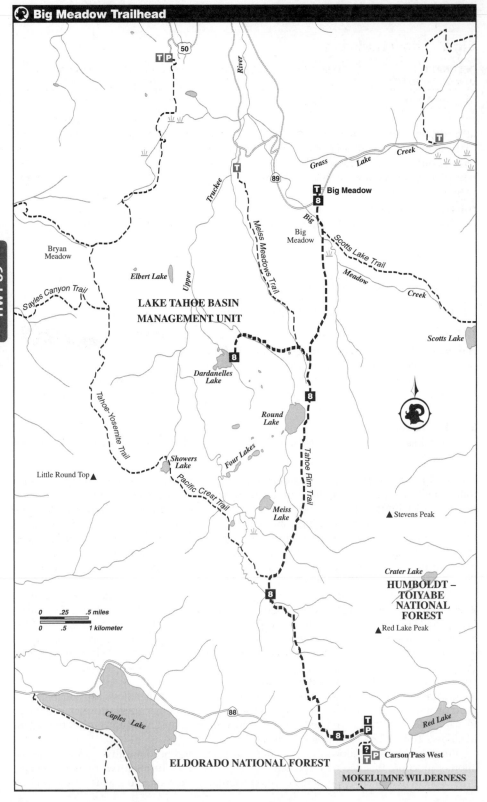

stream. Early in the season, search for logs upstream in order to avoid getting your feet wet. Away from the streams, stroll across a bench holding a small meadow and seasonal ponds.

Descend from the bench through dense forest of western white pines, red firs, and lodgepole pines and follow an alder-and-willow-lined stream down a canyon. The grade eases as the trail passes through meadow-like vegetation of grasses, wildflowers, and willows on the way to a boulder-hop of Round Lake's outlet. A short climb amid boulders and granite slabs leads to the east shore of Dardanelles Lake (7759'; 10S 758901 4294386), 1.3 miles from the TRT. Far enough off the thoroughfare of the TRT, you may be able to enjoy the relative seclusion of this lake. The lakeshore is shaded by light forest and dotted with boulders and slabs, and the picturesque cliffs of the Dardanelles loom above the south shore.

DAY 2 (Dardanelles Lake to Carson Pass West, 6.9 miles): Retrace your steps 1.3 miles back to the Meiss Meadows Trail junction, going right (southeast) at the last junction you passed and continuing to the next junction, where you turn right (south) onto the Meiss Meadows Trail/TRT.

From this junction, the TRT follows a steady climb through dense forest on sections of newly rerouted trail. After 0.6 mile, you crest the lip of Round Lake's basin above its northeast shore and reach an informal junction. From the junction, a use trail wraps around the lake's west shore, which is lined with rock outcrops and scattered forest, and then follows a cross-country route to Meiss Lake. You continue south on the TRT as it skirts the east shore of Round Lake below the ziggurat-like formation that towers over it and through thick forest, staying away from the lush meadows and thick willows that border the inlet at the south end.

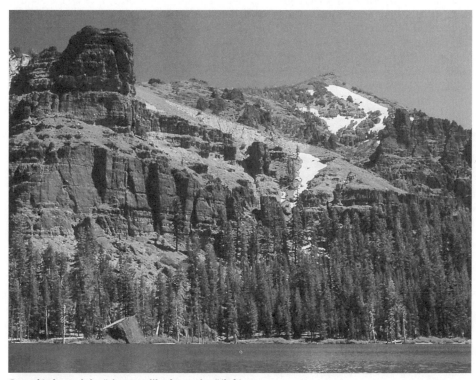

Round Lake and the "ziggurat-like formation" (left)

Beyond the lake, the TRT resumes its climb, soon reaching an extensive sloping meadow carpeted with willows, wildflowers, and other lush foliage, well watered by a thin, rock-lined rivulet spilling across the trail. Past the meadow, you reenter forest cover and hop across a pair of trickling rivulets. Eventually the grade eases to a mellow stroll where the trail breaks out into an open forest sprinkled with stands of aspen and swaths of drier groundcover, including sagebrush, currant, grasses, and drought-tolerant wildflowers.

Part of extensive Meiss Meadows soon appears through scattered lodgepole pines to the right of the trail, with Meiss Lake lying just a third of a mile to the west (an optional out-and-back detour). Leaving the meadow behind, hop across Round Lake's inlet and proceed to cross a creek that runs through a rocky channel 0.4 mile farther, where open terrain allows views of the rugged slopes leading up to 10,059-foot Stevens Peak. Continue on gently graded trail through lodgepole pines to the heart of Meiss Meadows and a well-signed junction with the PCT/TYT.

BYGONE DAYS

Near the junction, an old cabin harkens back to the days, not so long ago, when cattle were allowed to graze the lush grasses of picturesque and pastoral Meiss Meadows. This was once Meiss Cow Camp. Fortunately, the cows are gone, the trampling of the meadows is over, the cow pies have decomposed, and the trails have been left to wildlife and humans.

Turn left (south) on the PCT/TYT at the junction (also joining the last leg of the Tahoe-Yosemite Trail's Section 2) and stroll across the pleasant meadowlands, making several crossings of the young Upper Truckee River along the way. Eventually the terrain gets steeper as the trail begins a moderate climb of the narrowing gorge toward a saddle at the head of the canyon. Wildflowers grace the slopes below the saddle, and at the saddle there's a fine view north to Lake Tahoe and south to the jagged peaks of the Carson Pass area, including Elephants Back, Round Top, Sisters, Fourth of July Peak, and Thimble Peak. Red Lake Peak towers on your left.

Leaving the saddle, the trail descends past a lovely pond and drops steeply on open hillsides and across seasonal streams; these slopes are famed for their seasonal wildflower displays. Most of the trail is single-track, but there's a stretch that looks like old jeep road.

The final leg of the journey is through a light forest on a long traverse across the hillside above Hwy. 88. Early-season wildflowers are prevalent along this final stretch of trail, although highway noise may seem to detract from them. It's no surprise, therefore, when you reach a parking lot at the Carson Pass West Trailhead (8566'; 11S 239819 4287379 (field)) just off noisy Hwy. 88.

US HIGHWAY 50 TRIPS

Merely driving Hwy. 50 can be a treat, and for hikers, there's even more: the beauty of Desolation Wilderness north of the highway and of Meiss Country, the proposed Meiss Meadows Wilderness, south of it. We offer a trip from each of these trailheads (from west to east): Wrights Lake's Twin Lakes Trailhead north of the highway and into Desolation Wilderness, and the Echo Summit Trailhead south of the highway into Meiss Country on Section 2 of the TYT.

The scenic Wrights Lake area is a favorite gateway to western Desolation Wilderness. Despite this popularity, backpackers willing to step off the trail can still find peace and quiet amid the extraordinary scenery.

Meiss Country is the headwaters of the Truckee River and a beautiful region of wildflowers, streams, lakes, meadows, and peaks.

Note that this book has two Twin Lakes trailheads: this one, starting from Hwy. 50, and another from Hwy. 395.

TRAILHEADS: Twin Lakes
Echo Summit

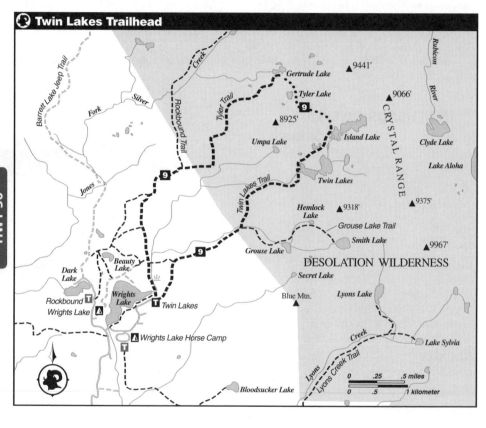

Twin Lakes Trailhead

6962'; 10S 740712 4303800 (field)

DESTINATION/ UTM COORDINATES	TRIP TYPE	BEST SEASON	PACE (HIKING/ LAYOVER DAYS)	TOTAL MILEAGE
9 Island Lake 10S 743700 4306729	Loop	Mid to late	2/0 Moderate, part cross-country	8

Information and Permits: Permits are available for a fee, either by advance reservation or on a first-come, first-served basis from Eldorado National Forest. For west-side entry, apply to or pick up your permit at Pacific Ranger District, located 4 miles east of Pollock Pines on Hwy. 50: 7887 Hwy. 50, Pollock Pines, CA 95726; 530-644-6048; www.fs.fed.us/r5/ eldorado/wild/deso/. During summer, the office is open seven days a week, 8 A.M. to 4:30 P.M. Reserved permits are currently mailed out.

Driving Directions: Approximately 4 miles west of Strawberry, turn north from Hwy. 50 onto FS Road 4 and, following signs for Wrights Lake, drive 8 miles on FS 4 past the Lyons Creek Trailhead and a junction with FS 32 to the vicinity of Wrights Lake. At a stop sign near the Wrights Lake Visitor Information Center, 0.1 mile past the entrance to the Equestrian Camp and Bloodsucker Lake Trailhead, turn right and proceed on a narrow, paved road 0.8 mile to the end of the pavement at the Twin Lakes Trailhead parking area. The trailhead, near the east end of Wrights Lake, is equipped with a pit toilet and bear-proof dumpster.

9 Island Lake

Trip Data: 10S 743700 4306729; 8 miles; 2/0

Topos: *Pyramid Peak, Rockbound Valley*

Highlights: Classic Desolation Wilderness scenery, including craggy peaks and glacier-scoured cirques harboring crystal-blue lakes, abounds on this trip into two tributary canyons of Silver Creek. While the maintained trails up both canyons are relatively short and accessible for scads of hikers and backpackers, the mile-long cross-country route over the ridge between is difficult enough to dissuade all but the hardy few from attempting this loop.

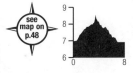

see map on p.48

HEADS UP! The cross-country leg on Day 2 is only for experienced backpackers with navigational and Class 2–3 climbing skills. Novice backpackers should return the way they came. Note that some maps are misleading: There is no trail directly to Tyler Lake; the maintained trail goes to Gertrude Lake.

DAY 1 (Twin Lakes Trailhead to Island Lake, 3.25 miles): From the parking lot, walk down a very short section of paved road past a black steel gate and a bridge over Wrights Lake's lazy inlet (don't cross the bridge) to the start of the Twin Lakes Trail, marked by a Desolation Wilderness signboard. Proceed on a wide, gently graded dirt path through a mixed forest canopy shading a lush understory of plants and flowers to a Y-junction with Trail 16E17 (signed LOOP). Turn right (northeast) and begin a stiff climb through alternating sections of open granite terrain and stands of mixed forest, crossing a trickling stream and the wilderness boundary on the way to a junction with the Grouse Lake Trail, marked by a post.

Following the directions for Twin Lakes, turn left (east) at the junction, immediately step across the seasonal outlet of Grouse Lake, and continue the ducked climb over granite slabs interspersed with scattered lodgepole pines. The stiff ascent is momentarily interrupted by an easy stretch of trail that leads near Twin Lakes' outlet creek. Following another section of steep, rocky climbing alongside the creek, the trail makes a brief descent

HWY 50

past a small pond, followed by a slightly rising ascent to the sparsely treed west shore of Lower Twin Lake, where the deep blue water picturesquely reflects the towering granite walls of the basin's cirque. Decent campsites can be found amid the glacier-polished terrain between the two Twin Lakes. Anglers can ply the waters in search of rainbow and brook trout.

Cross the outlet of Lower Twin Lake on the stone remains of an old dam, follow the trail around the west shore, and then make a short, rocky climb to skirt Boomerang Lake's south shore. Beyond the lake, proceed through a lush pocket meadow and past a cigar-shaped pond. A short, steep, rocky, and winding climb leads to austere Island Lake (8126; 10S 743700 4306729). As most parties seem content with either of the Twin Lakes as their destination, the open shoreline of rock-island-dotted Island Lake should offer campers a bit of peace and quiet. Because the fishing pressure is lower at Island Lake, anglers should do better here than at Twin Lakes. Mountaineers with a layover day could challenge themselves with a climb of 9975-foot Mt. Price.

DAY 2 (Island Lake to Twin Lakes Trailhead, 4.75 miles, part cross-country): From the west shore of Island Lake, leave the maintained trail and start climbing cross-country northwest up the steep slope above the lake, selecting a path that avoids the most brush en route to the crest of the ridge—aim for the low spot (about 8620'; 10S 743502 4306829) directly northeast of a tan-colored rock outcrop. A short section of Class 2–3 climbing just below the crest may be necessary in order to gain the ridge. Once at the top, views of both canyons are excellent.

The hardest part of the cross-country route is now over, as the climb from the crest down to Tyler Lake is less steep than the climb up from Island Lake. Initially, the way down travels roughly north over talus- and grass-covered slopes before an angling descent over granite slabs leads to the northeast shore of Tyler Lake (8233'; 10S 743035 4307275).

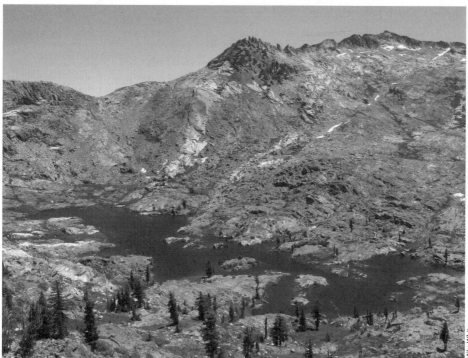

View of Island Lake from ridge

Shaded by a smattering of droopy-tipped hemlocks and upright pines, rimmed with low granite humps and angled slabs, and occupying a cirque with less severe walls, the shoreline of Tyler Lake offers visitors more of a pastoral, subalpine ambiance than that of the alpine-looking lakes in the previous canyon. Despite the less dramatic scenery, the lake does offer a reasonable opportunity for solitude because, contrary to what you'll see on some maps, there exists no maintained trail or boot-beaten path from Tyler Lake to Gertrude Lake, where most visitors prefer to stop.

Go around Tyler's northeast shore to begin the descent to Gertrude Lake, a descent that is short and straightforward. A light forest canopy obscures your view of Gertrude Lake for much of the trip, so pay close attention to where you're going as you descend northwest and then north to Gertrude's south side (8021'; 10S 742792 4307629). Gertrude Lake is a shallow, irregularly shaped body of water encircled by a mixture of grasses, slabs, and stands of conifers, offering limited campsites.

Finding the maintained trail from the vicinity of Gertrude Lake may be a bit of a challenge—look for a large cairn or a series of ducks on the granite bench south of the lake. Having located the ducks or cairn, follow a ducked course southwest on a moderate descent over granite slabs and through boulder- and conifer-sprinkled terrain. Where the trail passes through groves of light forest, the tread becomes easier to follow. The heather-lined path crosses several seasonal meltwater streams before a gentle ascent leads past a small pond. Then a short, steep climb leads to the apex of the ridge dividing the drainage of Jones Fork Silver Creek from the drainage of South Fork Silver Creek.

Breaking out of the trees to open views of Wrights Lake, the trail descends steeply before briefly moderating through a stretch of light forest, where lush vegetation carpets the forest floor. A moderately steep descent resumes down open, shrub-covered terrain that offers excellent views of the canyon holding Twin Lakes. Cross the signed Desolation Wilderness boundary and follow a gently graded path to a post marking a junction with the Rockbound Trail.

Turn left and head southwest on the Rockbound Trail, climb over a low hill, and proceed on the gradually descending trail to another junction, a half mile from the previous one. Here, turn left (south), leaving the Rockbound Trail to follow Trail 16E16 (follow signs to Wrights Lake at all junctions).

From the junction, follow the gently graded, sandy trail through open terrain until a steeper descent on rocky trail leads back into the forest. Pass by an unmarked junction with a short connector southwest to the Rockbound Trail and proceed to a major junction, where two side trails enter, the first from the right and the second from the left several yards farther on. Continuing straight ahead at both side-trail junctions, you soon see a large meadow through the trees to the left, where Wrights Lake's inlet follows a lazy, serpentine course toward the reservoir. An easy stroll eventually leads alongside this stream and shortly to the well-constructed bridge over the inlet, where you close the loop. From there, follow the paved access road a very short distance back to the trailhead parking lot (6940'; 10S 740712 4303800 (field)).

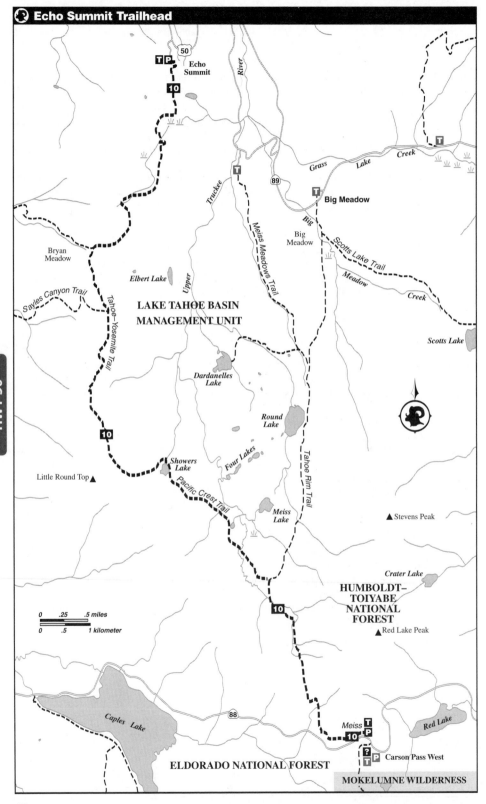

HWY 50

50
Echo Summit

Truckee River

Grass Lake Creek

89

Big Meadow

Big Meadow

Big Meadow

Scotts Lake Trail

Meadow Creek

Bryan Meadow

Elbert Lake

Upper

Meiss Meadows Trail

Scotts Lake

Sayles Canyon Trail

Tahoe-Yosemite Trail

**LAKE TAHOE BASIN
MANAGEMENT UNIT**

Dardanelles Lake

Round Lake

Little Round Top ▲

Showers Lake

Four Lakes

Meiss Lake

Tahoe Rim Trail

Pacific Crest Trail

▲ Stevens Peak

Crater Lake

**HUMBOLDT–
TOIYABE
NATIONAL
FOREST**

▲ Red Lake Peak

0   .25   .5 miles
0   .5   1 kilometer

Caples Lake

88

Meiss

Red Lake

Carson Pass West

ELDORADO NATIONAL FOREST

MOKELUMNE WILDERNESS

Echo Summit Trailhead

7389'; 10S 757559 4300186 (field)

T

DESTINATION/ UTM COORDINATES	TRIP TYPE	BEST SEASON	PACE (HIKING/ LAYOVER DAYS)	TOTAL MILEAGE
10 Carson Pass West 11S 239819 4287379 (field)	Shuttle	Mid to late	2/0 Moderate	13.4

Information and Permits: "Meiss Country" is the current term for the proposed Meiss Meadows Wilderness Area, highly deserving of wilderness status, in the Lake Tahoe Basin Management Unit. For information: USDA Forest Service, Lake Tahoe Basin Management Unit; 35 College Drive, South Lake Tahoe, CA 96150; 530-543-2600; www.fs.fed.us/r5/ltbmu/. No wilderness permits are required at this time, but you must have a California Campfire Permit to have a campfire or use a stove.

Driving Directions: Follow Hwy. 50 to Echo Summit, and from there go west to a paved access road on the south side of the highway, 0.2 mile west of Echo Summit. A sign reading SNO-PARK marks the turnoff. Proceed 0.2 mile to the large PCT parking lot.

10 Tahoe-Yosemite Trail Section 2: To Carson Pass West

Trip Data: 11S 239819 4287379 (field); 13.4 miles; 2/0 days

Topos: *Echo Lake, Caples Lake, Carson Pass*

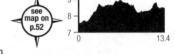

Highlights: This second leg of the TYT begins with an unpromising walk through a summer-dusty Sno-Park just south and west of Echo Summit (on Hwy. 50). But soon you leave this behind for the remarkable scenery of Meiss Country, where seasonal wildflowers from here to Carson Pass can be amazing. This section coincides with the PCT.

HEADS UP! *Hunters also favor this area: When hiking during deer season, wear bright clothing and stay near major trails.*

Shuttle Directions: To get to Carson Pass West, take Hwy. 88 to Carson Pass and go 0.3 mile west to a large parking lot on the highway's north side that serves this trailhead. There is a daily fee to park here.

DAY 1 (Echo Summit Trailhead to Showers Lake, 8.3 miles): First, walk a short way down the paved road (south) from the parking lot and then through the ski area to pick up the trail on the snow park's south edge. You've just passed through an old ski area, now a state Sno-Park in winter. The former ski lodge now houses a unit of the California Conservation Corps.

Start hiking through shrubs and low pines, immediately crossing a section of old paved roadway, and then making a moderate climb of the old ski hill. The route, well signed, levels, merges with an old road for a short distance, and then veers right (south) on well-marked, single-track trail. Follow the rocky trail up a shrub-covered slope to intersect a sandy road, and then turn right and climb up the road about 100 yards to the resumption of single-track trail at a TRT sign.

Swinging south, stroll along granite-dotted slopes sparsely covered by white firs and lodgepole and Jeffrey pines, with a generous understory of huckleberry oak bushes. Approximately 1 mile from the parking lot, a momentary descent leads past a lateral heading northeast to an unnamed pond; go right (west) here to Benwood Meadow, which can dry up by late season.

see map on p.52

HWY 50

Proceed through the forest around the edge of the boggy meadow and across a pair of seasonal streams to a wood-plank bridge over an alder-lined creek. After a moderate, winding climb from the bridge, the trail switchbacks and ascends into thinning forest, which allows periodic glimpses of Lake Tahoe over the next mile or so. Continue the moderate climb to the south past large granitic boulders.

Reach a saddle about 1.5 miles from Benwood Meadow, where an excellent view to the southeast includes the Upper Truckee basin and surrounding peaks as well as Elephants Back and Round Top. Past the viewpoint, continue climbing for another 0.3 mile, staying at the foot of a row of nearly vertical cliffs, and reach a tiny creek. Half a dozen people could camp on the flat above the creek's southeast bank. From the vicinity of this campsite, the trail switchbacks and climbs quite steeply to a hillside meadow with water and a campsite on a rise near the creek.

The grade soon eases upon entering a dense-to-moderate lodgepole forest as the trail crosses a ridge and descends gently to a shallow pass. Just beyond the pass, reach a junction with the Bryan Meadow Trail near the east end of the picturesque clearing. Nearby are several campsites with water plentiful in early season. Go left (ahead, south) here, staying on the PCT/TYT.

From Bryan Meadow, the trail leads south on sandy footing, undulating and then ascending gently to a minor summit, followed by a brief descent to a saddle and a junction with the Sayles Canyon Trail. Again, go left (ahead, south) here on the PCT/TYT.

A mile of gradually increasing ascent leads over the east ridge of Peak 9020, which separates the two branches of the headwaters of Sayles Canyon Creek. At the upper lobes of

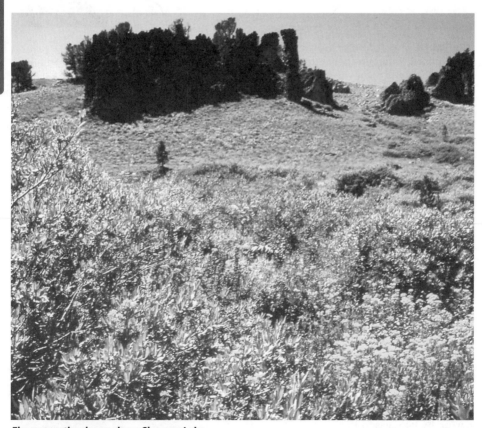

Flowers on the slopes above Showers Lake

a hillside meadow, there may be water into late season and campsites on a sandy rise near-by. At the first saddle beyond the ridge, a use trail crosses the PCT/TYT at right angles, and a short distance farther on is a junction with an infrequently maintained trail to Schneider's cow camp. Once more, go left (ahead, south) here on the PCT/TYT.

The trail next curves through a willow-covered meadow and crosses its larger, flower-covered neighbor; both may provide late-season water. Keen eyes will begin to notice how the character of the rocks begins to change from granitic to volcanic and the sandy tread turns pinkish.

A descent leads into a large bowl whose southwest rim may be draped with snow cornices for much of the summer. The slopes of this bowl are very open and laced with runoff streams, and they support lavish gardens of shrubs and flowers, including blue elderberry, rangers buttons (also called swamp whiteheads), mountain bluebells, green gentian, aster, wallflower, penstemon, cinquefoil, spiraea, corn lily, and columbine. This highly colorful bowl, harboring as-yet-unseen Showers Lake, offers photographers a great choice of hues, subjects, and compositions.

Make a gentle descent through the bowl, passing beneath a palisade-like outcropping below the cornice-laden rim. The trail, which here differs from the route shown on the topo, veers northeast and eventually drops below Showers Lake to cross the lake's outlet. Beyond the ford, zigzag steeply uphill south-southwest a short distance to Showers Lake (8647'; 10S 757728 4292385).

Day 2 (Showers Lake to Carson Pass West, 5.1 miles): Heading toward Hwy. 88, the trail climbs as it curves around the lake's east side to a junction at a small saddle above Showers Lake. Take the left fork southeast and away from the lake (the right fork is a seldom-used lateral to Schneider's cow camp). Descend a switchback and drop down a slope with vegetation and colors much like the previous bowl. This trail segment offers panoramic views of the large meadows around the headwaters of the Truckee River. The best views occur when there's just a bit of snow left on the west side of the Crystal Range.

Make a steady descent to traverse another meadow and reenter forest on the west slope of the upper Truckee Valley. The trail begins to resemble an old 4WD road, which it once was, on the way past a large pond. Just north of your first ford of the Truckee River, a use trail heads roughly north-northeast across Meiss Meadows a half mile to Meiss Lake. Reaching the lake in early season may be a bit of a challenge, as parts of the trail are quite mucky and the ford of the creek on the way to the lake will most likely be a wet one. You, however, stay on the main PCT/TYT and ford the young Truckee River.

> **MEISS MEADOWS**
>
> During the last Ice Age, a lake occupied all these meadows, which subsequently were filled with sediment—except for the small remnant of Meiss Lake. The meadows offer many attractions for the birder and also for those who wish to see the Belding ground squirrel. The house and barn are the remains of a former cow camp—thank goodness, grazing here was banned several years ago.

Near the buildings is a defunct stock gate and a well-signed junction with the Tahoe Rim Trail heading left (northeast) to Round Lake. *(Partial Recap: Trip 8, Day 2.)* Go ahead (south) to stay on the PCT/TYT. Beyond this junction, the PCT/TYT fords the river again and begins a final, moderate ascent to a saddle dividing the Truckee River and American River drainages. On the climb, increasingly fine views culminate at the saddle, with the Round Top complex dominating the scene immediately to the south, Lake Tahoe capturing the eye in the distance to the north, and Red Lake Peak towering immediately to the east (you're on its western slope).

From the saddle, the route descends past a lovely pond and then drops steeply on the rocky-dusty tread of a former jeep road. After several hundred yards, take a single-track trail that veers left (east) away from the road and follows a few switchbacks down sagebrush-covered slopes dotted with mule ears and other flowers. Follow the trail across a runoff stream and then around the nose of a ridge through a moderate forest cover of fir and pine.

Soon the sound of cars on Hwy. 88 below heralds the approach to Carson Pass West (also called Meiss Meadow Trailhead). The final leg takes longer than you'd expect because the trail curves well to the east before exiting at the trailhead parking lot (8566'; 11S 239819 4287379 (field)) just off the noisy road.

Backpackers continuing on the PCT/TYT must walk 0.3 mile uphill along the highway to pick up the next section of this trail—the southbound PCT/TYT—at Carson Pass proper (Carson Pass East).

STATE HIGHWAY 88 TRIPS

We feature five trailheads along scenic Hwy. 88. Four of them lead south into Mokelumne Wilderness; one leads north into Meiss Country.

South of Hwy. 88 lies 105,165-acre Mokelumne Wilderness, a wonderland of colorful volcanic peaks, contrasting granitic terrain, amazing wildflower displays, stunning canyons, and picturesque lakes. We visit Mokelumne Wilderness and its nearby areas from four trailheads along or just off of Hwy. 88 (from west to east): Silver Lake—Granite Lake Trailhead, Thunder Mountain Trailhead, Carson Pass East Trailhead, and Upper Blue Lake—Granite Lake Trailhead (a different Granite Lake from the earlier one).

Superb scenery, mixing volcanic and granitic rocks, is the hallmark of the region around Silver Lake and Thunder Mountain, particularly in Mokelumne Wilderness. During peak season, backpackers will experience some of the best flower displays in the entire Sierra. The trips from the Woods Lake Trailhead and the Carson Pass East Trailhead head into the extremely popular Carson Pass Management Area, famed for its peaks, lakes, and wildflowers. The beauty of the area is your reward for putting up with the poor campsites you're forced to use.

Off Blue Lakes Road, this highway section features a series of out-of-the-way reservoirs that lure campers, boaters, and anglers. The area beyond these reservoirs presents some equally attractive backcountry that is sure to please even the most discriminating of backpackers.

North of Hwy. 88 in the Carson Pass area lies wonderful Meiss Country, proposed for wilderness status and well deserving of it. Wide-ranging vistas, expansive meadows, and splendid wildflowers are just a few of the area's pleasures. From Hwy. 88, the Carson Pass West Trailhead, located in the west-to-east order between the Thunder Mountain and Carson Pass East trailheads, is your gateway to Meiss Country.

TRAILHEADS: Silver Lake–Granite Lake
Thunder Mountain
Woods Lake
Carson Pass West
Carson Pass East
Upper Blue Lake–Granite Lake

HWY 88

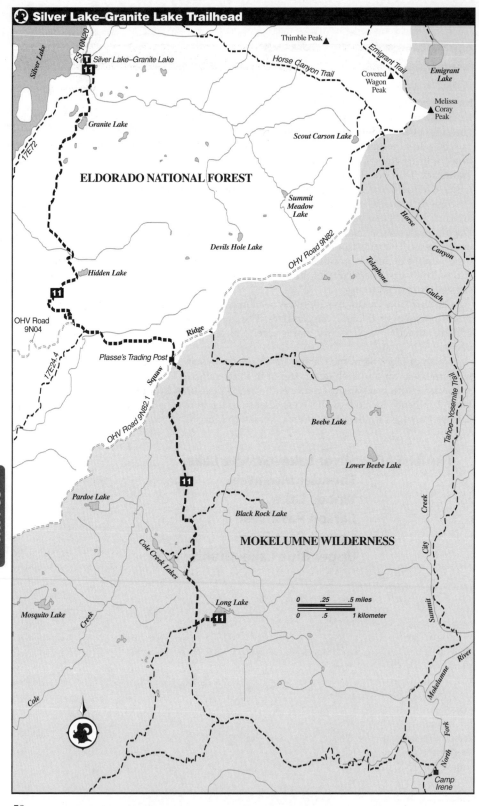

Thimble Peak ▲

Horse Canyon Trail

Emigrant Trail

Covered Wagon Peak ▲

Emigrant Lake

Melissa Coray Peak ▲

Silver Lake

FS 10N20

T Silver Lake–Granite Lake
11

1E72

Granite Lake

Scout Carson Lake

ELDORADO NATIONAL FOREST

Summit Meadow Lake

Horse

Devils Hole Lake

OHV Road 9N82

Canyon

Telephone

Gulch

11 Hidden Lake

OHV Road 9N04

Ridge

1TE24.4

Plasse's Trading Post

Squaw

OHV Road 9N82.1

Beebe Lake

Tahoe–Yosemite Trail

Lower Beebe Lake

11

Pardoe Lake

Black Rock Lake

MOKELUMNE WILDERNESS

Creek

City

Cole Creek Lakes

0   .25   .5 miles
0   .5   1 kilometer

Mosquito Lake

Long Lake **11**

Summit

Creek

Cole

Mokelumne

River

Fork

North

Camp Irene

Silver Lake–Granite Lake Trailhead

7347'; 10S 751532 4283031 (field)

DESTINATION/ UTM COORDINATES	TRIP TYPE	BEST SEASON	PACE (HIKING/ LAYOVER DAYS)	TOTAL MILEAGE (round trip)
I I Long Lake 10S 754220 4273544	Out & back	Mid	2/1 Moderate	18

Information and Permits: This trailhead is in Eldorado National Forest: 100 Forni Road, Placerville, CA 95667; 530-622-5061; www.fs.fed.us/r5/eldorado/wild/moke/index.html. For visitor information, call 530-644-6048.

Driving Directions: From Hwy. 88 near the north end of Silver Lake, leave the highway following signs east along the lake's north end for Kit Carson Resort. Continue past the resort to the east side of the lake and the small trailhead parking area, 1.4 miles from Hwy. 88.

I I Long Lake

Trip Data: 10S 754220 4273544; 18 miles; 2/1 days

Topos: *Caples Lake, Mokelumne Peak*

see map on p.58

Highlights: A hike full of wonderful views leads to one of the area's loveliest lakes, above which travelers will find campsites on granite benches that command spectacular views of the surrounding peaks.

DAY 1 (Silver Lake–Granite Lake Trailhead to Long Lake, 9 miles): Locate the trailhead on the left-hand side of the road marked by a sign reading MANKALO TRAIL 17E72, GRANITE LAKE 1, PLASSES 3. The trail begins on a gentle-to-moderate climb through a scattered forest of Jeffrey pines, lodgepole pines, and white firs. Proceed through granitic terrain dotted with aspens and manzanita past a seasonal pond/meadow and across a bridge over Squaw Creek. Beyond the bridge, reach a junction and turn left (south), following signed directions for Granite Lake. A steep climb leads up open terrain of granite slabs and shrubs to well-named Granite Lake, occupying a shallow basin of granite on a bench 550 feet above Silver Lake. Although the lake offers a few Spartan campsites sheltered by scattered conifers, the 1-mile distance from the trailhead ensures that these sites are heavily used and therefore not recommended.

Pass around the west shore of the lake and proceed through mixed forest past a stagnant pond and a flower-filled meadow. Continue straight ahead (south) at a T-junction, where the faint tread of a path heads right, providing an infrequently used connector to Plasse's Resort. Beyond the junction, a mostly gentle ascent leads through the forest to the crossing of a seasonal stream, followed by a short but steeper climb to Hidden Lake. Conifers shade the near lakeshore while the far shore is composed of meadows and clumps of willow backdropped nicely by granite cliffs. Good campsites will lure overnighters.

Climb out of Hidden Lake's basin around pockets of willow-and-flower-carpeted meadows to a signed junction on top of a low ridge. Veer left (south) at the junction to pass by a verdant meadow and then a spring on a hemlock-shaded climb to a divide between the American River and Bear River drainages. Descending from this view-packed ridge, cross a drift fence and in less than 100 yards turn left (east-southeast) onto a 4WD road.

Traveling along the road, the grade is level past the Allen Ranch and then across the seasonal headwaters of Bear River. Now ascending, cross some perennial trickles and then veer to the right, leaving the road just before a small creek. Rejoin the road on the crest of Squaw Ridge, where a sign indicates the former site of Plasse's Trading Post.

HWY 88

RAYMOND PLASSE

While traveling the Carson Emigrant Route, French immigrant Raymond Plasse fell in love with the area around Silver Lake. He established a trading post on Squaw Ridge in 1853 and ran it for many years before moving his family to the south end of the lake to raise cattle and operate a resort. No sign of the trading post exists today, but Plasse's Resort is in full operation each summer (www.plassesresort.com).

About 130 yards down from the ridge, leave the road by turning left (southeast) to enter Mokelumne Wilderness. In 1984, motorized vehicles were banned and the Mokelumne Wilderness was enlarged from 50,165 acres to the current 105,165 acres. At that point, this former roadbed began a process of rehabilitation. Just inside the wilderness boundary the route passes above Horse Thief Spring, which usually flows all year. Sadly, due to intense cattle grazing, the springs are mere remnants of their former glory, but fill up here anyway, as this may be the last water before Cole Creek Lakes.

Continuing south, the nearly level trail passes some long meadows and then joins a broad volcanic ridge where views extend south all the way into the Carson-Iceberg Wilderness. As the trail descends the ridge, continue ahead (south) at a junction with the faint, old, unmapped trail to Cole Creek Lakes. At the next junction, with the trail heading left (northeast) to Black Rock Lake, you go right (south).

Now on granite terrain, cross another view-blessed ridge, which includes a closer look at Mokelumne Peak. Descending the rocky ridge, you meet a signed trail right (southwest) to Cole Creek Lakes. A level, half mile stroll through the forest is followed by a brief descent to the southernmost Cole Creek Lake. From the lake's seasonal outlet, the trail makes a gentle descent southeast and then south for most of a mile before gradually ascending to the signed junction with the lateral to Long Lake.

Turn left (east-northeast) toward Long Lake, and in a short half mile, arrive at the south shore of many-bayed Long Lake (7831'; 10S 754220 4273544). People and cattle seemingly overuse the immediate lakeshore, but nice camping is available by skirting the south shore, crossing one of the tiny dams that enlarge this lake, and then heading east, away from the lake, onto open granite benches. Within several hundred yards of the lake are level, dry, cow- and mosquito-free campsites with fabulous views to the southeast over Wester Park to the headwaters of the Mokelumne River and the peaks around Ebbetts Pass.

DAY 2 (Long Lake to Silver Lake–Granite Lake Trailhead, 9 miles): Retrace your steps.

Thunder Mountain Trailhead

7939'; 10S 751533 4288072 (field)

DESTINATION/ UTM COORDINATES	TRIP TYPE	BEST SEASON	PACE (HIKING/ LAYOVER DAYS)	TOTAL MILEAGE (round trip)
12 Scout Carson Lake 10S 756354 4281829	Out & back	Mid	2/1 Leisurely	13
13 Summit City Canyon 10S 758438 4279583	Out & back	Mid	4/1 Leisurely	22
14 Mokelumne River 10S 757867 4272385	Out & back	Mid	6/1 Strenuous, part cross-country	33
15 Silver Lake– Granite Lake Trailhead 10S 751532 4283031 (field)	Shuttle	Mid	5/1 Strenuous, part cross-country	31.7

Information and Permits: This trailhead is on Eldorado National Forest: 100 Forni Road, Placerville, CA 95667; 530-622-5061; www.fs.fed.us/r5/eldorado/wild/moke/index.html. For visitor information, call 530-644-6048. **Note:** The Thunder Mountain Trailhead and the trail segment between it and the Horse Canyon Trail appear on the *Mokelumne Wilderness* map but not on the 7.5' topo.

Driving Directions: Follow Hwy. 88 to the roadside trailhead for the Thunder Mountain Loop near Carson Spur, 3.25 miles east of Silver Lake and 1.75 miles west of the Kirkwood Meadows junction, on the south side of the highway.

12 Scout Carson Lake

Trip Data: 10S 756354 4281829; 13 miles; 2/1 days

Topos: *Caples Lake*

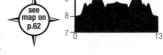

Highlights: A lovely, small, near-timberline lake is the goal of this trip, which passes through interesting geologic scenery along the way. An optional 1-mile round-trip detour to the 9408-foot summit of Thunder Mountain offers an expansive 360-degree vista of the Carson Pass region. The route continues with fine views of the surrounding volcanic battlements on the way to Scout Carson Lake.

HEADS UP! A 1.7-mile section of the Horse Canyon Trail between the junction with the Thunder Mountain Trail and the spur to Scout Carson Lake is open to motorcycles. However, they seldom travel that far up the trail from Silver Lake.

DAY 1 (Thunder Mountain Trailhead to Scout Carson Lake, 6.5 miles): Pass through a deteriorating cattle gate in a wire fence and proceed through a mixed forest of red firs, lodgepole pines, and western white pines, soon encountering a T-junction with a lightly used path that heads east to cross Hwy. 88 and then travels west to Castle Point. Continue straight ahead (southeast) on your main trail on a moderate climb, breaking out of the trees on a climb across a sagebrush-and-wildflower-covered hillside below Carson Spur, where the rocky crags of Two Sentinels spring into view. Briefly gain the crest at a saddle before a climb across the west side of the ridge leads into thickening forest. Following a pair of switchbacks, traverse below the pinnacles of Two Sentinels to an open saddle, where the peaks of the Carson Pass area burst into view, along with Kirkwood Meadows and Caples Lake below.

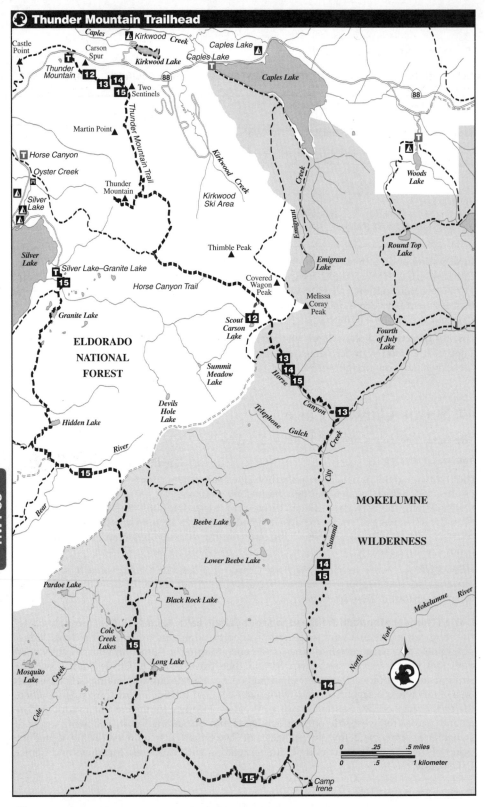

Caples
Castle
Point
Kirkwood Creek
Kirkwood
Carson Spur
Kirkwood Lake
Caples Lake
Caples Lake
Thunder Mountain
12
13 **14**
15
Two Sentinels
88
Caples Lake
88

Martin Point

Thunder Mountain Trail
Kirkwood Creek
T
Woods Lake

T Horse Canyon
Oyster Creek

Silver Lake

Thunder Mountain
Kirkwood Ski Area

Emigrant Creek
Round Top Lake

Silver Lake

Thimble Peak

Emigrant Lake

1 Silver Lake–Granite Lake
15

Covered Wagon Peak

Melissa Coray Peak

Fourth of July Lake

Horse Canyon Trail

Granite Lake

Scout Carson Lake
12

ELDORADO

NATIONAL

FOREST

Summit Meadow Lake

13
14
15

Horse Canyon

13

Devils Hole Lake

Telephone Gulch

City Creek

Hidden Lake

MOKELUMNE

River
15

Beebe Lake

WILDERNESS

Bear

Summit

Lower Beebe Lake

Pardoe Lake

14
15

Black Rock Lake

Mokelumne River

Cole Creek Lakes
15

North Fork

Mosquito Lake

Long Lake

14

Cole Creek

0   .25   .5 miles
0   .5   1 kilometer

15
Camp Irene

HWY 88

Head south along the ridge toward Martin Point, with additional eastward views along the way. A couple of switchbacks lead to an upward traverse around the east side of Martin Point, revealing the impressive profile of Thunder Mountain's north face, where the dark volcanic rock, punctuated with numerous clefts, gashes, pinnacles, and arêtes, creates a dramatic alpine scene. Continue the ascent along the ridgecrest toward Thunder Mountain. As you approach the northeast ridge of the peak, you make two more switchbacks and then a gentle traverse around the back of the ridge to a junction marked by a post, 3.5 miles from the trailhead.

THUNDER MOUNTAIN

Those who would like to bag a peak before continuing to Scout Carson Lake should turn right (southwest) at the junction and follow an ascending, westward traverse through scattered lodgepole pines, western white pines, mountain hemlocks, and whitebark pines. The trees diminish near the crest as the trail angles sharply to the east to follow the ridge to the summit. The top offers an incredible view in all directions, from the mountains of northern Yosemite in the south to the peaks of Desolation Wilderness in the north. Nearby landmarks include Silver and Caples lakes and Round Top.

To stay on or return to your main trail, turn left at the junction if you didn't go to Thunder Mountain, or right if you did, and in either case east. Head downhill across dry slopes through scattered to light timber to another junction, this one with a trail branching left (northeast) toward Kirkwood Meadows. Go right and continue the descent into thickening forest until breaking out of the trees onto open, flower-filled slopes that allow excellent views of Silver Lake and Horse Canyon. Reach a junction at the bottom of the descent with the Horse Canyon Trail.

Turn left (southeast) at the junction and climb an open hillside, drop briefly to cross an unnamed, year-round creek, and then climb a sagebrush-dotted slope. Now at 8800 feet, the trail follows a mile-long traverse across an open, flower-sprinkled bench on the south side of Thimble Peak. To the east of the peak are the tops of some of the ski lifts servicing Kirkwood Meadows in the next valley to the north. After passing an abandoned, overgrown path to Kirkwood Meadows, marked by an old post with a missing sign, ascend moderately through granite boulders to a signed junction in a sandy meadow.

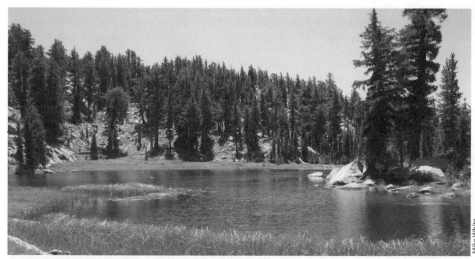

Mike White

Attractive Scout Carson Lake is Day 1's destination.

Turn right (southwest) and stroll an easy half mile on a winding ascent through stands of mixed forest and pocket meadows to Scout Carson Lake (8958'; 10S 756354 4281829) on the edge of, but not in, Mokelumne Wilderness. Perched on a small bench, ringed by meadow, and surrounded by a forest of lodgepole pine, western white pine, and mountain hemlock, diminutive Scout Carson Lake is a sweet example of Sierra Nevada charm. Perhaps not so charming are the numerous mosquitoes buzzing through the air until late season, and less charming still is the potential for cows with their clanking bells that may be heard as they graze the nearby meadows. You can reduce if not eliminate both annoyances by camping away from the meadow-fringed lakeshore in favor of drier and rockier terrain to the west. The lake supports a small but fat population of brook trout, which gratefully eat the mosquitoes. Emigrant Peak to the east is a straightforward climb offering a superb view from the summit of much of Mokelumne Wilderness.

DAY 2 (Scout Carson Lake to Thunder Mountain Trailhead, 6.5 miles): Retrace your steps.

13 Summit City Canyon

Trip Data: 10S 758438 4279583;
22 miles; 4/1 days

Topos: *Caples Lake*

see map on p.62

Highlights: Beyond Scout Carson Lake, this route crosses Squaw Ridge and descends isolated Horse Canyon to campsites along picturesque, remote, and lonely Summit City Creek.

DAY 1 (Thunder Mountain Trailhead to Scout Carson Lake, 6.5 miles): *(Recap: Trip 12, Day 1.)* At the trailhead, pass through a cattle gate and proceed to a T-junction with an eastbound path (left) to Castle Point. Go ahead (southeast) on a moderate climb, soon crossing a hillside below Carson Spur. Briefly gain the crest at a saddle and soon return to forest. Traverse below Two Sentinels to an open saddle and then head south along the ridge toward Martin Point. Traverse the east side of Martin Point and ascend a ridgecrest toward Thunder Mountain. At the junction with the trail up Thunder Mountain (optional excursion), stay on your main trail by turning left (east) and heading downhill across dry slopes to another junction, this one with a trail left (northeast) toward Kirkwood Meadows. Go right and continue the descent to the junction with the Horse Canyon Trail; turn left (southeast) at the junction to climb, then drop briefly to a year-round creek, and then climb to make a mile-long traverse of Thimble Peak's south side. Ignore an abandoned, overgrown path to Kirkwood Meadows, marked by an old post, and ascend through granite boulders to a signed junction in a sandy meadow. Turn right (southwest) and ascend a half mile to Scout Carson Lake (8958'; 10S 756354 4281829).

DAY 2 (Scout Carson Lake to Summit City Canyon, 4.5 miles): Return a half mile to the Horse Canyon Trail junction and turn right (south-southeast). The sometimes muddy trail ascends moderately through a thinning cover of trees almost to timberline, passing through upland meadows rife with flower color in early season. Approaching Squaw Ridge, cross a set of little-used jeep tracks and in 100 yards arrive at an unnamed pass and the boundary of Mokelumne Wilderness, where trails are generally maintained sufficiently for walkers but not for horses or mules.

The steep descent into Horse Canyon uses a great number of switchbacks that zigzag downslope among tall, elegant western white pines and past plentiful patches of flowers that include daisies, senecio, phlox, brodiaea, paintbrush, and whorled penstemon. At a natural overlook less than a mile down the trail, the far-gazing hiker can peer deep into the canyons of Summit City Creek and the North Fork Mokelumne River. Nowadays it's hard to imagine that 160 years ago stalwart emigrants brought their covered wagons up this canyon, winching them from tree to tree where it was too steep for their straining livestock to pull them.

Swinging east briefly, the trail descends more steeply to cross a creek at 8100 feet and pass two immense, centuries-old red firs. The sometimes faint trail descends grassy meadows and then, leaving the grazing cows behind, begins the final drop into Summit City Canyon. Now the views are open, revealing the trademark U-shaped gorge that characterizes glaciated canyons. Along a newer section of trail, brushy hillsides support a large population of chokecherries.

CHOKECHERRY

In late season, the chokecherry fruits grow in such abundance as to give a faint red tinge to this hillside when viewed from afar. Small and bitter, the origin of the name "choke" cherry presents little mystery, although the unlikely fruits produce a most exquisite syrup at the hands of an accomplished chef.

Meet the TYT at the forested canyon bottom and turn right (southwest). After an easy quarter mile, just before seasonal Horse Canyon Creek, pass an illegal campsite too close to the water, near where Summit City Creek makes an S-curve through a slot in the granite bedrock (6840'; 10S 758438 4279583) and search out legal campsites up- and downstream. Few people come this far down Summit City Canyon, and you're almost sure to have it to yourself.

DAYS 3–4 (Summit City Canyon to Thunder Mountain Trailhead, 11 miles): Retrace your steps.

14 Mokelumne River

Trip Data: 10S 757867 4272385; 33 miles; 6/1 days

see map on p.62

Topos: *Caples Lake, Mokelumne Peak*

Highlights: The largest wilderness river in the northern Sierra is the goal of this trip, where cathedral forests shade the cool, green river, brown trout often rise to the fly, and solitude is plentiful (with possible exceptions at river crossings).

HEADS UP! Consider as cross-country bushwhacking most of the route down Summit City Canyon beyond Telephone Gulch to the Mokelumne River. The Forest Service has seemingly given up on this route, as shown by the absence of a trail from the Mokelumne Wilderness map 1.5 miles beyond Telephone Gulch all the way to Camp Irene. Consider performing a little "vigilante trail maintenance" on this scenic route by using lightweight pruning shears to snip away some of the overgrowth.

Don't even consider a solo trip in this area! Attempt this route only if your party has experience in cross-country travel through chaparral and dense forest, experience in the use of map and compass, and bouldering skills—including the ability to make a few Class 2–3 moves with a full backpack. Wear durable, long-sleeved shirts and long pants through this overgrown section. Don't expect to find a lot of water late in the season or following dry winters—check with the Forest Service for current conditions. Given the difficulties above, an extra day or two of angling and idling along the Mokelumne River could be a well-deserved treat.

HWY 88

DAY 1 (Thunder Mountain Trailhead to Scout Carson Lake, 6.5 miles): *(Recap: Trip 12, Day 1.)* At the trailhead, pass through a cattle gate and proceed to a T-junction with an east-bound path (left) to Castle Point. Go ahead (southeast) on a moderate climb, soon crossing a hillside below Carson Spur. Briefly gain the crest at a saddle and soon return to forest. Traverse below Two Sentinels to an open saddle and then head south along the ridge toward Martin Point. Traverse the east side of Martin Point and ascend a ridgecrest toward Thunder Mountain. At the junction with the trail up Thunder Mountain (optional excursion), stay on your main trail by turning left (east) and heading downhill across dry slopes to another junction, this one with a trail left (northeast) toward Kirkwood Meadows. Go right and continue the descent to the junction with the Horse Canyon Trail; turn left (southeast) at the junction to climb, then drop briefly to a year-round creek, and then climb to make a mile-long traverse of Thimble Peak's south side. Ignore an abandoned, overgrown path to Kirkwood Meadows, marked by an old post, and ascend through granite boulders to a signed junction in a sandy meadow. Turn right (southwest) and ascend a half mile to Scout Carson Lake (8958'; 10S 756354 4281829).

DAY 2 (Scout Carson Lake to Summit City Canyon, 4.5 miles): *(Recap: Trip 13, Day 2.)* Return a half mile to the Horse Canyon Trail junction, turn right (south-southeast) on that trail, and descend steeply into Mokelumne Wilderness and to the bottom of Summit City Canyon, where you meet the TYT. Turn right (southwest, downstream) for about a quarter mile to the vicinity of seasonal Horse Canyon Creek (6840'; 10S 758438 4279583) and an illegal campsite; search out legal campsites nearby, up and down the creek.

DAY 3 (Summit City Canyon to Mokelumne River, 5.5 miles, mostly cross-country): If you haven't done so already in your search for a campsite, head downstream (generally southwest and then south) to cross seasonal Horse Canyon Creek—may be dry by midseason in a dry year. Continue winding down Summit City Canyon to cross Telephone Gulch. The main canyon narrows, but not so much as to force the path right next to the creek, as sandy duff tread leads across flats dotted with numerous lodgepole pines and aspens. The most common wildflower here, as has been the case since before you reached the floor of Summit City Canyon, is the pink-cupped sidalcea. The second-most common flower has been squaw root, also called yampa, with hundreds of tiny white flowers composing flat flowerheads that are more delicate and open than the dense flowerheads of yarrow.

Beyond Telephone Gulch, the trail descends Summit City Canyon, usually keeping a good distance away from the creek and heading generally south. Deadfalls are numerous through here, requiring frequent detours. A gentle descent crosses alternating sections of moist, shady areas and open, dry areas. The trail is usually obvious, although growing fainter, sometimes overgrown with thorny chaparral.

About 2.5 miles below Horse Canyon, the trail nears the bank where the creek leaves a shady flat to flow into a narrowing gorge of granite. Don't cross the creek here, as the trail, which is blasted out of the bedrock, continues along the west side of the creek a short distance and then abruptly ends. At a break in the granite—requiring bouldering skills in order to get you and your load up onto the next set of slabs—take some time to search for the best possible route. Continue along slabs and ledges above the creek, passing a campsite in a grove of Jeffrey pines, and after about another 200 yards, cross the creek just above where the creek flows through a narrow, steep-walled slot. The final descent to the creek is extremely steep—you may prefer to sit and scoot. The creek crossing can be wet or possibly even dangerous during periods of exceptionally high runoff. However, continuing on the west side of the creek would quickly become very steep and very brushy, so ford the creek you must.

The trail resumes on the east bank, climbs about 30 feet, and then continues down the canyon. The tread is usually noticeable beyond the creek crossing, except across stretches of bedrock, where ducks should help guide the way. Cross just such an area of bedrock a few hundred feet beyond the ford and then parallel the creek as it swings south. Descend near the creek for a short distance, and then climb high above the stream over the west shoulder of a small dome. Descend steeply past a smaller dome and reenter forest, encountering the first incense cedar along the way. The route is now separated from the creek by a low ridge, where the grade eases and then climbs onto some slabs. Descend the slabs toward (but not to) a small side stream on the left. At the bottom of the slabs, the trail heads down a steep notch toward the right (possibly requiring the removal of your pack) and presently draws near Summit City Creek again. Parallel Summit City Creek until the trail crosses the side stream just above its confluence with Summit City Creek.

Leave the forest again and climb very briefly onto an open, rocky slope. Continuing down the canyon, cross additional slabs, veering away from the creek. After several hundred yards, the trail enters a trail-crowding patch of waist- to shoulder-high huckleberry oak and manzanita. Staying mostly in brush, the route descends gently to a steeper, final slope down to the bottom of Mokelumne River Canyon, where views open up of the TYT ascending the south side of the canyon below Mt. Reba. Descend several hundred feet, veer left across a flat area, and then switchback downhill toward Summit City Creek, avoiding the tendency to cross the creek until reaching the valley floor. The trail descends ledges, at one point climbs a bit, and then drops through a cleft in the bedrock to the creek.

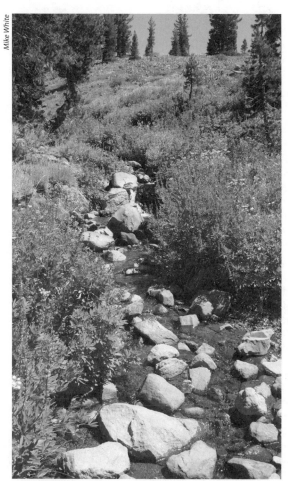

Mike White

Side stream in Horse Canyon

A faint trail leads to a ford of Summit City Creek's seasonal east channel and to a shady, seasonal island. Head downstream across the island to a point just above the confluence of the creek's seasonal and year-round main channels, and ford the main channel (with the help of rocks or logs, you hope). This ford can be wet or even dangerous during exceptionally high runoff. Get water here if you need it, as this may be your last chance before reaching North Fork Mokelumne River.

The trail becomes more distinct, but only briefly, as it scrambles up the bank and veers right (southwest) across a sandy flat with possible campsites and plenty of chaparral. Soon the path climbs over a low ridge past several large ponderosa pines and enters a thick forest that shows signs of a ground fire. Check your direction of travel, for it's easy to lose the trail completely here in the overwhelming amount of deadfall. (A reader reports that hikers have worn a path through the deadfall.) Pick your way carefully across this mess of giant pick-up sticks, heading toward the greenish light in a small clearing covered with bracken fern,

HWY 88

where defined trail reappears near a pair of huge pines. Faint, needle-covered trail continues to an open, rocky area where ducks resume. Before long, dense forest returns and giant pinecones scattered about the forest floor signal the presence of sugar pines, the largest species of pine in the world.

You presently meet the seasonal creek that drains Wester Park and Long Lake. North Fork Mokelumne River is just to the left, where overnighters could establish a primitive campsite (5388'; 10S 757867 4272385). Just below this tributary creek, the river makes a bend, and there's a long, deep pool; the tranquil waters beautifully reflect the cathedral forest towering above. This must have been the sort of scene that inspired the 19th Century painter Albert Bierstadt to create his famous images of supernatural wonder. Beneath the surface of this mysterious pool dwell many fat trout.

DAYS 4–6 (Mokelumne River to Thunder Mountain Trailhead, 16.5 miles): Retrace your steps.

15 Silver Lake–Granite Lake Trailhead

Trip Data: 10S 751532 4283031; 31.7 miles; 5/1 days

Topos: *Caples Lake, Mokelumne Peak*

Highlights: This tour visits examples of all the landscapes of the Carson Pass region—volcanic

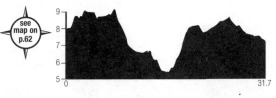

peaks, rounded granite domes, deep-cut river canyons, and lake-dotted plateaus. Anyone in good condition possessing basic cross-country skills will enjoy this long shuttle trip.

HEADS UP! *Consider as cross-country bushwhacking most of the route down Summit City Canyon beyond Telephone Gulch to the Mokelumne River. The Forest Service has seemingly given up on this route, as shown by the absence of a trail from the* Mokelumne Wilderness *map 1.5 miles beyond Telephone Gulch all the way to Camp Irene. Consider performing a little "vigilante trail maintenance" on this scenic route by using lightweight pruning shears to snip away some of the overgrowth.*

Don't even consider a solo trip in this area! Attempt this route only if your party has experience in cross-country travel through chaparral and dense forest, experience in the use of map and compass, and bouldering skills—including the ability to make a few Class 2–3 moves with a full backpack. Wear durable, long-sleeved shirts and long pants through this overgrown section. Don't expect to find a lot of water late in the season or following dry winters—check with the Forest Service for current conditions. Given the difficulties above, an extra day or two of angling and idling along the Mokelumne River could be a well-deserved treat.

Shuttle Directions: From Hwy. 88 near the north end of Silver Lake, leave the highway following signs east along the lake's north end for Kit Carson Resort. Continue past the resort to the east side of the lake and the small trailhead parking area, 1.4 miles from Hwy. 88.

DAY 1 (Thunder Mountain Trailhead to Scout Carson Lake, 6.5 miles): *(Recap: Trip 12, Day 1.)* At the trailhead, pass through a cattle gate and proceed to a T-junction with an eastbound path (left) to Castle Point. Go ahead (southeast) on a moderate climb, soon crossing a hillside below Carson Spur. Briefly gain the crest at a saddle and soon return to forest. Traverse below Two Sentinels to an open saddle and then head south along the ridge toward Martin Point. Traverse the east side of Martin Point and ascend a ridgecrest toward Thunder Mountain. At the junction with the trail up Thunder Mountain (optional excursion), stay on your main trail by turning left (east) and heading downhill across dry slopes to another junction, this one with a trail left (northeast) toward Kirkwood Meadows. Go right and continue the descent to the junction with the Horse Canyon Trail; turn left (southeast) at the junction to climb, then drop briefly to a year-round creek, and then climb to make a mile-long traverse of Thimble Peak's south side. Ignore an abandoned, overgrown path to Kirkwood Meadows, marked by an old post, and ascend through granite boulders to a signed junction in a sandy meadow. Turn right (southwest) and ascend a half mile to Scout Carson Lake (8958'; 10S 756354 4281829).

DAY 2 (Scout Carson Lake to Summit City Canyon, 4.5 miles): *(Recap: Trip 13, Day 2.)* Return a half mile to the Horse Canyon Trail junction, turn right (south-southeast) on that trail, and descend steeply into Mokelumne Wilderness and to the bottom of Summit City Canyon, where you meet the TYT. Turn right (southwest, downstream) for about a quarter mile to the vicinity of seasonal Horse Canyon Creek (6840'; 10S 758438 4279583) and an illegal campsite; search out legal campsites nearby, up and down the Summit City Creek.

DAY 3 (Summit City Canyon to Mokelumne River, 5.5 miles, mostly cross-country): *(Recap: Trip 14, Day 3.)* If you haven't done so already, head downstream (generally southwest and then south) to cross Horse Canyon Creek—may be dry by midseason. Continue down-canyon to cross Telephone Gulch and follow the tread across some flats. Beyond Telephone Gulch, the track usually stays away from the creek and heads generally south. Deadfalls are numerous, requiring frequent detours. The trail, though faint, is usually obvious but sometimes overgrown by thorny chaparral.

About 2.5 miles below Horse Canyon, the creek flows into a narrowing granite gorge. Don't cross the creek here, as the trail, blasted out of the bedrock, continues along the creek's west side a short distance and then abruptly ends. At a break in the granite—requiring bouldering skills in order to get you and your load up onto the next set of slabs—take some time to search for the best possible route. Continue along slabs and ledges above the creek, and after about another 200 yards, cross the creek just above a narrow, steep-walled slot. The final descent to the creek is extremely steep, and the crossing can be wet or possibly even dangerous during high runoff.

The trail resumes on the east bank, climbs about 30 feet, and then continues down the canyon. The tread is usually noticeable except across stretches of bedrock, where ducks may help. Cross just such an area of bedrock a few hundred feet beyond the ford and then parallel the creek as it swings south. Briefly descend near the creek, and then climb high above the stream over the west shoulder of a small dome. Descend steeply past a smaller dome and reenter forest; your route is now separated from the creek by a low ridge, where the grade eases and then climbs onto some slabs. Descend the slabs toward (but not to) a small side stream on the left. At the bottom of the slabs, the trail heads down a steep notch toward the right and then nears Summit City Creek again. Parallel Summit City Creek until the trail crosses the side stream just above its confluence with Summit City Creek.

Leave the forest again and climb very briefly onto an open, rocky slope. Continue down-canyon across more slabs, leaving the creek. After several hundred yards, the trail enters waist- to shoulder-high chaparral. Staying mostly in brush, descend gently to a steeper, final slope down to the bottom of Mokelumne Canyon, where views open up of the TYT ascending the south side of the canyon below Mt. Reba. Descend several hundred feet, veer left across a flat area, and then switchback downhill toward Summit City Creek. Don't cross until you hit the valley floor. The trail descends ledges before dropping through a cleft in the bedrock to the creek.

Faint trail leads to a ford of Summit City Creek's seasonal east channel and to a shady, seasonal island. Head downstream across the island to a point just above the confluence of the creek's seasonal and year-round main channels, and ford the main channel—wet or even dangerous during high runoff. Get water here if you need it, as this may be your last chance before reaching North Fork Mokelumne River.

The trail briefly becomes more distinct as it scrambles up the bank and veers right (southwest) across a sandy flat to climb over a low ridge and enter dense, fire-scorched for-

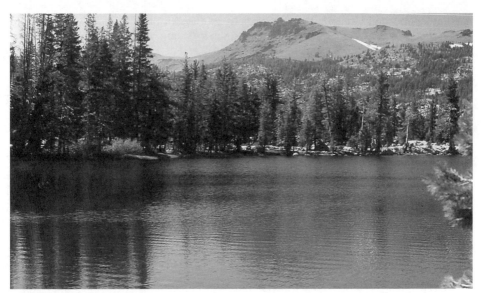

Granite Lake (out of Silver Lake)

est. Check your direction of travel, for it's easy to lose the trail completely here in the dead-fall. Pick your way across this mess, heading toward a greenish light in a small clearing covered with bracken fern, where defined trail reappears near a pair of huge pines. Faint, needle-covered trail continues to an open, rocky area where ducks resume.

Soon you're back in dense forest that includes huge sugar pines. You presently meet the seasonal creek that drains Wester Park and Long Lake. North Fork Mokelumne River is just to the left, where you can camp (5388'; 10S 757867 4272385).

DAY 4 (Mokelumne River to Long Lake, 6.2 miles): From the seasonal creek that drains Wester Park and Long Lake, head west and soon begin climbing the 3000 vertical feet out of the Mokelumne River Canyon. Even though water is readily available during the first 1800 feet, an early start is recommended to beat the heat on a typically hot summer day. Following ducks, climb 200 feet onto a bench, leaving the last of the extra-huge sugar pines behind. Another steep, 200-foot climb leads over a granite ridge with good views behind of the stately forested canyon bottom and the large expanses of glaciated granite. Curving west, the trail undulates through a mixed forest of oaks, pines, and cedars to the unsigned junction (although a square post may still be present) with the TYT heading left (southeast) down to Camp Irene. If the trail ahead appears to drop steeply through a shallow slot of broken rock, don't go that way: Look for *your* trail, which goes to Munson Meadow and Long Lake, half hidden under leaf litter on the right and heading uphill west and then southwest.

From the junction, make a steep, 200-yard climb on rocky-dusty tread. Beyond, the trail continues on a moderate-to-steep switchbacking climb that is generally well shaded. The trail crosses several perennial streams offering chances to fill water bottles on the seemingly unrelenting ascent. These all-year streams are shaded by alders, willows, and aspens, and the banks are lined with bracken fern and a bounty of wildflowers, including tiger lily, columbine, groundsel, and white yarrow.

You eventually leave shade and water behind as the steep, sandy trail becomes completely exposed to the intense summer sun. Trudging up long switchbacks, beleaguered hikers can at least enjoy the expansive views across the canyon. The grade eases a tad where the tread becomes rocky and dusty again, and a sparse cover of red firs offers a welcome bit of shade. Beyond the brutal 3000-foot climb out of the canyon, the reward is an easy, mile-long stroll northwest across a forested plateau to Munson Meadow. The green, sloping meadow has the first flowing water since the initial climb out of the Mokelumne River Canyon. On your way, you may spot a junction with a faint trail going left (southward); ignore it and forge ahead on your main trail.

Leave the vicinity of Munson Meadow on gently graded trail that receives more frequent maintenance than the previously hiked leg from the Mokelumne River. The trail veers north on a gradual descent toward a junction with the lateral to Long Lake. Beneath a dense forest of fir and pine, many rivulets lace this slope in midseason, and their courses are fertile growing grounds for lavender shooting stars and other meadow flowers. Reach the Long Lake junction and turn right, which leads to the south shore of the many-bayed lake in a half mile (7831'; 10S 754220 4273544). Skirt the south shore, cross a dam, and head east, away from the lake, onto open granite benches to campsites with fabulous views to the southeast over Wester Park to the headwaters of the Mokelumne River and the peaks around Ebbetts Pass.

DAY 5 (Long Lake to Silver Lake–Granite Lake Trailhead, 9 miles): Retrace your steps a half mile from Long Lake to the junction with the main trail. *(Recap in Reverse: Trip 11, Day 1.)* Turn right (north) and follow gradual trail to the east shore of the southernmost Cole Creek Lake. Beyond, follow the trail a half mile to a junction with a signed trail on the left to Cole Creek Lakes. Continue ahead (north) and climb a rocky ridge whose top offers great views.

At junctions with the maintained trail right (east) to Black Rock Lake and an abandoned path to Cole Creek Lakes on the left, stay on your main trail generally northward toward Hidden and Granite lakes. After a steady, 0.75-mile climb along a ridge with superb views, leave the ridgecrest and eventually stroll by some long meadows. Pass above Horse Thief Spring, soon exiting Mokelumne Wilderness.

Beyond the wilderness boundary, turn right (north) onto an old road and make a short climb to the crest of Squaw Ridge, former site of Plasse's Trading Post. Here, turn left (north and west) off the ridge, leaving the road for a time before rejoining it on a mile-long descent toward Allen Ranch. Pass by the ranch on a stretch of level road. Away from the ranch, gently rising road leads to a trail junction where you turn right (northwest) and follow the single-track trail on a winding climb to a ridgetop. After descending from the ridgetop, you presently reach a junction on a low ridge.

Turn right (generally northeast), following signs to Hidden Lake, and begin a moderate descent to the lake's southeast shore (campsites). Past the lake, a winding descent from it leads to a seasonal-stream crossing, beyond which you continue north toward Granite Lake. Midway between Hidden and Granite lakes, at junction with a little-used connector trail to Silver Lake, continue ahead (generally north) toward overused Granite Lake and its few, fair campsites.

A moderate, rocky descent from the lake leads to a junction where you turn right (northeast), cross a bridge, pass a meadow, and shortly reach the Silver Lake–Granite Lake Trailhead (7347'; 10S 751532 4283031 (field)).

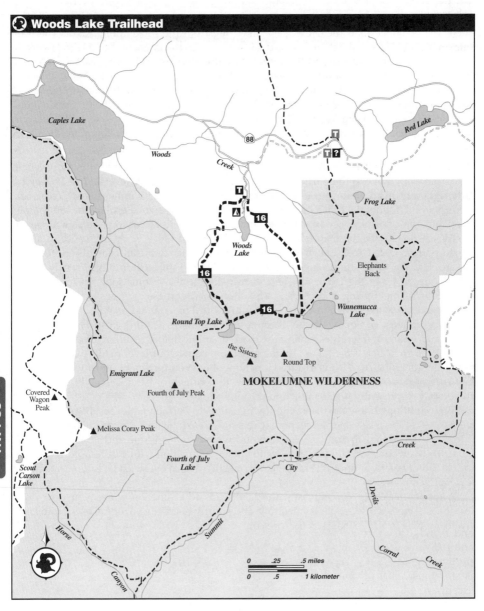

Woods Lake Trailhead

Caples Lake

Red Lake

88

Woods

Creek

Frog Lake

Woods
Lake

16

Elephants
Back

16

Round Top Lake

16

Winnemucca
Lake

the Sisters

Round Top

MOKELUMNE WILDERNESS

Emigrant Lake

Fourth of July Peak

Covered
Wagon
Peak

Melissa Coray Peak

Fourth of July
Lake

City

Creek

Scout
Carson
Lake

Devils

Horse

Summit

Corral   Creek

Canyon

0   .25   .5 miles

0   .5   1 kilometer

Woods Lake Trailhead

8220'; 10S 760130 4286760 (field)

DESTINATION/ UTM COORDINATES	TRIP TYPE	BEST SEASON	PACE (HIKING/ LAYOVER DAYS)	TOTAL MILEAGE
16 Round Top Lake 10S 759988 4284263	Loop	Mid	2/0 Leisurely	5

Information and Permits: Camping in the Carson Pass Management Area (CPMA) is allowed only in the designated sites at Winnemucca, Round Top, and Fourth of July lakes. Permits for camping in these sites are only issued on a first-come, first-served basis at the Carson Pass Information Station, which is open seven days a week in the summer. The Carson Pass Information Station is located at the top of Carson Pass on Hwy. 88, 6 miles east of the Kirkwood Mountain Resort. See www.enfia.info/carson.htm for details. Campfires are prohibited within the CPMA at all times. There's a fee to park at the trailhead, which is in the Eldorado National Forest: 100 Forni Road, Placerville, CA 95667; 530-622-5061; www.fs.fed.us/r5/eldorado/wild/moke/index.html. For visitor information, call 530-644-6048.

Driving Directions: Turn off Hwy. 88 at the signed Woods Lake access road, 1.7 miles west of Carson Pass. Follow paved road for 0.8 mile to a junction and turn right, proceeding another 0.1 mile to the Woods Lake Trailhead, where motorists must cough up a nominal fee for parking. Toilets, water.

16 Round Top Lake

Trip Data: 10S 759988 4284263; 5 miles; 2/0 days

Topos: *Caples Lake, Carson Pass*

see map on p.72

Highlights: Two picturesque lakes backdropped by craggy volcanic summits provide the main highlights on this very popular loop trip through Mokelumne Wilderness. Midsummer visitors will have the added bonus of a number of wildflower-laden meadows. Ambitious peakbaggers can make a side trip to the summit of Round Top.

DAY 1 (Woods Lake Trailhead to Round Top Lake, 2 miles): From the trailhead parking lot, walk a short distance on the access road toward Woods Lake Campground and find the official start of the Round Top Lake Trail just past a bridge (don't cross the bridge). Stroll along on dirt trail through mixed forest, soon rising above Woods Lake Campground, where single-track trail merges with an old roadbed. Follow the road on a stiff, winding climb to the signed Lost Cabin Mine Trailhead, a half mile from the parking lot.

Now on single-track again, make a moderate climb with filtered views of Round Top and Woods Lake through the trees. Hop across boulder- and willow-lined Woods Creek and follow a switchbacking climb above the old structures of the Lost Cabin Mine, which produced gold, silver, copper, and lead before shutting down in the early 1960s. The mine is still considered private property, so resist the urge to trespass. Continue the steady ascent, roughly following the west branch of Woods Creek. The grade eventually eases near the signed Mokelumne Wilderness boundary as the volcanic summits of Round Top and the Sisters come into view. The canyon broadens farther upstream amid more open vegetation of willow, heather, and wildflowers, which allows even better views. Reach a junction with the Fourth of July Lake Trail near the north shore of Round Top Lake (9352'; 10S 759988 4284263), 2.2 miles from the parking lot.

Round Top is a stunningly scenic lake rimmed with stands of whitebark pines and backdropped by the broodingly dark slopes of Round Top and the Sisters. To promote revegetation of the shoreline, overnighters are limited to six designated, mostly hard-to-find campsites on the northwest side of the lake, available by reservation only.

CLIMBING ROUND TOP

Competent peakbaggers can climb nearby Round Top (10,381'). Near Round Top Lake, leave the trail and travel southeast on a well-defined use trail up the prominent gully located between the east Sister and Round Top. Initially, the route heads toward the saddle between the two peaks, but higher up the slope, it veers left of the saddle to a prominent notch in Round Top's northwest ridge. Follow the backside of the ridge to a false summit that should satisfy most non-climbers as their ultimate destination. The true summit is only a few feet higher and is separated from the false summit by a steep cleft of loose rock that should be negotiated only by skilled mountaineers, as the exposure is quite significant. Both summits offer spectacularly expansive views of the northern Sierra.

OPTIONAL HIKES

Emigrant Lake: From the junction near the north shore of Round Top Lake, turn onto the Fourth of July Lake Trail and follow an arcing traverse around the west shoulder of the Sisters to the crest of a divide. From there, experienced cross-country travelers can access Emigrant Lake by traversing west to a notch directly southeast of Point 9020, as shown on the *Caples Lake* quadrangle, and then dropping steeply to the lake's outlet.

Fourth of July Lake: From the crest mentioned above, continue on the Fourth of July Lake Trail on a switchbacking descent that loses 1000 feet of elevation on the way to Fourth of July Lake. (Avoid the old, knee-wrenching, straight-down descent.) Colorful wildflowers should cheer midsummer hikers along the descent. Fourth of July Lake is quite scenic, cradled in a rocky amphitheater between Fourth of July Peak and peaks 9795 and 9607. A mixture of open meadows, pockets of willow, and stands of white fir and western white pine ring the shoreline. Six designated campsites are scattered around the lake, one near the outlet, two on a forested rise above the northeast shore, and three near the edge of the meadow on the northwest side.

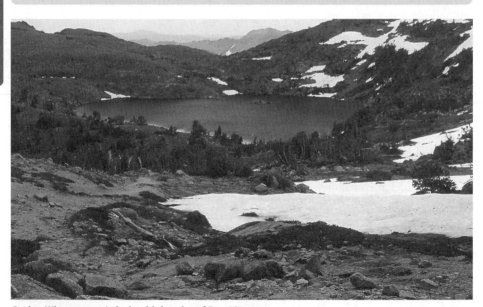

Seeing Winnemucca Lake is a high point of Day 2's route.

DAY 2 (Round Top Lake to Woods Lake Trailhead, 3 miles): Return to the junction with the trail (on your right) that you took to get up to Round Top Lake. Here, go ahead (east toward Winnemucca Lake) on a gradually rising ascent over a granite ridge peppered with wind-battered whitebark pines and ground-hugging shrubs. Once across the crest, follow the trail downslope through open terrain and across the outlet of Winnemucca Lake to its west shore and a junction.

Windswept Winnemucca Lake sits majestically at the base of Round Top Peak's north face, with the rounded hump of Elephants Back a mile to the northeast. The mostly open terrain is broken by scattered clumps of whitebark pine that shelter three designated camp-sites above the north shore.

At a junction at Winnemucca's west end, turn left (north) toward Woods Lake and follow the trail along the course of the east branch of Woods Creek through sagebrush, willows, and a fine assortment of wildflowers in season. Exit Mokelumne Wilderness about a half mile from the lake and continue the steady descent into mixed forest. Nearing the trailhead, pass a lateral on the left to Woods Lake, stroll across a wood bridge, walk across the paved access road, and walk a short distance to the parking area.

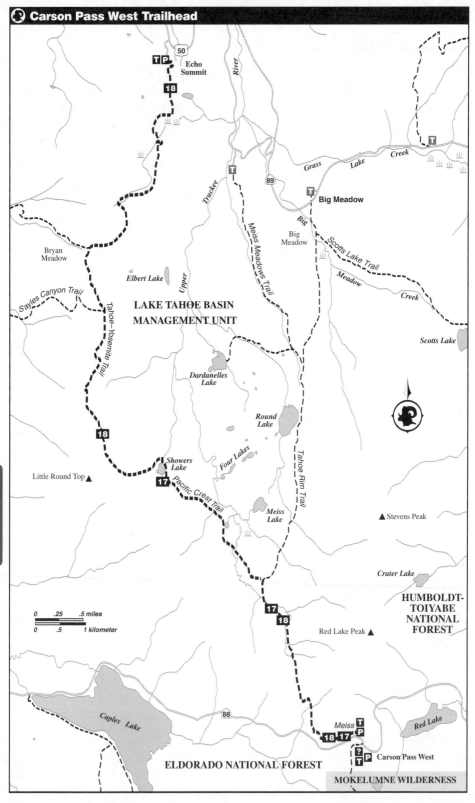

50
T P Echo
Summit
18

River

Grass Lake Creek

T

89

Truckee

T Big Meadow

Big Meadow

Big

Meiss Meadows Trail

Bryan
Meadow

Elbert Lake

Upper

Scotts Lake Trail

Meadow

Creek

Sayles Canyon Trail

**LAKE TAHOE BASIN
MANAGEMENT UNIT**

Tahoe–Yosemite Trail

Scotts Lake

Dardanelles
Lake

Round
Lake

18

Tahoe Rim Trail

Showers
Lake

Four Lakes

Little Round Top ▲

17 Pacific Crest Trail

Meiss
Lake

▲ Stevens Peak

Crater Lake

0   .25   .5 miles
0   .5   1 kilometer

17
18
Red Lake Peak ▲

**HUMBOLDT-
TOIYABE
NATIONAL
FOREST**

Caples Lake

88

Meiss T
P
18 17
? P
T Carson Pass West

Red Lake

ELDORADO NATIONAL FOREST

MOKELUMNE WILDERNESS

HWY 88

Carson Pass West Trailhead

8557'; 11S 239819 4287379 (field)

DESTINATION/ UTM COORDINATES	TRIP TYPE	BEST SEASON	PACE (HIKING/ LAYOVER DAYS)	TOTAL MILEAGE
I7 Showers Lake 10S 757728 4292385	Out & back	Mid	2/1 Moderate	10.2
I8 Echo Summit Trailhead 10S 757559 4300186 (field)	Shuttle	Mid	2/1 Moderate	13.4

Information and Permits: Wilderness permits aren't required in Meiss Country as yet, but you must have a California Campfire Permit to have a campfire or use a stove. There's a fee to park at the trailhead, which is in the Eldorado National Forest: 100 Forni Road, Placerville, CA 95667; 530-622-5061; www.fs.fed.us/r5/eldorado/wild/moke/index.html. For visitor information, call 530-644-6048.

Driving Directions: From Carson Pass on Hwy. 88, drive 0.3 mile west to the Carson Pass West Trailhead (also known as the Meiss Meadow Trailhead) and the parking lot on the north side of the road. There is a daily fee to park here.

I7 Showers Lake

Trip Data: 10S 757728 4292385; 10.2 miles; 2/1 days

Topos: *Caples Lake*

see map on p.76

9
8
0   10.2

Highlights: Showers Lake is one of the best camping areas between Hwy. 50 and Hwy. 88, with numerous campsites and good angling for brook trout. En route, the trail passes through the Upper Truckee River drainage, offering panoramic views of immense volcanic formations.

HEADS UP! *There is a daily fee to park at the Carson Pass West (Meiss Meadow) Trailhead.*

DAY 1 (Carson Pass West Trailhead to Showers Lake, 5.1 miles): *(Recap in Reverse: Trip 10, Day 2.)* Leave the parking lot and curve left (west) to follow the single-track trail above the highway. Soon the trail veers north on a stiff ascent with few switchbacks toward the prominent saddle above.

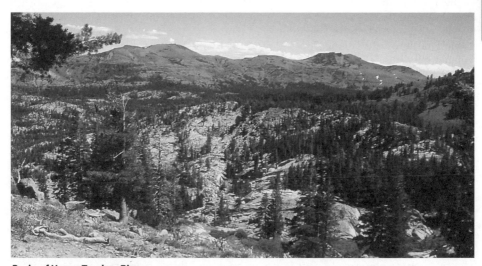

Basin of Upper Truckee River

Nearly level trail passes a pond before a moderate descent leads through open terrain toward the headwaters of the Upper Truckee River, crossing the nascent stream a few times before reaching the canyon floor. Follow an old jeep road on an easy stroll to another river crossing before passing some old cabins on the left (west). A short distance beyond the cabins is a well-signed junction of the TRT right (northeast) to Round Lake and the PCT/TYT.

Turn left (northwest) at the junction and follow the PCT/TYT to ford the river again (wet in early season). Near the crossing, a faint use trail heads right (northeast) a very soggy half mile to Meiss Lake. From the river crossing, stay on the pleasantly graded PCT/TYT. Beyond a shallow pond and a ford of the stream draining Dixon Canyon, the trail starts an increasingly steep climb northwestward toward the broad crest above Showers Lake. At the top, at an unmarked X-junction, turn right (north) and follow a realigned section of the PCT/TYT that descends to the northeast shore of Showers Lake (8647'; 10S 757728 4292385).

DAY 2 (Showers Lake to Carson Pass West Trailhead, 5.1 miles): Retrace your steps.

18 Echo Summit Trailhead

Trip Data: 10S 757559 4300186; 13.4 miles; 2/1 days

Topos: *Caples Lake, Echo Lake*

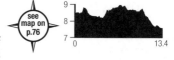

Highlights: Reversing Trip 10 and following a section of the renowned PCT/TYT, this journey between Hwy. 88 and Hwy. 50 exposes hikers to a variety of scenery, including dense forests, verdant meadows, lovely Showers Lake, and grand views of the Upper Truckee River drainage.

Shuttle Directions: To access the take-out trailhead, take Hwy. 50 to Echo Summit and go west to a paved access road on the south side of the highway, 0.2 mile west of Echo Summit. A sign reading SNO-PARK marks the turnoff. Proceed 0.2 mile to the large PCT parking lot. The drive between the Carson Pass West and Echo Summit trailheads is approximately 25 miles long.

DAY 1 (Carson Pass West Trailhead to Showers Lake, 5.1 miles): *(Recap in Reverse: Trip 10, Day 2.)* Leave the parking lot and curve left (west) to follow the single-track trail above the highway. Soon the trail veers north on a stiff ascent with few switchbacks toward the prominent saddle above.

Nearly level trail passes a pond before a moderate descent leads through open terrain toward the headwaters of the Upper Truckee River, crossing the nascent stream a few times before reaching the canyon floor. Follow an old jeep road on an easy stroll to another river crossing before passing some old cabins on the left (west). A short distance beyond the cabins is a well-signed junction of the TRT right (northeast) to Round Lake and the PCT/TYT.

Turn left (northwest) at the junction and follow the PCT/TYT to ford the river again (wet in early season). Near the crossing, a faint use trail heads right (northeast) a very soggy half mile to Meiss Lake. From the river crossing, stay on the pleasantly graded PCT/TYT. Beyond a shallow pond and a ford of the stream draining Dixon Canyon, the trail starts an increasingly steep climb northwestward toward the broad crest above Showers Lake. At the top, at an unmarked X-junction, turn right (north) and follow a realigned section of the PCT/TYT that descends to the northeast shore of Showers Lake (8647'; 10S 757728 4292385).

DAY 2 (Showers Lake to Echo Summit Trailhead, 8.3 miles): *(Recap in Reverse: Trip 10, Day 1.)* Make a short, steep drop from the lake, crossing its outlet, and then make a short, steep climb up the opposite bank before the grade eases. The trail soon offers views over the Upper Truckee River canyon as it traverses northwest through an open bowl. At the far end of the traverse, climb to a ridgetop and descend through a pair of meadows to a T-junction, where you go right (ahead, north) on the PCT/TYT to descend to a shallow gap where paths on either side of the PCT/TYT lead several hundred feet to passable campsites with water available nearby, at least until midsummer.

After a brief climb away from the gap, a rocky descent leads to a soggy meadow and a stream crossing. A short climb away from the creek, followed by a longer descent, delivers hikers to a junction with the Sayles Canyon Trail, 1.3 miles from T-junction. Turn right (ahead, north) to stay on the PCT/TYT. Presently, an increasingly steep descent leads to a junction in Bryan Meadow. Go right (east) at the junction and climb to a forested saddle.

Following a brief descent, the trail climbs to a ridgetop and makes a long, steep descent toward Benwood Meadow, fording a creek three times, the last time on a wood-plank bridge. After another 0.2 mile of steep descent, the trail levels near Benwood Meadow, visible to the right. Skirt the west edge of the meadow, passing a path into the meadow and soon reaching a post marking an unmaintained 0.4-mile trail on the right to the unnamed pond directly north of Benwood Meadow. Go left (north) here on single-track trail through mixed forest to a jeep road and turn right.

The remaining distance to the Echo Summit Trailhead follows a variety of old jeep roads and sections of single-track trail. The route is well marked with TRT and PCT emblems and arrows at all junctions. Soon the trail intersects another road and the descent continues across an old ski run. A section of single-track trail leads to a 40-yard stretch of jeep road before a final piece of trail to the Echo Summit PCT parking lot (7389'; 10S 757559 4300186 (field)).

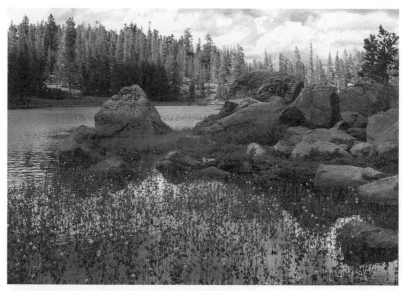

Pretty Meiss Lake is an easy detour from Day 1's route.

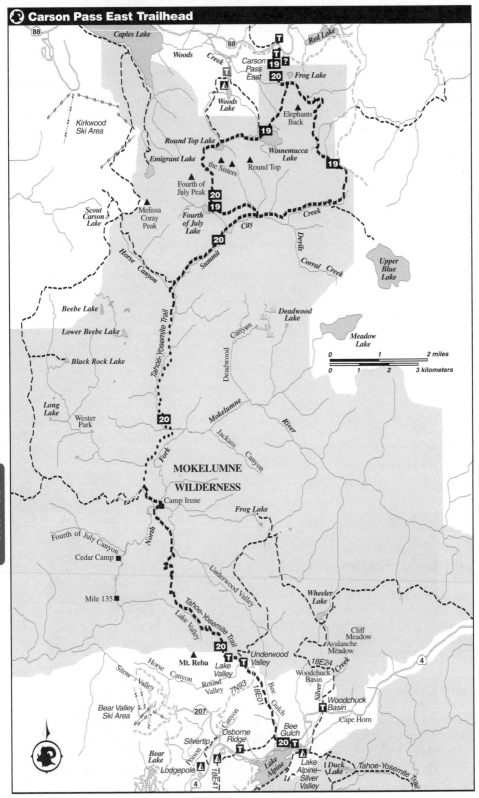

Carson Pass East Trailhead

8595'; 11S 240024 4287145 (field)

DESTINATION/ UTM COORDINATES	TRIP TYPE	BEST SEASON	PACE (HIKING/ LAYOVER DAYS)	TOTAL MILEAGE
19 Fourth of July Lake 10S 759726 4282215	Semiloop	Mid to late	2/1 Moderate	14
20 Tahoe-Yosemite Trail Section 3: To Lake Alpine– Silver Valley Trailhead 11S 239527 4263329 (field)	Shuttle	Mid	4/1 Strenuous, part cross-country	26.6

Information and Permits: Camping in the Carson Pass Management Area (CPMA) is allowed only in the designated sites at Winnemucca, Round Top, and Fourth of July lakes. Permits for camping in these sites are only issued on a first-come, first-served basis at the Carson Pass Information Station, which is open seven days a week in the summer. The Carson Pass Information Station is located at the top of Carson Pass on Hwy. 88, 6 miles east of the Kirkwood Mountain Resort. See www.enfia.info/carson.htm for details. Campfires are prohibited within the CPMA at all times. There's a fee to park at the trailhead, which is in the Eldorado National Forest: 100 Forni Road, Placerville, CA 95667; 530-622-5061; www.fs.fed.us/r5/eldorado/wild/moke/index.html. For visitor information, call 530-644-6048.

Driving Directions: The trailhead is right at Carson Pass on Hwy. 88, on the highway's south side, where you'll also find the Carson Pass Information Station. The trailhead is on the station's west side.

19 Fourth of July Lake

Trip Data: 10S 759726 4282215; 14 miles; 2/1 days

Topos: *Caples Lake, Carson Pass*

Highlights: Backpackers who don't mind regaining lost elevation will appreciate this semiloop trip through the northeast section of Mokelumne Wilderness, which includes several ponds and lakes, wildflower-covered slopes, sweeping vistas, and a deep canyon.

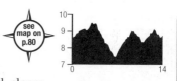

see map on p.80

DAY 1 (Carson Pass East Trailhead to Fourth of July Lake, 5.5 miles): Find this section of the PCT/TYT on the west side of the Carson Pass Information Station, and head south on the wide, well-traveled path through a mixed forest of lodgepole pines, mountain hemlocks, and western white pines. The gradually descending trail leads past a small pond surrounded by willows before making a gentle-to-moderate ascent as the trail crosses the Mokelumne Wilderness boundary and switchbacks toward the Sierra Crest. The forest thins on the approach to a ridge, allowing glimpses of the volcanic summits of Round Top

JOHN C. FRÉMONT

With Kit Carson as his scout, John C. Frémont made the first winter crossing of the Sierra somewhere on this plateau in February of 1844. From an encampment in Faith Valley a few miles to the east, Frémont, along with his chief cartographer, Charles Preuss, climbed Red Lake Peak, just north of Carson Pass. From the summit, they were the first Europeans to see the great mountain lake we now know as Tahoe. The climb of Red Lake Peak was the first recorded ascent of an identifiable Sierra mountain.

HWY 88

and the Sisters. On a plateau, reach an unmarked junction with a short use trail left (north-east) to Frog Lake (no camping), which fills a shallow depression in an open bowl dotted with widely scattered pines.

> ### WHITEBARK PINES
>
> Stands of high-altitude-loving whitebark pine provide nesting places for hundreds of Clark's nutcrackers, which swoop back and forth over the heads of hikers. Like the Native Americans, these birds eat lots of whitebark-pine nuts. The Clark's nutcracker's fondness for these nuts is probably one of the main reasons that whitebarks expand their territory. These large, noisy, crow-like, gray-and-white birds are messy eaters and drop seeds to the ground while picking the cones apart, thus propagating new pines.

From the unmarked junction to Frog Lake, go ahead (south) a short way to a junction and turn right (south-southeast), leaving the PCT behind to follow the TYT as it descends open slopes on the west side of Elephants Back. Cross shrubby slopes dotted with small groves of whitebark and lodgepole pines on a mile-long descent toward Winnemucca Lake, enjoying excellent views of hulking Round Top. Seasonally, a meadow near Winnemucca offers an unbelievable wildflower display. Cruise picturesque Winnemucca's west shore beneath Round Top to a junction, marked by a post, with a trail to Woods Lake.

Go ahead (south-southwest) from the junction, ford the lake's outlet, and begin a moderate climb up a gully covered with pockets of willow, heather, and grasses to the crossing of a stream. Continue the ascent to a saddle and then make a short descent to a junction near the north shore of Round Top Lake. The junction is with another trail to Woods Lake.

Go left (southwest) from the junction and follow an arcing traverse around the west shoulder of the Sisters to the crest of a divide. On the far side of Round Top Lake, the steep cliff is a mélange of grays, greens, and browns, and the surrounding talus slopes vary in color according to which bedrock yielded up which talus blocks. All the rock outcroppings in this region are dark colored. Volcanic rocks are normally dark, but even the granite here

HWY 88

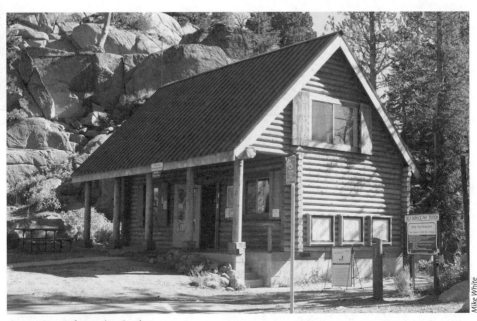

Mike White

Carson Pass Information Station

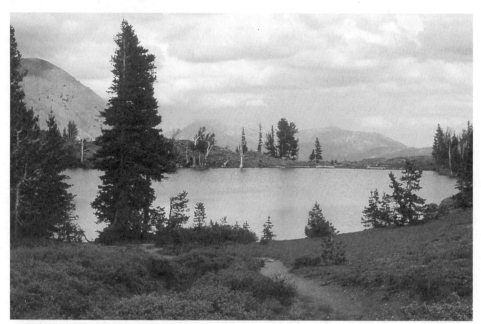

You'll pass little Frog Lake on Day 2 of this scenic trip.

is much darker than the shining granites found in Desolation Valley. Along this stretch of trail, views are excellent (scanning from east to north to west) of Markleeville Peak, Hawkins Peak, the Crystal Range, the slopes above Caples Creek, and Caples Lake.

Soon the TYT descends to a saddle, leaving the basin of the American River and entering the Mokelumne River drainage. From the crest, avoid a use trail to Fourth of July Peak and follow the main trail as it descends almost 1000 feet on gradual-to-moderate switchbacks through a handsome bowl and toward Fourth of July Lake. Ignore the knee-killing old trail that plunges straight down. Colorful wildflowers should cheer midsummer hikers along the descent.

At a junction abreast of Fourth of July Lake, turn right (west) to the lake (8201'; 10S 759726 4282215), which is quite scenic, cradled in a rocky amphitheater between Fourth of July Peak and peaks 9795 and 9607. A mixture of open meadows, pockets of willow, and stands of white fir and western white pine ring the shoreline. Your campsite is one of the six designated sites at this pretty lake.

DAY 2 (Fourth of July Lake to Carson Pass East Trailhead, 8.5 miles): From Fourth of July Lake, the trail heads south to follow a switchbacking course through mixed forest before veering northeast and emerging onto open, brush-covered slopes that allow expansive views of Summit City Canyon. A long, descending traverse across these slopes leads down toward the floor of the canyon and into lodgepole pine forest on the way to a junction with the trail on the canyon's floor. Here, the TYT turns right (west, then southwest) and this trip turns left (east) to head through the trees, passing a campsite and soon reaching a second junction, marked by a post.

Take the left fork, following signed directions generally east to the PCT, and begin a 3-mile climb, initially through a lodgepole pine forest with a lush understory of plants and flowers. A steady ascent on the sometimes rocky trail leads away from the floor of Summit City Canyon, where the groundcover soon disappears beneath a dense forest of red firs and western white pines. After a few long switchbacks, the trail emerges from the forest and onto brush-covered slopes that allow for fine views of the canyon, rimmed by impressive-looking mountains to the south. The shrubs are quite thick in places, threatening to overgrow the trail in spots and at times reaching over-the-head heights. Well-watered slopes farther up harbor ferns, willows, alders, young aspens, and an assortment of wild-flowers, including tall alpine knotweeds. Sagebrush heralds the approach to Forestdale Divide and a junction with the PCT.

Turn left (west) onto the PCT at the junction and make a short climb over the crest of Forestdale Divide, cross the Mokelumne Wilderness boundary, and begin a winding descent to a bench harboring a group of subalpine ponds near the head of Forestdale Creek's canyon. Although the ponds are never more than knee deep, the sweeping views extending from Elephants Back to Hope Valley create a picturesque setting quite suitable for a lingering break.

Continue the descent away from the bench to cross a branch of Forestdale Creek. Past the creek, a stiff, winding climb begins across flower-covered slopes on the east side of Elephants Back, where amateur botanists will see a diverse assortment of wildflower species during the height of the season. The 900-foot ascent leads to the crest of Elephants Back's north ridge and back into Mokelumne Wilderness, topping out south of Frog Lake. A descent leads shortly to the junction with the TYT on its way from Carson Pass East (right) to Winnemucca Lake (left). You close the loop here and turn right (ahead, first west and then north), retracing your steps along the PCT/TYT to the Carson Pass East Trailhead.

20 Tahoe-Yosemite Trail Section 3: To Lake Alpine–Silver Valley Trailhead

Trip Data: 11S 239527 4263329; 26.6 miles; 4/1 days

Topos: *Carson Pass, Caples Lake, Mokelumne Peak, Tamarack, Spicer Meadow Reservoir*

see map on p.80

Highlights: The fine scenery in the Carson Pass Management Area (CPMA) is a splendid begin-ning to this TYT section, while the rough, lonely, part cross-country descent of Summit City Canyon to the North Fork Mokelumne River and Camp Irene gives the TYT a definite edge over the JMT in terms of adventure.

HEADS UP! This is a tough section of the TYT. Backpackers who decide they'd rather not deal with the difficulties of this section should skip it altogether and pick up the route again at the Lake Alpine–Silver Valley Trailhead off Hwy. 4. Consider as cross-country bushwhacking most of the route down Summit City Canyon beyond Telephone Gulch to the Mokelumne River. The Forest Service has seemingly given up on this route, as shown by the absence of a trail from the Mokelumne Wilderness map 1.5 miles beyond Telephone Gulch all the way to Camp Irene. Consider performing a little "vigi-lante trail maintenance" on this scenic route by using lightweight pruning shears to snip away some of the overgrowth.

Don't even consider a solo trip in this area! Attempt this route only if your party has experience in cross-country travel through chaparral and dense forest, experience in the use of map and compass, and bouldering skills—including the ability to make a few Class 2–3 moves with a full backpack. Wear durable, long-sleeved shirts and long pants through this overgrown section. Don't expect to find a lot of water late in the season or following dry winters—check with the Forest Service for current condi-tions. Given the difficulties above, an extra day or two of angling and idling along the Mokelumne River could be a well-deserved treat.

HWY 88

Shuttle Directions: To get to the take-out trailhead at Lake Alpine–Silver Valley from Ebbetts Pass on Hwy. 4, drive 16.4 miles west toward Lake Alpine. Just east of the lake, turn south on East Shore Road and go 0.3 mile more to the Silver Valley/Highland Lakes Trailhead. There's no parking at the trailhead, so park on the shoulder as best you can.

DAY 1 (Carson Pass East Trailhead to Fourth of July Lake, 5.5 miles): If you've just stepped off the PCT/TYT at the Carson Pass West Trailhead on the north side of Hwy. 88, get to this next section of the TYT by turning left and walking along the highway shoulder 0.3 mile southeast to the Carson Pass East Trailhead on the south side of Hwy. 88 next to the Carson Pass Information Station. Get your permit to camp in the CPMA here unless you can make it all the way down to the floor of Summit City Canyon today.

(Recap: Trip 19, Day 1.) From the trailhead, begin just beyond the Carson Pass Information Station, where the PCT/TYT briefly drops and then climbs to Frog Lake's plateau, entering Mokelumne Wilderness. At an unsigned junction with a path left (northeast) to Frog Lake, go right (ahead) on the PCT/TYT, leaving behind a forest of western white and lodgepole pines, junipers, and mountain hemlocks to enter the realm of whitebark pines.

Find the start of this section of the PCT/TYT on the west side of the Carson Pass Information Station, and head south. On a plateau, reach an unmarked junction with a short use trail left (northeast) to Frog Lake (no camping). Go ahead (south) a short way to a junction and turn right (south-southeast), leaving the PCT behind to follow the TYT as it makes a mile-long descent toward Winnemucca Lake. Follow Winnemucca's west shore beneath Round Top to a junction, marked by a post, with a trail to Woods Lake.

Go ahead (south-southwest) from the junction, ford the lake's outlet, and climb up a gully to a saddle. Descend to a junction near the north shore of Round Top Lake (the junction is with another trail to Woods Lake). Go left (southwest) from the junction. Soon the TYT descends to a saddle. Follow the main trail as it swings down gradual-to-moderate switchbacks through a handsome bowl and toward Fourth of July Lake. Ignore the knee-killing old trail that plunges straight down.

At a junction abreast of Fourth of July Lake, turn right (west) to the lake (8201'; 10S 750726 4282215) and find your assigned site. Campfires are prohibited.

DAY 2 (Fourth of July Lake to Summit City Canyon, 6.3 miles, part cross-country): *(Partial Recap: Trip 19, Day 2, from Fourth of July Lake to the junction in Summit City Canyon with the Summit City Canyon Trail.)* Follow the switchbacking trail as it leaves the lake, leaves forest, and descends into Summit City Canyon. At the bottom of the canyon, find a junction with the trail on the canyon's floor and turn right (west) on the TYT, leaving the Day 2 route of Trip 19.

From here, the TYT descends gently under a canopy of dense lodgepole pine, passing a very built-up campsite, crossing Fourth of July Lake's outlet, and passing a USFS marker reading LOWER SUMMIT CITY 1862–1867. The sandy footpath begins a steady descent, as the forest cover becomes moderate to sparse and a few Jeffrey pines start intermixing with the other conifers. Crossing open slopes, excellent views abound of the towering granite walls of the canyon that rise 2000 feet above. Green fingers of brush poke upward between granite outcrops, and the black lichen against the granite is reminiscent of the walls of Yosemite Valley. The trail, ill-maintained, is occasionally overgrown by chaparral or overlain by deadfalls. If you find these trail conditions difficult, turn around now, because they will only worsen.

As the trail reenters a moderate forest cover, some white fir appears along with the red fir, lodgepole and Jeffrey pine, and an occasional aspen. Beyond a junction with the signed Horse Canyon Trail is Horse Canyon Creek, which may be dry by midseason in drought years. (At the junction with the Horse Canyon Trail, you meet trips 13, 14, and 15 at the end of those trips' Day 2.) Look for campsites up- and downstream along Summit City Creek in this area (6840'; 10S 758438 4279583).

DAY 3 (Summit City Canyon to Camp Irene, 5.5 miles, mostly cross-country): *(Partial Recap: Trip 14, Day 3, from Summit City Canyon to the seasonal creek draining Wester Park.)* If you haven't done so already, head downstream (generally southwest and then south) to cross Horse Canyon Creek (may be dry by mid season). Continue down-canyon to cross Telephone Gulch and follow the tread across some flats. Beyond Telephone Gulch, the track usually stays away from the creek and heads generally south. Deadfalls are numerous, requiring frequent detours. The trail, though faint, is usually obvious but sometimes overgrown by thorny chaparral.

About 2.5 miles below Horse Canyon, the creek flows into a narrowing granite gorge. Don't cross the creek here, as the trail, blasted out of the bedrock, continues along the creek's west side a short distance and then abruptly ends. At a break in the granite—requiring bouldering skills in order to get you and your load up onto the next set of slabs—take some time to search for the best possible route. Continue along slabs and ledges above the creek, and after about another 200 yards, cross the creek just above a narrow, steep-walled slot. The final descent to the creek is extremely steep, and the crossing can be wet or possibly even dangerous during high runoff.

The trail resumes on the east bank, climbs about 30 feet, and then continues down the canyon. The tread is usually noticeable except across stretches of bedrock, where ducks may help. Cross just such an area of bedrock a few hundred feet beyond the ford and then parallel the creek as it swings south. Briefly descend near the creek and then climb high above the stream over the west shoulder of a small dome. Descend steeply past a smaller dome and reenter forest; your route is now separated from the creek by a low ridge, where the grade eases and the trail climbs onto some slabs. Descend the slabs toward (but not to) a small side stream on the left. At the bottom of the slabs, the trail heads down a steep notch toward the right and then nears Summit City Creek again. Parallel Summit City Creek until the trail crosses the side stream just above its confluence with Summit City Creek.

Leave the forest again and climb very briefly onto an open, rocky slope. Continue down-canyon across more slabs, leaving the creek. After several hundred yards, the trail enters waist- to shoulder-high chaparral. Staying mostly in brush, descend gently to a steeper, final slope down into North Fork Mokelumne River Canyon, where views open up of the TYT ascending the south side of the canyon below Mt. Reba. Descend several hundred feet, veer left across a flat area, and then switchback downhill toward Summit City Creek (don't cross until you hit the canyon floor). The trail descends ledges before dropping through a cleft in the bedrock to the creek.

A faint trail leads to a ford of Summit City Creek's seasonal east channel and to a shady, seasonal island. Head downstream across the island to a point just above the confluence of the creek's seasonal and year-round main channels, and ford the main channel (wet or even dangerous during high runoff). Get water here if you need it, as this may be your last chance before reaching North Fork Mokelumne River.

The trail briefly becomes more distinct as it scrambles up the bank and veers right (southwest) across a sandy flat to climb over a low ridge and enter dense, fire-scorched forest. Check your direction of travel, for it's easy to lose the trail completely here in the dead-fall. Maintaining your direction of travel as best you can, pick your way through this mess, heading toward the greenish light in a small clearing covered with bracken fern, where defined trail reappears near a pair of huge pines. Faint, needle-covered trail continues to an open, rocky area where ducks resume.

Soon you're back in dense forest that includes huge sugar pines. You presently meet the seasonal creek that drains Wester Park and Long Lake, and you could bear left here to find a campsite near the Mokelumne River. This is the destination of Day 3 of trips 14 and 15.

Leaving the Day 3 route of Trip 14, you pick up the Day 4 route of Trip 15, from the seasonal creek to the junction with the trail to Munson Meadow and Long Lake. From the seasonal creek, head west toward Camp Irene. Following ducks, climb 200 feet onto a bench. Beyond, another steep, 200-foot climb leads over a granite ridge, where a backward glance reveals a fine view of the stately, forested canyon and the large expanses of glaciated granite. Veer west and follow a quarter-mile undulating route through a mixed forest of oaks, pines, and cedars to an unsigned junction, where the trail to the right heads uphill and west toward Munson Meadow (the route of Trip 15), and the TYT continues ahead to Camp Irene.

Now you leave the route of Trip 15. Proceed ahead from the junction to drop steeply through a shallow slot of broken rock, descending to an unnamed stream. The trail follows this stream generally southeast back to North Fork Mokelumne River. Pass by a 1974 burn just before reaching the north bank of North Fork Mokelumne River at the ford called Camp Irene (5316'; 10S 758129 4271068). Camp Irene is complete with a sandy beach, fine granite slabs, lovely pools—and sometimes other campers. You can also camp up- or downstream for more privacy or ford the river (may be dangerous in early season) to the flat opposite. This ford is the lowest point on the TYT, and fishing here should be good for brown or rainbow trout.

DAY 4 (Camp Irene to Lake Alpine–Silver Valley Trailhead, 9.3 miles): The trail for this day is easier to follow than that of Day 3. However, the brutal, exposed, 3400-foot climb out of the North Fork Mokelumne River Canyon to a ridge east of Mt. Reba, followed by a sometimes very steep, 1400-foot drop to Lake Alpine, makes for a very long, very strenuous day. Before you leave the river, know that by late season of an average year or midseason of a dry year, the river may be your last opportunity for water before you're almost at Hwy. 4 and Lake Alpine. Streams along the way may be dry by midseason in a dry year. Carry plenty of extra water just in case—perhaps enough for a dry bivouac.

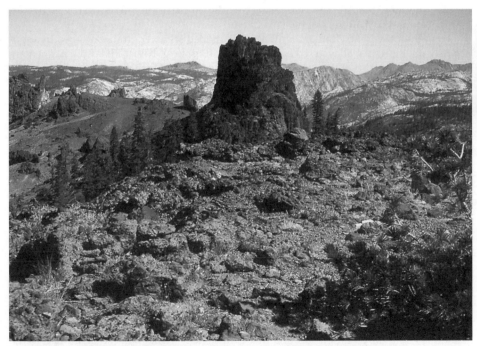

Last overlook of Mokelumne Wilderness from the shoulder of Mt. Reba on Day 4

If you haven't already done so, resume your TYT adventure with a ford of North Fork Mokelumne River (most likely very wet; may be dangerous in early season). Past the ford, the trail climbs the sandy south bank, passes through a large and shady packer campsite that's too close to the water, and curves downstream through dense forest and more dead-fall. Once again, the trail becomes very faint as it follows the river downstream for a few hundred yards. Soon the trail veers left, generally southeast away from the river, and starts a moderate-to-steep, nearly mile-long climb through the same kind of forest as the one you passed through on your way between the last junction and Camp Irene.

Presently, you reach open slopes where a few black oaks dot a hillside composed of granite slabs and boulders and pockets of huckleberry oak and manzanita. Here, hikers encounter the first in a long series of blasted granite areas that leave the impression that the Forest Service had a little too much fun with its use of dynamite. The going is often steep and can be very hot along this section of trail, made even more difficult by the presence of dynamited rocks and overgrowing brush. On these open slopes, the first several switchbacks take you near the seasonal Underwood Valley stream. A few more switchbacks zigzag back and forth toward its banks before the trail veers southwest away from the stream for a while and makes some more switchbacks.

You then reach a ducked route up open granite slabs. The route presently meets the stream again and parallels it for about 50 yards to a switchback overlooking the stream, which is only 7 yards away. This may be your last chance for water for about 2 miles during mid and late season in a normal year.

Beyond this pool, the trail switchbacks again near a flat area with some fair campsites not far from the creek. When it's running, this is probably your last chance for a legal campsite with access to water—but it may also be too soon to stop. After passing below a cliff to the southwest and negotiating more switchbacks, the trail heads southeast on a route on which you struggle toward the last and highest cliff visible along this section of trail. Then, veering to the right, head southwest for about a quarter mile and descend slightly to an overlook of the Mokelumne River Canyon in the west, with the "Mokelumne Tetons" and rusty Mokelumne Peak rising grandly on the north canyon wall. The breath-taking view is worth all the trouble to get here!

From the viewpoint, climb up a moderately graded section of trail, bordered by thousands of wildflowers well watered by dozens of springs in early to mid season. A few more switchbacks deliver southbound TYT hikers to a modest but illegal campsite right next to the trail that, during early and mid season in a normal year, overlooks the first easily obtainable water. In another quarter mile, reach a larger but equally illegal campsite beside the Lake Valley stream, which may be dry by mid season in a dry year but which may otherwise offer the first water in several miles for *northbound* TYT hikers. There seems to be no legal, accessible campsites in Lake Valley; if you must bivouac here, please do your best to protect the stream from your wastes.

Climbing slightly from the campsite, the route passes just above a former lakebed (hence "Lake Valley") and then begins a long series of switchbacks up the east wall of Lake Valley. The wall is capped by dark, volcanic outcroppings from which boulders have broken off and rolled down to the trail and beyond. At the final switchback, on a ridge graced by young hemlocks, there's a sweeping and heartstopping vista over the rugged backcountry soon to be left behind. Ahead to the south is a panoramic view that includes the Dardanelles, a striking volcanic formation, as well as a couple of big, blue reservoirs.

On an 8750-foot shoulder east of Mt. Reba, leave Mokelumne Wilderness. Now following a dirt road open to motor vehicles, stroll past what could be the world's largest field of mule ears. In early season, the large yellow flowers and very large green leaves present a chromatic wonder. In mid to late season, the dry leaves rattle fiercely in the stiff breezes that seem always to blow here in the afternoon. At the first intersection beyond the wilderness boundary—an intersection that is unsigned—remain on the main road to the right (northbound hikers should take the left-hand route). Several dirt roads weave through here; stick to the main road. Grazing cattle may be present here as well. Approximately 0.75 mile from the boundary, the road-trail forks at a low point. Take the branch to the left (east) that heads uphill 30 yards to a saddle. (The other branch ahead also heads uphill but to the south.) Step across another dirt road onto single-track trail at a sign marked TRAIL.

Beyond the road, the trail goes straight downhill for about 200 yards, then veers right and makes a very steep, dusty, loose, and exposed descent of Bee Gulch. Hikers should beware of mountain bikers on this section of trail! The dry surroundings are made more bearable by good views of volcanic towers to the east and, after early summer, by a profusion of wildflowers. The hillside is blessed with extensive areas of pennyroyal, which emit a very pleasant and pungent scent in the warm afternoon sun. After a mile-long descent, you make an easy crossing of a perennial stream. For the next 0.75 mile, a shady, moderate descent leads to a junction where a trail signed ALPINE BYPASS heads to the right (southwest) and another sign reads TAHOE YOSEMITE TRAIL.

Continue straight ahead on the signed TYT from the junction, also following a sign indicating that Hwy. 4 is a half mile away, passing a wooden water tank, and stepping over a seasonal stream. Now walk a well-used and dusty trail up one low ridge and down another, higher one, before making an eastward traverse that climaxes with a descent to State Route 4 opposite a paved road to a backpackers' campground (fee), two car-campgrounds, and restrooms with running water. The next TYT trailhead is 0.3 mile ahead on that paved road at the Silver Valley Trailhead immediately east of Lake Alpine (7386′; 11S 239527 4263329 (field)).

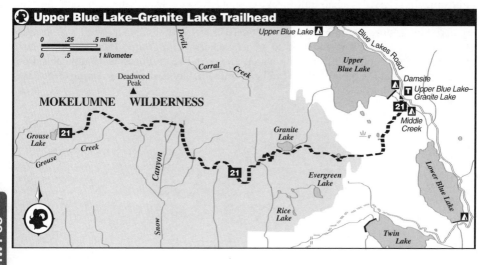

Upper Blue Lake–Granite Lake Trailhead

0   .25   .5 miles
0   .5   1 kilometer

Upper Blue Lake

Blue Lakes Road

Upper
Blue Lake

Damsite

Upper Blue Lake–
Granite Lake

21

Middle
Creek

Devils

Corral   Creek

Deadwood
Peak

MOKELUMNE   WILDERNESS

Granite
Lake

Grouse
Lake   **21**

Creek

Grouse

Canyon

Evergreen
Lake

Lower Blue Lake

21

Rice
Lake

Snow

Twin
Lake

Upper Blue Lake–Granite Lake Trailhead   8155'; 11S 244064 4279573 (field)

DESTINATION/ UTM COORDINATES	TRIP TYPE	BEST SEASON	PACE (HIKING/ LAYOVER DAYS)	TOTAL MILEAGE
21 Grouse Lake 10S 760731 4279178	Out & back	Mid to late	2/1 Leisurely	12

Information and Permits: As with other Mokelumne Wilderness destinations off Hwy. 88, this trailhead is in the Eldorado National Forest: 100 Forni Road, Placerville, CA 95667; 530-622-5061; www.fs.fed.us/r5/eldorado/wild/moke/index.html. For visitor information, call 530-644-6048.

Driving Directions: Leave Hwy. 88 at 6.3 miles east of Carson Pass and head south on Blue Lakes Road through Hope Valley and over a divide to a junction with the road to Lower Blue Lake, 10.3 miles from the highway. Continue straight ahead for another mile and turn right at the Mokelumne Hydro Project. Proceed past Middle Blue Lake to a small parking area on the left, just below the spillway of Upper Blue Lake, 13 miles from Hwy. 88.

21 Grouse Lake

Trip Data: 10S 760731 4279178; 12 miles; 2/1 days

Topos: *Carson Pass, Pacific Valley, Mokelumne Peak*

Highlights: Nestled into a little-traveled corner of Mokelumne Wilderness, Grouse Lake sits high above Summit City Canyon. Requiring only modest effort, this hike offers both the spectacular scenery of sweeping vistas and the intriguing beauty of geologic diversity.

DAY 1 (Upper Blue Lake–Granite Lake Trailhead to Grouse Lake, 6 miles): The Grouse Lake Trail begins just south of the Middle Creek Campground. Cross the seasonal channel of the spillway overflow, turn south into lodgepole pine forest and descend briefly to ford the perennial outflow from Upper Blue Lake. The nearly level trail leads past an unsigned lateral to the campground (ignore it) before your trail swings west on a gentle ascent with tree-shrouded views of the surrounding peaks, including Round Top. The grade eases

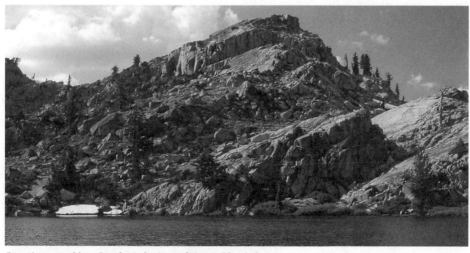

Day 1's route skims Granite Lake (out of Upper Blue Lake).

momentarily at the signed crossing of the Mokelumne Wilderness boundary. Continuing west, skirt a small pond, cross its outlet, climb northwest to a shoulder, and go west through small meadows and past tarns. Climb a small ridge and descend to swing west-southwest next to the flower-lined, seasonal outlet from Granite Lake (another one, not the Granite Lake near Silver Lake or Bayview). Soon the lake springs into view, cradled in a small basin surrounded by weathered granite outcrops. The coarse grains of disintegrating granite rock, called *grus*, come almost to the meadow-fringed shore.

Skirt the south shore of the lake past campsite laterals and veer left over a low ridge. Beyond the lake, you leave most dayhikers behind as the trail winds west for most of a mile through the weathered granite landscape, passing pockets of mixed forest and a small, flower-lined creek. Farther on, a very steep climb on deteriorating tread leads to a stunning vista: Clockwise from the east is the Carson Range (in Nevada); dark, volcanic Raymond Peak; metamorphic Highland, Stanislaus, and Leavitt peaks; and the polished, light granite of the deep cleft of North Fork Mokelumne River Canyon.

Continue through open terrain past an old gravesite, followed by a gradual descent across a verdant, flower-dotted meadow. Beyond the meadow, a lengthy ascent leads across several gullies to a sloping bench bisected by several spring-fed rills.

GEOLOGY LESSON

On the sloping bench, notice how light granite overlies dark volcanic bedrock. A slope change typically occurs at such a contact zone, as the overlying volcanic rock is softer and more easily eroded than granite. The numerous spring-fed rills indicate that the volcanic rock above holds more water than the granite below.

Descend west to a small creek, remaining on the north side, and climb through willows a short distance past the source of the creek. Continue climbing as the trail fades on an open slope. A ducked route levels off and contours northwest for a quarter mile, until multiple paths descend a flower-filled gully dotted with boulders, where Grouse Lake appears several hundred feet below. Eventually the paths merge into a single trail that continues the descent into thickening forest to the shore of the secluded lake (8560'; 10S 760731 4279178). On a hot day, Grouse Lake provides a wonderful wilderness swimming pool. Nearby viewpoints offer glimpses of Summit City Canyon below to the west, down which TYT hikers may be struggling as you gaze. Golden eagles, which traditionally nest in the canyon, may occasionally be seen riding thermals to dizzying heights above.

DAY 2 (Grouse Lake to Upper Blue Lake–Granite Lake Trailhead, 6 miles): Retrace your steps.

STATE HIGHWAY 4 TRIPS

Hwy. 4 over Ebbetts Pass is something of an anomaly. It's a fine, two-lane mountain highway from the town of Arnold on the west to Lake Alpine. Just past Lake Alpine, it shrinks to a narrow, winding, one-lane road with steep drops and climbs and demanding hairpin turns as it climbs over Ebbetts Pass and descends eastward to a junction with Hwy. 89.

Your reward for putting up with this is spectacular scenery in Carson-Iceberg Wilderness, a wilderness area that we're happy to report is so lightly visited beyond day-hiking range that you may wonder if anyone but you knows it's there. From Hwy. 4, we offer trips from three major trailheads, from west to east: Lake Alpine–Silver Valley Trailhead and the Mosquito Lakes Trailhead on the west side of Ebbetts Pass, and the High Trail Trailhead on the east side of Ebbetts Pass. Note that for trail information, the USDA/USGS *Carson-Iceberg Wilderness* map is usually more accurate than the topos.

The Lake Alpine–Silver Valley Trailhead features Section 4 of the TYT, which heads through Carson-Iceberg Wilderness. While Lake Alpine and hiking trails near it attract a majority of the visitors to this general area, far fewer visitors press on from the west or come up from the east to see the beautiful backcountry around Mosquito Lakes and Wolf Creek (the High Trail).

TRAILHEADS: Lake Alpine–Silver Valley
Mosquito Lakes
High Trail

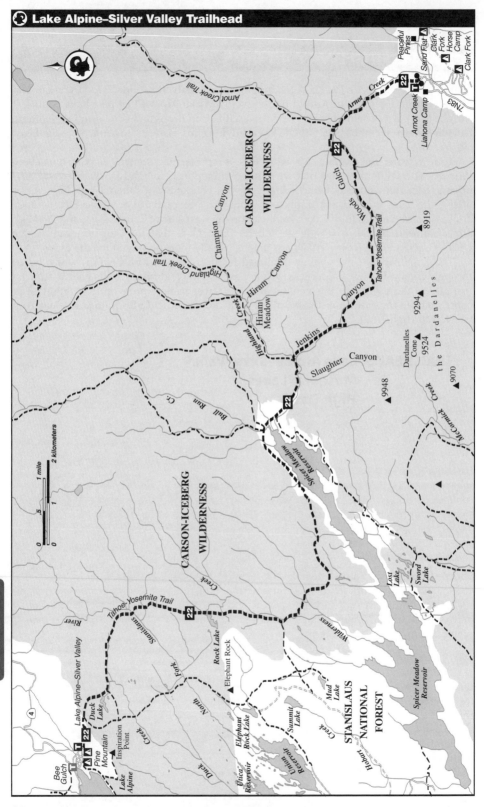

Lake Alpine–Silver Valley Trailhead   7384'; 11S 239528 4263335

DESTINATION/ UTM COORDINATES	TRIP TYPE	BEST SEASON	PACE (HIKING/ LAYOVER DAYS)	TOTAL MILEAGE
22 Tahoe-Yosemite Trail Section 4: To Clark Fork 11S 255434 4254423	Shuttle	Mid to late	3/0 Moderate	19.8

Information and Permits: You must have a wilderness permit for overnight visits to this part of Carson-Iceberg Wilderness. This trip is in the Stanislaus National Forest: Calaveras Ranger District, P.O. Box 500, Hathaway Pines, CA 95233; 209-795-1381; www.fs.fed.us/r5/stanislaus/visitor/carson.shtml.

Driving Directions: Lake Alpine is about 50 miles east of Angels Camp and 16.4 miles west from Ebbetts Pass on Hwy. 4. Near the east end of Lake Alpine, turn south on East Shore Road and go 0.3 mile more to the Silver Valley Campground entrance and the Silver Valley Trailhead. Along East Shore Road, you will find a backpacker's campground near Hwy. 4, Pine Marten Campground to the west, and Silver Valley Campground just west of the trailhead. There is no parking lot; park along the shoulders as best you can.

22 Tahoe-Yosemite Trail Section 4: To Clark Fork

Trip Data: 11S 255434 4254423; 19.8 miles, 3/0 days

Topos: *Spicer Meadow Reservoir, Dardanelles Cone*

Highlights: This section of the TYT is the most timbered and has the least elevation change per mile. After wild and woolly Section 3, Section 4's peaceful, wooded scenery and real trails come as a pleasure and a relief.

HEADS UP! Along this section of the TYT, long, dry stretches of trail are common in mid- and late summer. Note, too, that the topos in this area are way out of date. Spicer Meadow Reservoir has been considerably enlarged, drowning Gabbott Meadow and making the TYT traverse high above its north shore. Also, there's now a direct trail from the Silver Valley Trailhead to Rock Lake. You'll get better trail information from the Carson-Iceberg Wilderness map than from the topos. Note: The given mileage does not include the 3.7 miles on Clark Fork Road between the bridge over Arnot Creek and the road's end at Iceberg Meadow.

Shuttle Directions: To access the take-out location, follow the ill-signed turnoff from Hwy. 108 to paved Clark Fork Road, 17.1 miles west of Sonora Pass and on the north side of the road. Turn northeast on Clark Fork Road and follow it to a left turn onto a dirt road between 5.1 and 5.2 miles. After turning left on that dirt road, continue by going right where a spur goes left to a camp. Follow the road about 0.9 mile to a parking lot at its end.

DAY 1 (Lake Alpine–Silver Valley Trailhead to Rock Lake, 4 miles): A trail signed SILVER VAL-LEY TRAILHEAD heads south between two large boulders. Ascend this trail gently for a quarter mile through a red fir and lodgepole pine forest dotted with flowering meadows to a low, timbered ridge. Enter Carson-Iceberg Wilderness and follow the ridge northeast through a stock gate. About 200 yards down the far side of the ridge, the road makes a sharp bend and leaves the ridge. This dusty segment, now a foot trail, descends gently to moderately under a forest cover of Jeffrey pines with a mixture of western junipers and white firs. Soon the path levels and then passes about 100 yards from the north end of very shallow Duck Lake, barely visible through a forest of lodgepole pines. Wind through a boggy flat—a haven for mosquitoes in early season—and proceed to a junction with the Highland Creek Trail, signed DUCK LK. LOOP, STAN. RIVER, LK. ALPINE.

Go left (east-northeast) on the Highland Creek Trail at the junction, heading toward North Fork Stanislaus River, as the TYT climbs gently to a saddle overlooking the river. You immediately make a moderate, half-mile descent under red fir, lodgepole, and juniper to the river and ford here; during early-season high water, explore upstream for better places to ford. By late summer, the "river" may be barely more than a creek. There are campsites on both sides of the ford.

Beyond the river, the TYT climbs south for 400 vertical feet in two stages—a short, steep, stony one followed by a long one—to a gently sloping ridge with undistinguished views to the west and an attractive display of seasonal wildflowers. Then, via a two-stage descent of more modest proportions, the trail wanders south to marshy little Rock Lake (7315'; 11S 242683 4260034) and a junction with a trail heading west-southwest to Elephant Rock Lake. There are some good campsites on Rock Lake's southeast shore amid thick stands of fir and pine, and swimmers will find this lake to be one of the warmer spots for a dip along the TYT.

DAY 2 (Rock Lake to Highland Creek Campsite, 7.5 miles): If you camped at Rock Lake, retrace your steps to the last junction and turn right (south); if continuing past Rock Lake, go ahead (south) at the junction.

Continuing south in either case, the trail beyond Rock Lake's outlet (may be dry by late season) ascends gently for a short distance and then drops almost to the banks of Wilderness Creek, where water is usually available until late summer. Veer southwest away from the stream and cross an open, dry, sandy flat carpeted with mat lupine and bordered by red firs and junipers. About 1.25 miles from Rock Lake, you pass a junction with the Sand Flat Trail heading right (northwest) to Summit Lake. Go left (southwest) at the junction and descend on pleasant duff underfooting to a ford of Wilderness Creek, where there are a few fair campsites nearby, made somewhat less desirable if cattle happen to be grazing in the vicinity.

Beyond the ford, make a short climb to a minor saddle, drop to the crossing of two Wilderness Creek tributaries (poor campsites in the rocks above the second tributary), and then climb moderately up to a larger, essentially viewless saddle, although photogenic slopes of gray, granitic bedrock appear to the northeast. Descend briefly south, traverse east through a seasonally boggy area, and then climb gently east for a half mile to a viewpoint. Across Highland Creek canyon are the chocolate-colored, layered volcanic formations called the Dardanelles on the southern horizon. Eastward, up the canyon of Highland Creek, Hiram, Airola, and Iceberg peaks reach above timberline to nearly 10,000 feet. Far below, Spicer Meadow Reservoir's long northeast arm sparkles in the summer sun.

HWY 4

THE DARDANELLES

This monumental ridge, composed of lava hundreds of feet thick, is only a small remnant of a long, ancient lava flow that originated near Bridgeport, California. From the source, it flowed about 100 miles down-canyon, stopping at the western edge of the Sierra foothills. The walls of the canyon the lava flowed down were eventually eroded away, while the buried canyon bottom was preserved beneath the flow. Glacial attacks further eroded the surrounding landscape until the granitic floor of Highland Creek lay a good 1000 feet below the base of the Dardanelles. Visible up-canyon are Iceberg, Airola, and Hiram peaks—all volcanic summits but none of them related to the Dardanelles flow.

Beyond the viewpoint, the trail threads two minor gaps and then descends moderately above the reservoir to a junction where paths go right (northeast) to the reservoir and ahead (left, north) to Highland Lakes. Go ahead to traverse—with a slight climb—the steep slopes high above the reservoir. The narrow trail crosses a few seasonal streams. Eventually, the trail enters a forested area where there may be a few campsites. Next, you ascend gently to ford Bull Run Creek and meet the Bull Run Peak/Pacific Valley Trail. Continue ahead to ford another stream and then follow the descending trail that curves southwest. Glimpses of the reservoir appear as the forest thins.

At a junction signed HORSE FORD with a trail right to Spicer Meadow Reservoir, go left toward Sword, Lost, and Highland lakes. Climb to another junction where a trail on the right heads southwest to Sword and Lost lakes, and a trail on the left heads southeast to Highland Lakes, Jenkins Canyon, and Bull Run Creek. Go left on rocky and sandy trail that skirts below Point 7635 and follows Highland Creek upstream into the forest. You meet a junction (6615'; 11S 247145 4258427) with the Jenkins Canyon Trail (ahead, east) where yet another path, this one quite faint, heads left (north) to Highland Lakes. Camping in the area is poor and marginally legal, but the nearby creek offers a chance for a refreshing splash.

DAY 3 (Highland Creek Campsite to Clark Fork Road, 8.3 miles): From the last junction, go ahead (east) on the Jenkins Canyon Trail, bound for Woods Gulch, and arrive in 60 yards at the west bank of Highland Creek at a ford above its confluence with Jenkins Canyon Creek. The trail resumes on the east bank, climbing steeply through heavy forest cover before it becomes level and contours along the canyon slope above the stream. On this stretch of trail there is an unusual sight: Within a few yards of one another are specimens of every tree found anywhere along this section of the TYT—Jeffrey, western white, and lodgepole pines; red and white firs; and western juniper, aspen, and black cottonwood.

Shortly after beginning another moderate ascent, broken volcanic rock lying on the ground offers evidence of the great volcanic outpourings that created the Dardanelles and Dardanelles Cone. The trail crosses the east fork of Jenkins Canyon Creek and then ascends moderately to a series of beautiful wet meadows. The grass in this quarter-mile-long area is interrupted by stands of young red firs and willows that turn flame-yellow in September. A moderate half-mile ascent leads to a saddle on the northeastern ridge of the Dardanelles, a ridge that divides Jenkins Canyon from Woods Gulch. If there's a stock gate here, be sure you close it after you pass through.

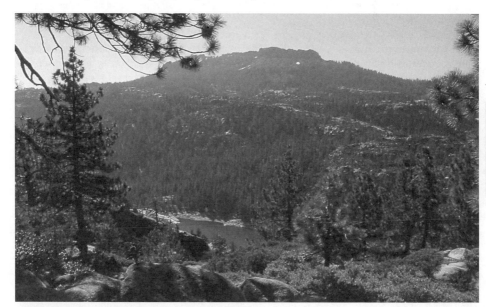

The Dardanelles above Spicer Meadow Reservoir

As the descent into Woods Gulch begins, the vegetation changes markedly, with the appearance of huckleberry oak, chinquapin, and sagebrush, followed by a beautiful dry meadow, perhaps made a bit less stunning if grazing cattle are present. Beyond the meadow, the south-facing slope is covered with scads of aromatic sagebrush interspersed with the yellow flowers of thousands of mule ears. Across this little valley, the north slope is thoroughly shaded by red firs and lodgepole pines.

Sandy trail descends moderately and then gently, crossing the unnamed streams that drain Woods Gulch; you may find a few campsites near these streams. As the red fir forest cover thickens, the descent quickens, becoming first moderate and then steep. After switchbacking 350 rocky feet down eroded and dusty tread, the trail levels and crosses the main stream in Woods Gulch. Just beyond the ford, the trail curves east to descend gently beside the stream under a moderate cover of white fir, incense cedar, and aspen. After less than a half mile, you reach a junction and turn right (south) onto the Arnot Creek Trail, arriving in 100 yards at a final ford of Woods Gulch Creek.

Follow the tread of an old jeep road, initially passing a few campsites. These are the last wilderness campsites before you end this day at Clark Fork Road. Continue along the jeep road for almost 2 miles from the ford of Woods Gulch Creek, fording Arnot Creek twice; the second ford is broad and bouldery and can be wet. Exiting Carson-Iceberg Wilderness and finally reaching a gate, you find a trail that arcs southeast to a trailhead parking lot (6184'; 11S 255434 4254423), where this TYT section ends. Those who have left a car or who are being picked up should find their ride here.

GETTING TO TYT SECTION 5

Many hikers choose to continue on to the next TYT section immediately. From the lot, such hikers can take the dirt road (7N13) about 0.1 mile south to the point where the road angles southwest. From here, descend on use trail to Arnot Creek and follow its forested bank to a bridge where Clark Fork Road crosses Arnot Creek. Climb up to the road near here. There is no continuous footpath between the point where you meet Clark Fork Road and the beginning of the next trail section (TYT Section 5) at Iceberg Meadow, so your best bet is to walk the easy 3.7 miles generally east on the lightly used road to the roadend at Iceberg Meadow. After all, you won't want to miss the cross-country excitement and beauty of Section 5!

If you are ending this day on Clark Fork Road, you can walk to riverside Clark Fork Campground or to Sand Flat Campground. These campgrounds offer your best opportunity for a comfortable campsite between here and your next opportunity for a legal campsite, the area where Boulder Creek and Clark Fork Stanislaus River meet, about 8.4 miles of road and then of trail from the bridge over Arnot Creek. If you exit near the bridge where Clark Fork Road crosses Arnot Creek, Sand Flat Campground is nearer and is on the way east toward Iceberg Meadow.

HWY 4

Mosquito Lakes Trailhead
8054'; 11S 245850, 4267004 (field)

DESTINATION/ UTM COORDINATES	TRIP TYPE	BEST SEASON	PACE (HIKING/ LAYOVER DAYS)	TOTAL MILEAGE
23 Stanislaus Meadow Trailhead 11S 243825 4265830	Shuttle	Mid	3/0 Leisurely	8

Information and Permits: You must have a wilderness permit for overnight visits to this part of Carson-Iceberg Wilderness. This trip is in the Stanislaus National Forest: Calaveras Ranger District, P.O. Box 500, Hathaway Pines, CA 95233; 209-795-1381; www.fs.fed.us/r5/stanislaus/visitor/carson.shtml.

Driving Directions: From the east end of Lake Alpine, travel 6 miles northeast up Hwy. 4, or, from Ebbetts Pass, drive 8.4 winding miles west, to the west end of Mosquito Lakes (a single lovely pond at high water, or a pair of attractive ponds at low water) and the signed trailhead. There's a toilet in the Mosquito Lakes Campground across the highway.

23 Stanislaus Meadow Trailhead

Trip Data: 11S 243825 4265830; 8 miles; 3/0 days

Topos: *Pacific Valley, Spicer Meadow Reservoir*

Highlights: You'll visit two of the better, scenic, trout-stocked lakes off Hwy. 4 on this easy hike. Dayhikers and anglers may choose to hike only to Heiser Lake via the Heiser Lake Trail (Mosquito Lakes Trailhead), or only to larger Bull Run Lake via the Bull Run Trail (Stanislaus Meadow Trailhead), thereby avoiding the short car shuttle.

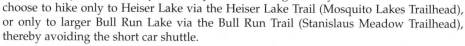

Shuttle Directions: Access the take-out location at the Stanislaus Meadow Trailhead from the east end of Lake Alpine by traveling 4 miles northeast up Hwy. 4. Or, from Ebbetts Pass, drive 10.4 miles west. From either location, come to a spur road branching right and signed STANISLAUS MDW, BULL RUN TRAIL. With 4WD, you can follow this road a half mile to the end. Otherwise, park after 0.3 or 0.4 mile and, on your way out, walk that extra distance to the trailhead.

Day 1 (Mosquito Lakes Trailhead to Heiser Lake, 2 miles): Head briefly south on the Heiser Lake Trail, almost immediately meeting a junction with the Emigrant Trail on the right heading west to Lake Alpine (not shown on the topo). Step across the Emigrant Trail and continue ahead (south), remaining on the Heiser Lake Trail and curving around the western Mosquito Lake before beginning a steep climb up a moraine south of the lake through moderate-to-sparse forest. Gaining the ridge at last, descend the sandy trail and enter Carson-Iceberg Wilderness near the half-mile mark. Continue generally southeast through forest interrupted by a pair of small meadows and then, at 0.75 mile, climb up the next moraine.

On fresh-looking, glacially scoured rock, descend the moraine and follow a winding route that takes the path of least resistance down rock slabs. After leveling off in deep forest, climb 0.3 mile to a small flat and a junction where tomorrow's route will turn right (southwest) down a creekside trail. For today, you turn left (east) at the junction and make a quarter-mile ascent to a switchback and then climb south over the low granitic ridge that hides shallow Heiser Lake (8340'; 11S 246495 4264722). Dotted with several small granite islands, the conifer-fringed lake presents anglers with a picturesque distraction while they contemplate a meal of fresh trout. Campsites lie on the north and south shores under a pleasant canopy of red firs, lodgepole pines, western white pines, and mountain hemlocks.

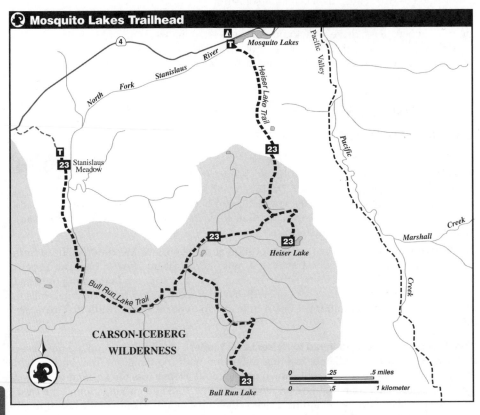

Mosquito Lakes Trailhead

DAY 2 (Heiser Lake to Bull Run Lake, 2.5 miles): First, retrace your steps a quarter mile to the trail junction. From here, the route, usually well-blazed and ducked, leads southwest to the brink of a rocky slope and then down the slope on very steep switchbacks. Paralleling Heiser Lake's outlet, head west across a flat basin shaded by mountain hemlocks. Approaching the basin's west edge, cross four closely spaced branches of a tributary that joins the outlet creek just south of the trail. After a brief climb west, the trail turns south and leads to a signed junction with the Bull Run Trail.

Turn left (east) at the junction and almost immediately ford Heiser Lake's outlet, a ford that could present a problem in early season when the creek is a small torrent of whitewater. After following a nearly level granite bench for 0.3 mile, the route angles south to cross the first of many small rivulets. The winding route climbs and gyrates up toward Bull Run Lake from one granite slab to another. Broken into two distinct ascents, the first climb trends southeast up and around a secondary ridge; the second trends southwest past a trailside pond before approaching the outlet and then ascending alongside it to the lake's bedrock dam (8333'; 11S 245739 4263315).

Although not large by Sierra standards, this popular lake can accommodate a large number of campers, particularly on the spacious flats shaded by large red firs. Swimming in the lake is comfortable by early August, and fishing is reported to be good for brook trout.

DAY 3 (Bull Run Lake to Stanislaus Meadow Trailhead, 3.5 miles): Backtrack to the trail junction west of Heiser Lake's outlet and turn left (southwest) onto the Bull Run Trail. Descend, steeply at times, 350 vertical feet down rock slabs covered with lodgepole and western white pines, red firs, and mountain junipers, staying well above the outlet creek from both lakes before the grade eases in a shady flat. A short, forested traverse leads to a crossing of this creek, which may entail a cold, wide, knee-deep ford in early season. Beyond the ford, follow the course of the creek on a shady, long 0.3 mile to a ford of the twin-branched outlet, which may also present early-season challenges. Beyond the ford the trail maintains a westbound course for 100 yards to an even wider ford of the headwaters of North Fork Stanislaus River. A search for logs across this stream may result in a quicker and drier crossing.

Immediately beyond the North Fork, cross a seasonally dry wash before turning north and roughly paralleling the river upstream. A wide path leads up a moderate grade to Stanislaus Meadow, where a chorus of cowbells may herald the presence of cattle munching away on the verdant grasses. A fence helps to keep the cattle in the meadow while the trail follows an easy route through the trees near the west edge for 0.3 mile to the Stanislaus Meadow Trailhead (7739'; 11S 243825 4265830).

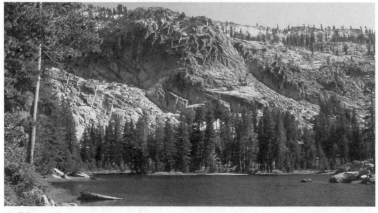

Bull Run Lake

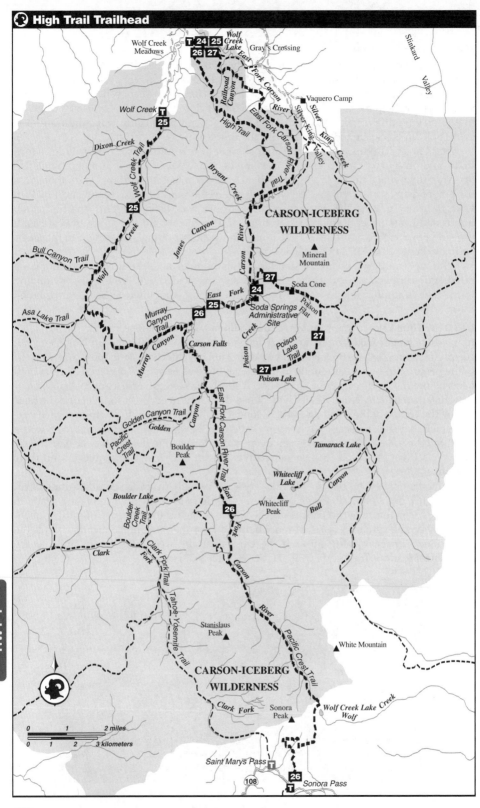

High Trail Trailhead

6406'; 11S 266210, 4275931 (field)

DESTINATION/ UTM COORDINATES	TRIP TYPE	BEST SEASON	PACE (HIKING/ LAYOVER DAYS)	TOTAL MILEAGE
24 Soda Springs 11S 268656 4265493	Semiloop	Mid	2/1 Moderate	20.5
25 Wolf Creek Meadows 11S 265040 4273180	Shuttle	Mid or late	2/0 Strenuous	24
26 Sonora Pass 11S 269685 4245685	Shuttle	Mid	3/0 Strenuous	30
27 Poison Lake 11S 268627 4262383	Semiloop	Mid	4/0 Moderate	36.5

Information and Permits: Wilderness permits are required here, but there are no quotas, so you can get one on demand. You can also issue one to yourself at the trailhead. The High Trail Trailhead trips are in the Humboldt-Toiyabe National Forest: Carson Ranger District, 1536 South Carson St., Carson City, NV 89701, (775) 331-6444; www.fs.fed.us/r4/htnf/ recreation/wilderness/carson_iceberg.shtml.

Driving Directions: From the junction of Hwy. 4 and Hwy. 89 south of Markleeville and east of Ebbetts Pass, drive about 2.5 miles south on Hwy. 4 and then turn southeast on the signed Wolf Creek Road. Proceed 3.3 miles to a fork, turn left following signed directions for the High Trail and Carson River Trailhead, and descend northeast around the north end of Wolf Creek Meadows. Past the meadows, the road climbs through the trees and, at 0.6 mile from Wolf Creek Road, reaches a spur road heading southeast a short distance to the trailhead.

24 Soda Springs

Trip Data: 11S 268656 4265493; 20.5 miles; 2/1 days

Topos: *Wolf Creek, Disaster Peak*

see map on p.102

Highlights: Backpackers acquire a good feeling for eastside Sierra flora and geology on this trip, as the landscape is viewed from two very different perspectives: a crest route and a canyon route.

HEADS UP! Much of this route is not shown, or is shown incorrectly, on either the 7.5' topos or the Carson-Iceberg Wilderness map. Also note that in the vicinity of Soda Springs Administrative Site, the 7.5' topo and the wilderness map both show two routes leading eastward up out of the river canyon toward the Soda Cone and Poison Flat—a southern route that seems more direct and a northern one. The routes are shown as joining west of the Soda Cone. The southern route does not exist. Soda Springs Guard Station is now the Soda Springs Administrative Site (no staff).

DAY 1 (High Trail Trailhead to Soda Springs, 9.5 miles): At the edge of a volcanic slope covered with sagebrush, bitterbrush, and mule ears, the High Trail climbs upward into an open forest of Jeffrey pine and white fir to a junction of the High Trail and the East Fork Carson River Trail. The latter trail is nearer East Fork Carson River—it's the one that runs by Wolf Creek Lake—but that trail is not named on the maps (the High Trail is named). We call the unnamed trail that's nearer the river the East Fork Carson River Trail. On this trip, you'll make the loop part out on the High Trail, and your return is partly on the East Fork Carson River Trail.

Turn right (south) at the junction onto the High Trail, experiencing brief views of Wolf Creek Meadows. Leaving the views of the meadows behind, enjoy the shade provided by the forest on this steep section. Beyond a large split boulder and the surrounding mountain mahogany bushes, the trail parallels the ridge up to a level crest and then climbs steeply to a small, grassy flat. Past the flat, the trail makes an uphill traverse across a grassy, gentle slope containing a curious combination of water-loving, white-barked aspens almost next to drought-resistant, mangy-barked junipers. Jeffrey pines, white firs, willows, sagebrush, and mule ears complete the cast of principal plants.

Climb shady slopes for about a half mile beyond the meadow until the steep grade of the trail eases and then levels across an open slope. Here, the trail provides a brief view of the Vaquero Camp buildings in the east, down in Silver Valley, and views in the northwest of the granitic Freel Peak area, beyond whose summits lies Lake Tahoe.

AUTOBRECCIATED LAVA FLOW

Along this short, open traverse is a good exposure of a blocky volcanic rock common to this "land of fire and ice" and known as an autobrecciated (self-broken) lava flow. Geologists speculate that from the middle Miocene epoch through the late Pliocene epoch, thick andesitic lava flows poured from summits that were perhaps similar to the Oregon Cascades of our time. These lava flows covered an area of the Sierra Nevada from Sonora Pass north to Lassen Park and from east of the present Sierra Crest westward to the Central Valley. Flowing along their downward paths, the thick lava flows cooled and became less and less able to move, particularly on the rapidly cooling edges that eventually solidified. Pressure from the still-flowing internal areas fractured the edges, creating the broken-up texture seen today.

"Autobrecciated lava flow" is a mouthful. The Hawaiians, who live intimately with volcanoes, call such flows *aa*, pronounced "Ah! Ah!" and equivalent to "Ow! Ow!," which is what you might say if you walked on *aa* in bare feet. We'll use *aa* instead of "autobrecciated lava flow."

At the base of some *aa* decorated with vine maples, enter a shady white fir forest and find a refreshing, flowery, mossy, spring-fed rivulet. From this delightful watercourse, the trail climbs moderately eastward and then descends slightly to a low knoll covered with ragged mountain mahogany. Leaving the knoll, pass through a forest of pines and firs and descend steeply south into two seasonal, parallel creeklets that drain Snowslide Canyon. Volcanic rocks give way to granitic ones as you leave the broad, brushy canyon behind on a descent through forest, around a jagged, granitic ridge, and to another seasonal stream.

A quarter mile beyond this creek, the trail tops out at a bedrock saddle along a ridge above the East Fork Carson River's canyon. From there, short switchbacks lead steeply down a brushy slope covered with huckleberry oak and manzanita; then the trail diagonals southwest down to a gentle slope and the crossing of an unsigned, east-west trail. You soon reach the crossing of a bubbling creek and continue a mere 90 yards to a ford of East Fork Carson River. Before mid-July, the river is usually waist deep, about 50°F at most, and swift, but by Labor Day, hikers can expect a knee-deep ford.

FISH IN THE EAST FORK CARSON RIVER

A likely catch for anglers is the mountain whitefish, which resembles a cross between a trout and a sucker. A small mouth on the lower part of its head is the sucker characteristic, but the presence of an adipose fin on the lower back identifies it as a close relative of trout and salmon. As with those two fish, the whitefish is good to eat. The river also is home to the Tahoe sucker, whose protractile mouth on the bottom of its head is ideally suited for scavenging the river bottom. Although bony, the Tahoe sucker is quite tasty.

Across the river, the High Trail ends in 80 yards at a signed junction with the East Fork Carson River Trail—a former jeep road. Turn right (south, upstream) on it. The old road parallels the river for 0.3 mile upstream to the north edge of a sagebrush flat, where the river angles west but the road heads south through dense sagebrush. Reaching a dry wash debouching from a small, very bouldery gorge, you climb up the wash to a low bedrock saddle. From the saddle, make a short descent past a small, steep cliff on the right and then reach a larger, longer, steeper cliff on the left.

Parallel the cliff southeast and then continue to three closely spaced Jeffrey pines in a sagebrush flat. From between the west and south pines, your main route goes 200 yards southwest to a ford of East Fork Carson River and then south along jeep tracks through a shady forest to a refording of the river 1 mile farther. This ford occurs at the "bottom" (south) curve of a large meander, where the west half dries up in late summer when the lower river shoots directly east 150 yards to the ford (see the accompanying map). Eventually, the meander will disappear as the river establishes a more efficient, more direct course. About 250 yards south of this ford, in a field of granitic boulders left by a glacier, an indistinct trail heads east-southeast through the grass another 250 yards to Poison Creek. Just beyond the east bank is a path that leads south 300 yards to Soda Springs Administrative Site.

> **AVOID THE FORDS**
>
> Most hikers, when they arrive at the three Jeffrey pines, will prefer not to ford and reford East Fork Carson River, even though these two fords are considerably easier than the High Trail ford. For them there is a dry route to the Soda Springs Administrative Site. After leaving the south and east pines, follow a path south-southeast for 100 yards. Bend south and reach a granitic cliff that plunges down to East Fork Carson River only a quarter mile due south of the three pines. Once around the bouldery base of this small cliff, an easy, open walk southward parallels the river. About 0.75 mile beyond, the river bends west and the trail follows alongside through sagebrush to the northeast corner of the large meander mentioned in the main route's description, above. From this corner, a set of jeep tracks leads southeast 0.2 mile across a flat to a signed junction with the Poison Flat Trail, just within forest cover. Turn south, up-canyon, and follow the jeep tracks, which quickly dwindle to a path in the 100 yards it takes to reach the first of as many as a half a dozen distributaries of Poison Creek.

The main route and the route that avoids the fords meet between a couple of Poison Creek's distributaries. A little beyond, find the fenced-in compound around Soda Springs Administrative Site (6784′; 11S 268656 4265493). Backpacker campsites are available by multibranched and misnamed Poison Creek—the water isn't poisonous—or near a small creek 0.3 mile along the trail west of the guard station. Camping is prohibited in the administrative site's immediate vicinity; read and follow all posted regulations.

DAY 2 (Soda Springs to High Trail Trailhead, 11 miles): First, retrace your steps down-canyon 2.75 miles north to the signed High Trail junction.

From the junction, don't take the High Trail left to the ford. Instead, go right (northeast) briefly away from the river on a jeep road and then quickly curve right around an open flat. In 0.4 mile from the junction, you arrive at an East Fork Carson River ford that is almost as difficult as the High Trail ford.

Ford the river, pick up the jeep road, and take it northeast across a flat where the road is nearly cut in two by a meander of the river that has eroded deeply into the flat. Beyond the meander, a traverse across an equally long flat ends at East Fork Carson River a mile below the High Trail junction.

Look for two large Jeffrey pines just to the north, between which a barbed-wire gate marks the start of a trail. From the gate, this trail remains on the west side of East Fork

Carson River (despite what the maps show), paralleling the river at first, and then gradually veering away. Cross two long but not high moraines and then cross a seasonal rivulet that is only about 70 yards west of the river. The trail then parallels the river to a junction with some jeep tracks.

Turn left and follow the jeep tracks north almost a half mile up to a low ridgecrest of a rocky moraine. Atop this moraine is a barbed-wire fence across the jeep tracks. The challenging route leaves the jeep tracks atop the moraine, follows the fence west (left) about 300 yards to a gate, descends to the entrance of a gorge, and follows the west side of the river through this gorge for 2.5 miles.

The difficulty of this gorge route varies, the hardest part occurring in the scenic first half. When the water is low—usually after Labor Day—walking along the river's edge is possible, but earlier in the season it may be necessary to climb above the river in several places. Nevertheless, a rope is unnecessary. First, pass by impressive, deeply cut cliffs of *aa*. Farther downstream, you may see columnar flows—lava flows that cooled and cracked into vertical columns. Campsites in this isolated gorge are plentiful, but the best ones unfortunately seem to be on the opposite bank. Your west-bank route ends where it meets the East Fork Carson River Trail, which fords East Fork Carson River at Gray's Crossing, directly west of a low gap. You go left (west) here to stay on the west side.

From this junction, the East Fork Carson River Trail heads west and then climbs steeply up to gentler slopes above the river. Pass through a gate and gradually curve westward into Railroad Canyon. Hike up this canyon, seemingly for too long a period to actually be on the correct route, and then cross the canyon's stream. From here, the last permanent source of water, the trail climbs north out of the canyon, circles the edge of a flat-topped *aa* flow, and then traverses 0.3 mile northwest to the south tip of shallow Wolf Creek Lake (not the better-known Wolf Creek Lake at the east base of Sonora Peak).

From the lake, the trail climbs west up to the base of steep volcanic slopes and then ascends a ridge to the junction with the High Trail coming in on the left (south). Go ahead (west) on the joined trails to a saddle from which you make a steep descent to the trailhead (6406'; 11S 266210, 4275931 (field)).

25 Wolf Creek Meadows

Trip Data: 11S 265040 4273180; 24 miles; 2/0 days

Topos: *Wolf Creek, Disaster Peak*

Highlights: This trip starts as a scenic crest route and then proceeds through parts of three glaciated canyons. Plenty of campsites near creeks await anglers.

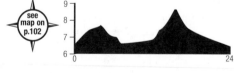

HEADS UP! *Much of this route is not shown, or is shown incorrectly, on either the 7.5' topos or the Carson-Iceberg Wilderness map. Also note that in the vicinity of Soda Springs Administrative Site, the 7.5' topo and the wilderness map both show two routes leading eastward up out of the river canyon toward the Soda Cone and Poison Flat—a southern route that seems more direct and a northern one. The routes are shown as joining west of the Soda Cone. The southern route does not exist.*

Shuttle Directions: Driving to the take-out at the Wolf Creek Meadows Trailhead begins as for driving to the High Trail Trailhead: From the junction of Hwy. 89 and Hwy. 4 south of Markleeville and east of Ebbetts Pass, drive about 2.5 miles south on Hwy. 4 and then turn southeast onto Wolf Creek Road. Proceed 3.3 miles to a fork. Avoiding the left fork (which leads to the High Trail Trailhead), continue ahead (south) on Wolf Creek Road 1.5 miles to where the road bends sharply left. The signed Wolf Creek Meadows Trail is on the right immediately after the bend.

DAY 1 (High Trail Trailhead to Murray Canyon Trail Junction, 12 miles): *(Partial Recap: Trip 24, Day 1, to Soda Springs Administrative Site.)* From the trailhead, climb to the High Trail-East Carson River Trail junction and turn right (south) onto the High Trail. Follow it over forested and volcanic terrain to the ford of East Fork Carson River (campsites nearby). Following the principal route rather than any alternate ones, ford here (may be dangerous in early season), pick up the High Trail again, and in 80 yards meet the East Fork Carson River Trail. Turn right (upstream) on it to a flat with three closely spaced Jeffrey pines. From between the west and south pines, go 200 yards southwest to ford the river again and then head south along jeep tracks to yet another ford at the "bottom" (south) curve of a large meander. After fording, go about 250 yards south to an indistinct trail east-southeast and follow it another 250 yards to Poison Creek. Just beyond the creek's east bank is a path that leads south 300 yards to Soda Springs Administrative Site (6784'; 11S 268656 4265493). (From the three closely spaced Jeffrey pines, there's an alternate route that goes south and southeast from the south and east pines. This route lets you remain on the river's east side—with no river fords—to a signed junction with the Poison Flat Trail, on which you turn right, south, to the administrative site.) If you decide to camp here, there are a number of sites in the area, but camping is prohibited in the administrative site's immediate vicinity; read and follow all posted regulations.

Leaving the administrative site and the Day 1 route of Trip 24, hike west on a jeep trail, and after 0.3 mile, cross a spring-fed stream. Just beyond is a well-used campsite shaded by lodgepole pines, 20 yards downslope. Immediately below this campsite is a trail coming from a large meander. Westward, this trail parallels the jeep trail before dying out in a grassy meadow. An easy, half-mile route along the jeep trail passes through sagebrush before dying out in the same meadow as the trail. The jeep tracks quickly reappear at the northwest end of the meadow and continue 200 yards northwest to a wide ford of East Fork Carson River.

Ford the river and follow the trail northwest from the ford to an unsigned junction with a path that heads east along the base of the canyon's north wall to another ford of the river. Turn left and take the generally westbound trail from the junction, beyond which the trail is often a multilane cowpath for the next 1.5 miles. The trail tends to stay away from the river on a gentle ascent through Jeffrey pine forest. After the canyon bends south, the trail emerges on the edge of large, cow-infested Falls Meadow. On the northwest side of the meadow, cross Murray Creek. About 50 yards beyond the crossing of Murray Creek, there's a signed junction with the Murray Canyon Trail (6923'; 11S 265768 4264430). Several fair campsites can be found near the cottonwoods along the creek. Both the creek and the river offer fair-to-good fishing.

DAY 2 (Murray Canyon Trail Junction to Wolf Creek Meadows, 12 miles): At the signed trail junction, take the right fork generally westward, leaving the East Fork Carson River Trail, and climb, steeply at times, up more than a dozen switchback legs that lead high up a brushy, open-forested slope and into Murray Canyon.

MURRAY CANYON GLACIER

Like virtually every tributary of East Fork Carson River upstream of Soda Springs, Murray Canyon held a glacier at the same time as a glacier occupied the East Fork Carson River's canyon. However, being much smaller, the Murray Canyon glacier was unable to keep pace with the tremendous excavating power of East Fork Carson River's glacier, which was estimated to be as thick as 800 feet in this area. As a result, the glacier cut deeper, leaving Murray Canyon as a hanging valley—the same valley hikers enter at the top of the upcoming switchbacks.

From the top of the switchbacks, travel 200 yards to a crossing of lushly lined and crystal-clear Murray Canyon Creek. After 100 steep yards, a moderate grade resumes that leads past the first of many flower-lined rivulets. Pass through the gate of a cattle fence 0.3 mile from the creek crossing, and continue up the flowery path. Where the canyon splits, the trail forks; go right (generally west) and climb steeply west up the canyon.

About a quarter mile up from the junction, cross a perennial creek lined with willows and alders; ford another stream a quarter mile farther. The route becomes steeper past the stream, following a few short switchbacks up a granitic slope. Talus from volcanic formations above has buried much of the granite bedrock, becoming very widespread where the grade eases and the trail enters a small gully flowered with mule ears. Beyond this gully, climb steadily north for a half mile to a crest saddle and come to a junction a few hundred yards northwest of the actual crest.

From the junction, the left fork eventually connects with the PCT, but you go right on switchbacking trail that heads northwest down open volcanic slopes toward a flat-topped ridge composed of several thick, horizontal lava flows with a huge talus slope below. Reach the floor of Wolf Creek's canyon at the bottom of the descent and pass through the gate of a cattle fence, as the single-track trail widens to a jeep road. About 100 yards past an intersection with a jeep spur from the south—you go ahead (west)—there is a signed junction with a trail left (southwest) to Asa Lake.

You go right (north) on an old jeep road for the remainder of this trip and soon reach a ford—usually a wet one—of Wolf Creek. Across the creek, amble along an easy 0.3 mile to a meadow and another junction, where you go ahead (generally northeast).

Continue northeast around the fenced meadow, descend to a small stream, and then parallel Wolf Creek for a short distance, staying above the small gorge that the creek has cut through the volcanic rock. Small, tempting pools appear in the creek, particularly just before a gate on a low, descending ridge. Beyond this gate, the route descends very steeply to a crossing of Bull Canyon Creek, a wet ford except in late season. Near this alder-lined stream, granitic bedrock once again is evident, becoming more abundant farther down the canyon. You may notice a junction with a trail that goes left (southwest) up Bull Canyon. Whether you notice it or not, you continue your journey ahead and generally northeast.

Heading down-canyon to Dixon Creek, the trail approaches and veers away from Wolf Creek several times. A long, wide, rocky streambed has formed behind a constriction in the canyon created by a prominent granitic ridge on the east and Dixon Creek's alluvial fan on the west. Continue to Dixon Creek, which usually runs too high to ford without getting wet feet—the last such ford en route to the trailhead. Beyond the ford, the jeep road first parallels and then veers northwest away from the creek. Skirt a grove of aspens and cottonwoods and then curve east around a well-weathered granite knob. From here, an easy 1-mile stroll leads to the Wolf Creek Meadows Trailhead (6550'; 11S 265040 4273180) just outside the wilderness boundary.

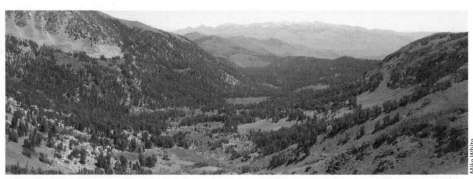

View of Wolf Creek's canyon

26 Sonora Pass

Trip Data: 11S 269685 4245685;
30 miles; 3/0 days

Topos: *Wolf Creek, Disaster Peak,
Sonora Pass*

Highlights: One of the longest and
deepest canyons east of the Sierra

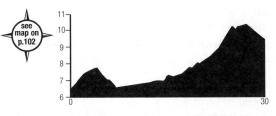

Crest, the East Fork Carson River's
canyon at times contained glaciers up to 19 miles long. The trip follows this canyon to its
end and beyond Sonora Peak to Sonora Pass.

*HEADS UP! Your trip starts in the north near one Wolf Creek and one Wolf Creek Lake and ends far to
the south near an entirely different Wolf Creek and Wolf Creek Lake. From its junction with the Golden
Canyon Trail south to the PCT junction, your route is on an officially unmaintained trail and may be
hard to follow.*

Shuttle Directions: This take-out trailhead, a PCT trailhead, is at Sonora Pass, the highest
point on Hwy. 108, 67 miles northeast of the town of Sonora and 15 miles east of Hwy. 395.
The parking lot is on the north side of the highway.

DAY 1 (High Trail Trailhead to Murray Canyon Trail Junction, 12 miles): *(Partial Recap: Trip
24, Day 1, to Soda Springs Administrative Site.)* From the trailhead, climb to the High Trail-
East Fork Carson River Trail junction and turn right (south) onto the High Trail. Follow it
over forested and volcanic terrain to the ford of East Fork Carson River (campsites nearby). Following the principal route rather than any alternate ones, ford here (may be dangerous in early season), pick up the High Trail again, and in 80 yards meet the East Fork
Carson River Trail. Turn right (upstream) on it to a flat with three closely spaced Jeffrey
pines. From between the west and south pines, go 200 yards southwest to ford the river
again and then head south along jeep tracks to yet another ford at the "bottom" (south)
curve of a large meander. After fording, go about 250 yards south to an indistinct trail east-
southeast and follow it another 250 yards to Poison Creek. Just beyond the creek's east
bank is a path that leads south 300 yards to Soda Springs Administrative Site (6784'; 11S
268656 4265493). (From the three closely spaced Jeffrey pines, there's an alternate route that
goes south and southeast from the south and east pines. This route lets you remain on the
river's east side—with no river fords—to a signed junction with the Poison Flat Trail, on
which you turn right, south, to the administrative site.) If you decide to camp here, there
are a number of sites in the area, but camping is prohibited in the administrative site's
immediate vicinity; read and follow all posted regulations.

Leaving the administrative site and the Day 1 route of Trip 24, hike west on a jeep trail,
and after 0.3 mile, cross a spring-fed stream. Just beyond is a well-used campsite shaded
by lodgepole pines, 20 yards downslope. Immediately below this campsite is a trail coming from a large meander. Westward, this trail parallels the jeep trail before dying out in a
grassy meadow. An easy, half-mile route along the jeep trail passes through sagebrush
before dying out in the same meadow as the trail. The jeep tracks quickly reappear at the
northwest end of the meadow and continue 200 yards northwest to a wide ford of East
Fork Carson River.

Ford the river and follow the trail northwest from the ford to an unsigned junction with
a path that heads east along the base of the canyon's north wall to another ford of the river.
Turn left and take the generally westbound trail from the junction, beyond which the trail
is often a multilane cowpath for the next 1.5 miles. The trail tends to stay away from the
river on a gentle ascent through Jeffrey pine forest. After the canyon bends south, the trail
emerges on the edge of large, cow-infested Falls Meadow. On the northwest side of the

HWY 4

meadow, cross Murray Creek. About 50 yards beyond the crossing of Murray Creek, there's a signed junction with the Murray Canyon Trail (6923'; 11S 265768 4264430). Several fair campsites can be found near the cottonwoods along the creek. Both the creek and the river offer fair-to-good fishing.

DAY 2 (Murray Canyon Trail Junction to Wolf Creek Lake, 13 miles): Your goal today is the Wolf Creek Lake east of Sonora Peak, not the one near the High Trail-East Fork Carson River Trail off Hwy. 4.

From the Murray Canyon Trail junction, go left (south), briefly along Murray Canyon Creek. In early season, you may need to wade the creek's high waters for several yards downstream in order to pick up the trail on the river's west side. Once across the creek, follow the west bank for approximately 200 yards to where the creek bends east to join the meandering East Fork Carson River. Immediately south of this bend, rejoin the main path of the trail. (This path, obvious to northbound hikers, fords Murray Canyon Creek four times and, due to willows and grass, is difficult for southbound hikers to locate).

Staying along the west edge of Falls Meadow, follow the trail for about a half mile south to a usually flowing creek, cross a very low ridge, and make a very steep but short, 200-yard climb to a junction. From the junction, a quarter-mile-long alternate route leads east to Carson Falls before turning south and rejoining the main route. Since both routes are equally strenuous, the more scenic Carson Falls route (left fork) is recommended. Follow the short Carson Falls Trail to near the midpoint and descend briefly to almost level granite slabs near the lip of the river's gorge.

CARSON FALLS

With backpack removed, you can cautiously explore the falls and pools of this gorge. Over a period of thousands of years, large potholes have been drilled into the bedrock, while strong currents have swirled large boulders round and round. At low water, some of these potholes make for brisk and invigorating swimming holes. The top of an almost isolated granitic mass just downstream provides the best view of the main falls, provided you can make the climb.

Where the Carson Falls Trail rejoins the main trail, walk through a flat that shows evidence of beaver activity. Entering an aspen grove at the edge of this flat, the trail curves southwest along a granitic base just above the sometimes-swampy flat and soon reaches a ford of East Fork Carson River. If fording here looks too tough, find a wide and shallow ford of the river downstream. A short half mile farther, where the river, trapped in a small gorge, turns abruptly west, the trail leaves the river and goes up-canyon to a junction with the Golden Canyon Trail. At this junction, go left as the route curves southeast and quickly becomes a steep and brushy 400-vertical-foot climb to the top of a granitic mass that has withstood repeated efforts at eradication by glaciers. Leaving the southeast end of the mass, the trail follows a rollercoaster route for a half mile and touches upon a river meander just before the start of a fairly long climb.

The winding climb crosses a few creekbeds before going south up the gully of a north-flowing seasonal creek. Beyond the top of this gully, junipers together with Jeffrey, lodgepole, and western white pines are momentarily left behind on a descent into a red fir forest, home of the red squirrel, or chickaree. The path levels at a year-round creek and then parallels the East Fork—usually at a small distance away—for 3 miles upstream. The shady stream crosses many rivulets on a gentle-to-moderate grade on the way up the canyon. Glimpses of the high cliffs along the canyon's east side provide periodic visual interest. At the south end of the cliffs, a descending ridge forces the route across the East Fork, which can be a slippery and wet ford in early and midseason. Once on the west bank, head south for about 150 yards to the trail's end a T-junction with the PCT.

Turn left (southeast) onto the PCT and continue upstream, crossing the path of a major avalanche about a mile from the junction. The avalanche carried so much force on the descent of the west slope that it swept across the snow-covered floor of the canyon and knocked down trees on the east slope. Continue along the trail past a second avalanche swath and enter a forest of mature lodgepole pines. A 0.6-mile walk leads to a crossing of a perennial stream (tricky in early season). Beyond the crossing, the grade grows steeper as you continue climbing toward a windswept saddle at the head of the canyon. Whitebark pines and even late-season snow patches start to appear on the final push. The struggle eventually ends at the 10,240-foot saddle, where a view northward down the U-shaped canyon of the East Fork Carson River is a fine reward for the effort. You may notice a use trail going left (southwest) to Sonora Peak; ignore it to continue this trip.

From the saddle, the PCT leads southwest along Sonora Peak's northeast slopes, but you leave the PCT and descend cross-country, possibly on use trail, 0.3 mile south to campsites at the west edge of the grassy, frog-inhabited meadow harboring shallow, serene Wolf Creek Lake (10,090'; 11S 270857 4248798). A moderately steep descent leads to the lake, which pops into view after 200 yards. Continue down to the lake, which provides chilly swimming and no fish.

DAY 3 (Wolf Creek Lake to Sonora Pass, 5 miles): Retrace your steps from the lake to the saddle and head south on the PCT. Winding among fractured granite blocks, reach a steep, conspicuous ramp, which the trail is forced to climb without the aid of switchbacks. To add to the difficulty, snow patches can obscure parts of this climb well into August. Emerging from the climb, encounter a couple of rivulets on a slope covered with wind-cropped willows. Peakbaggers seeking to scale Sonora Peak, the highest peak between Hwy. 108 and Mt. Shasta far to the north, can leave the trail in this vicinity for a stiff but technically easy 1000-foot climb to the expansive vista atop the summit.

Granitic bedrock gives way to volcanic rocks and talus on a traverse south along the east slopes of Sonora Peak. Dwarf whitebark pines, reduced to the height of shrubs by winter's freezing winds, are common along this easy stretch of trail.

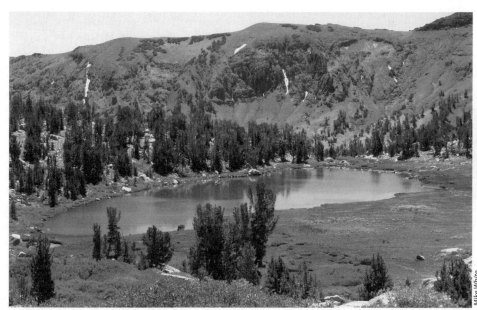

Mike White

The Wolf Creek Lake near Sonora Pass

THE SIGHTS HERE

To the east, the effects of glaciation are evident in the canyon of Wolf Creek (not the Wolf Creek near this trip's start but the outlet stream of the Wolf Creek Lake where you spent last night). You may see camouflaged Marines on maneuvers from the nearby Mountain Warfare Training Center east of Sonora Pass. From the saddle southeast of Sonora Peak, the high peaks along the Yosemite border are visible on the southeast horizon.

The now well-graded trail winds in and out of bleak gullies before coming to the bleak tops of a conspicuous group of volcanic pinnacles that sit right on the Alpine County-Mono County line. A 30-yard scramble south to one of their summits permits a sweeping panorama. More gullies lie ahead as the trail descends west and goes a half mile to a ridge, where the trail doubles back eastward. You cross more gullies, typical of the eroded volcanic landscape, as the trail heads south along the crest. Several of these gullies have reliable water all year. The sunny slopes are covered with sagebrush, mule ears, creambush, and a smattering of lodgepole and whitebark pines. Clark's nutcrackers flap and caw overhead, while red-tailed hawks wheel and soar through the typically clear Sierra sky. A final, gentle descent leads to the PCT parking lot just north of Hwy. 108's Sonora Pass crossing.

27 Poison Lake

Trip Data: 11S 268627
4262383; 36.5 miles;
4/0 days

Topos: *Wolf Creek, Coleville, Disaster Peak, Lost Cannon Peak*

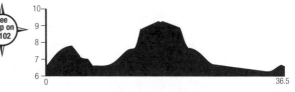

Highlights: Good fishing and swimming await hikers who backpack into Poison Lake, which isn't poisonous at all. Along the way they'll enjoy numerous panoramas of large, glaciated canyons and visit several carbonate and soda springs.

DAY 1 (High Trail Trailhead to Soda Springs, 9.5 miles): *(Recap: Trip 24, Day 1.)* From the trailhead, climb to the High Trail-East Fork Carson River Trail junction and turn right (south) onto the High Trail. Follow it over forested and volcanic terrain to the ford of East Fork Carson River (campsites nearby). Following the principal route rather than any alternate ones, ford here (may be dangerous in early season), pick up the High Trail again, and in 80 yards meet the East Fork Carson River Trail. Turn right (upstream) on it to a flat with three closely spaced Jeffrey pines. From between the west and south pines, go 200 yards southwest to ford the river again and then south along jeep tracks to yet another ford at the "bottom" (south) curve of a large meander. After fording, go about 250 yards south to an indistinct trail east-southeast and follow it another 250 yards to Poison Creek. Just beyond the creek's east bank is a path that leads south 300 yards to Soda Springs Administrative Site (6784'; 11S 268656 4265493). (From the three closely spaced Jeffrey pines, there's an alternate route that goes south and southeast from the south and east pines. This route lets you remain on the river's east side—with no river fords—to a signed junction with the Poison Flat Trail, on which you turn right, south, to the administrative site.) If you decide to camp here, there are a number of sites in the area, but camping is prohibited in the administrative site's immediate vicinity; read and follow all posted regulations.

DAY 2 (Soda Springs to Poison Lake, 8 miles): The topo and wilderness map are wrong; they show a trail from the administrative site that goes almost directly east up the river's east canyon wall toward the Soda Cone, but this trail doesn't exist. So, from the campsites at Soda Springs Administrative Site, head north and retrace your steps a quarter mile to the signed junction with the Poison Flat Trail. Take the right fork northward at the junction and follow the Poison Flat Trail as it hugs the east edge of Dumonts Meadows and then begins to climb the river canyon's east wall. The canyon's west wall looms impressively on this moderate-to-steep climb up a few switchbacks to a ridgetop. Atop the ridge, head east toward a small exfoliating dome that at first glance appears to resemble those of Yosemite but upon closer inspection seems to be volcanic in nature. The grade eases past the dome, and you pass the Soda Cone, which is about 100 yards away on the south bank of Poison Flat's creek.

SODA CONE

The Soda Cone is misnamed: A "soda [sodium bicarbonate] cone" it is not. It's largely a deposit of calcium carbonate, formed when underground water was heated by a nearby magma body and then rose to the surface bearing dissolved calcium. When the water reached the surface as a spring, the calciumå in the water reacted with carbonates to form calcium carbonate. (Around Mono Lake, this stuff is better known as tufa and forms the lake's famous tufa towers.) The calcium carbonate built this cone, and a spring still issues from its top. Besides calcium, this spring's water also contains dissolved arsenic and traces of uranium and manganese, making it a nasty and perhaps cattle-poisoning brew that may have given the name "Poison" to so many nearby features.

Beyond the Soda Cone, you soon enter Poison Flat's multilobed meadow (may be dry by late season in a dry year), where the trail's tread may occasionally fade out. Just keep going, and you'll shortly pick up the tread again. Cattle sometimes graze here. The trail traces the meadow's north side before angling across the meadow to its south side at a barely discernable rise. Beyond the rise, you continue along the meadow's south (or sometimes west) side to a signed junction with the Silver King Trail. On your left, the northeast-bound Silver King Trail's tread may be invisible under the meadow's mud. You continue ahead (southeast) on the joined Poison Flat and Silver King trails. At the meadow's east end, you pass through a barbed-wire stock gate (may be down by late season) and an aspen grove, climbing over a steep little ridge and dropping to a signed junction with the Poison Lake Trail near another stock gate. Silver King Creek is 100 yards ahead on the left fork here (the Silver King Trail) if you need water, and you may find a legal campsite there if you need to stop for the day. Otherwise, you make a hard right turn onto the southwest-bound trail to Poison Lake.

The trail to Poison Lake begins steeply and then eases on a climb up to a ridgecrest, remaining on the ridge for the next mile. At the end of the ridge, near the base of a steep slope, climb steeply southwest to a minor ridge that provides a major, sweeping view of rounded hills in the north, granitic cliffs in the east, Silver King Canyon in the south, and the ragged Sierra Crest in the southwest. From the ridge, the trail continues to climb through thick brush. Soon, short, very steep switchbacks lead up into forest shade once again as the gradient becomes pleasant.

Another climb leads to a small, rocky flat densely covered with sagebrush and bitterbrush. At the south end of the flat is a good view up the canyon into Lower Fish Valley, Upper Fish Valley, and Fourmile Canyon. From the flat, the trail makes an undulating traverse west toward a small canyon, nearly reaching its top. Here, the trail turns northwest and goes past several meadows before leveling off on a broad ridge above Poison Lake. A short, steep descent down this ridge leads to the lake's willow-clad south shore (9176'; 11S 268627 4262383). Good campsites lie beneath lodgepole pines and hemlocks on the northwest shore. Fishing may be good for brook trout.

HWY 4

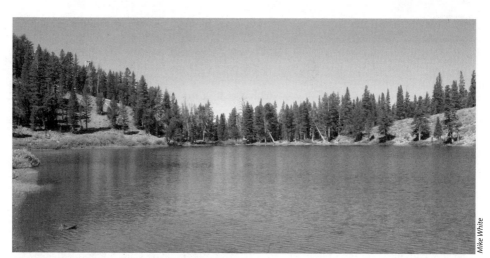
Mike White

Poison Lake is lovely and not poisonous at all.

DAY 3 (Poison Lake to Soda Springs, 8 miles): Retrace your steps of Day 2 to Soda Springs (6784'; 11S 268656 4265493).

Day 4 (Soda Springs to High Trail Trailhead, 11 miles): This is the loop part of your trip; optionally, you could forgo the loop and retrace your steps of Day 1 to the High Trail Trailhead.

(Recap: Trip 24, Day 2.) Otherwise, retrace your steps down-canyon 2.75 miles north to the signed High Trail junction. From the junction, don't take the High Trail left to the ford. Instead, go right (northeast) on a jeep road and around an open flat. In 0.4 mile from the junction, ford East Fork Carson River (this is as difficult as the High Trail ford). Pick up the road and go northeast across a flat and past a meander that nearly cuts the flat in two. Make a traverse across an equally long flat to the East Fork Carson River a mile below the High Trail junction. Look for two large Jeffrey pines just to the north, between which a barbed-wire gate marks the start of a trail.

From the gate, this trail remains on the west side of the East Fork Carson River, paralleling it before veering away over a couple of long moraines and then crossing a seasonal rivulet. The trail then parallels the river to a junction with some jeep tracks. Follow the jeep tracks north almost a half mile to the crest of a rocky moraine and a barbed-wire fence across the tracks. Leave the tracks and follow the fence west (left) about 300 yards to a gate, descend to a gorge, and follow the west side of the river through the gorge for 2.5 miles. At low water, usually after Labor Day, you can walk along the river's edge; otherwise, you must climb above the river at times. Campsites are plentiful here, but the best ones are on the opposite bank. Your west-bank route ends where it meets the East Fork Carson River Trail, which fords the East Fork Carson River at Gray's Crossing, directly west of a low gap. You go left (west) here to stay on the west side.

From this junction, the East Fork Carson River Trail heads west, climbs above the river, passes through a gate, and curves west into Railroad Canyon. Hike up this canyon and cross its stream (last reliable water). From here, climb north out of the canyon, circle the edge of some *aa*, and then traverse 0.3 mile northwest to the south tip of shallow Wolf Creek Lake (not the one near Sonora Peak). From the lake, climb west up to the base of steep volcanic slopes, ascends a ridge to a junction with the High Trail coming in on the left, go ahead (west) on the joined trails to a saddle, and descend steeply to the trailhead (6406'; 11S 266210, 4275931 (field)).

STATE HIGHWAY 108 TRIPS

South of Hwy. 108 and west of Sonora Pass, lake-filled Emigrant Wilderness unfolds southward toward northern Yosemite National Park. Except for Emigrant Wilderness's lack of high granite peaks, the scenery is hard to beat anywhere in the Sierra. We explore this wilderness from trailheads that are, from west to east, Crabtree Camp, Gianelli Cabin, and Kennedy Meadow. From the Crabtree Camp Trailhead on the western edge of Emigrant Wilderness, we offer two journeys to some of the wilderness's more delightful spots. The Gianelli Cabin Trailhead, also on Emigrant Wilderness's west side, is a gateway to many of the wilderness's most beautiful and dramatic spots, and we present five exciting trips from there. From the Kennedy Meadow Trailhead, major trails lead into Emigrant Wilderness as well as into northern Yosemite National Park. The TYT continues its course through here, from Kennedy Meadow through Emigrant Wilderness and northern Yosemite to its end at Tuolumne Meadows.

Also south of Hwy. 108 and east of Sonora Pass, we visit the beautiful proposed Hoover Wilderness Additions from Leavitt Meadows Trailhead, a gateway to a string of subalpine lakes set like jewels in a long bracelet of handsome peaks.

North of Hwy. 108 lies Carson-Iceberg Wilderness. Section 5 of the TYT starts from the Iceberg Meadow Trailhead and explores some of Carson-Iceberg Wilderness's most remote and beautiful country. In terms of west-to-east order on Hwy. 108, the Iceberg Meadow Trailhead lies between the Gianelli Cabin and Kennedy Meadow trailheads.

TRAILHEADS: Crabtree Camp
Gianelli Cabin
Iceberg Meadow
Kennedy Meadow
Leavitt Meadows

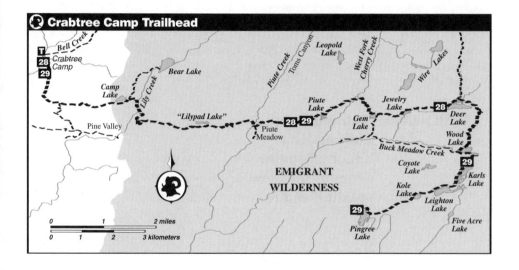

Crabtree Camp Trailhead

7153'; 11S 245407 4229620

DESTINATION/ UTM COORDINATES	TRIP TYPE	BEST SEASON	PACE (HIKING/ LAYOVER DAYS)	TOTAL MILEAGE
28 Deer Lake 11S 257676 4227795	Out & back	Mid or late	4/2 Leisurely	22.6
29 Pingree Lake 11S 254940 4224516	Out & back	Mid or late	6/2 Moderate, part cross-country	35.6

Information and Permits: Emigrant Wilderness is in Stanislaus National Forest, and wilderness permits are required, but there are no quotas. For permit reservations, contact Stanislaus National Forest: Supervisor's Office, 19777 Greenley Road, Sonora, CA 95370; 209-532-3671; www.fs.fed.us/r5/stanislaus/visitor/emigrant.shtml. For on-demand permits, visit the Summit Ranger District: #1 Pinecrest Lake Road, Pinecrest, CA 95364; 209-965-3434. Bear canisters and stoves are strongly recommended. No campfires above 9000 feet, and no campfires within a half mile of Emigrant Lake. One-night camping limit per trip at the following lakes: Bear, Camp, Grouse, Powell, and Waterhouse.

Driving Directions: From the west, from the junction of highways 108 and 120 west of Sonora, go 33.5 miles northeast on Hwy. 108 to Cold Springs (east of Long Barn, west of the Pinecrest Y). Continue 1.2 miles east of Cold Springs and turn right on signed Crabtree Road. Or, from the east, drive west on Hwy. 108 over Sonora Pass to the Pinecrest Y. Continue about 2 miles more to signed Crabtree Road, onto which you turn left. From this turnoff, follow this paved road 6.8 miles (do not turn onto the road to the Dodge Ridge Ski Area) to a junction just before a pack station. Go straight ahead onto dirt road and drive 2.6 miles to a junction. Go right and then ahead 0.7 miles to the trailhead parking lot beside Bell Creek.

28 Deer Lake

Trip Data: 11S 257676 4227795; 22.6 miles; 4/2 days

Topos: *Pinecrest, Cooper Peak*

Highlights: Not only is fishing and swimming good at Deer Lake itself, a basecamp at Deer Lake offers access to dozens of other fishable and swimmable lakes within a 2-mile radius.

DAY 1 (Crabtree Camp Trailhead to Lilypad Lake, 5.1 miles): Leaving the Crabtree Camp Trailhead going south, you hop Bell Creek and quickly come to a junction with the Chewing Gum Lake Trail (shown on the *Emigrant Wilderness* map but not on the 7.5' topo) to your left (north). Your route continues ahead (south) and curves east on a moderate ascent to a junction with a lateral trail to the right (south) to Pine Valley. Continue ahead (east) from this junction.

You next pass the Emigrant Wilderness boundary and in 400 yards reach the west end of shallow, green Camp Lake (7590'), where camping is poor and swimming is invigorating. At a saddle just past Camp Lake, the trail to popular Bear Lake takes off to the left (north); you go ahead (northeast).

The trail soon curves south to an easy ford of Lily Creek, where there are mosquito-plagued campsites just west of the stream. Beyond the ford, switchbacks lead to a lengthy traverse that passes through meadows south of black-streaked granite outcrops, and you soon reach long, narrow "Lilypad Lake" (7856'; 11S 250121 4227345), not named on the 7.5'

HWY 108

topo or on the wilderness map and much larger than it appears on either map. The water is covered with Indian pond lilies and still supports a noisy population of yellow-legged frogs. There is good camping to the south, above the trail.

DAY 2 (Lilypad Lake to Deer Lake, 6.2 miles): After a short climb east of Lilypad Lake, you reach a point overlooking large Piute Meadow in the east, dome-guarded Toms Canyon in the north, Groundhog Meadow below in the southeast, and, on the far eastern horizon, Bigelow Peak and the jutting prominence of Tower Peak.

Keeping to the trees south of the willowed west arm of Piute Meadow, the route passes a small campsite; then, where the route crosses Piute Creek, many unpleasant campsites lie among the trees just to the north. This rest stop is heavily used by packers and stock. Only yards after Piute Creek, the unsigned Groundhog Meadow spur trail comes in from the right (south); you continue ahead, eastward.

Now a slog brings you to tiny, 2-acre Piute Lake (7865') and the good campsites on its north side. From Piute Lake onward (east) on this route, you can choose among many beautiful lakes and campsites.

From Piute Lake, the trail drops to ford West Fork Cherry Creek and then steeply ascends a rocky, washed-out section to an overlook just above Gem Lake (8224'). There is limited camping to the north and a few sites on the lake's south side. Just after rounding Gem Lake, ignore a lateral right (south) to Buck Meadow Creek. Your route continues straight ahead (east), and then climbs and skirts the north side of the meadow fringes surrounding Jewelry Lake (8399'). Camping is very poor, but fishing for rainbow is fair to good in the lake and the lagoons around the inlet.

From the east end of Jewelry Lake, it is a short mile to the excellent campsites on the north side of Deer Lake (8482'; 11S 257676 4227795), where there is a junction with one trail north to the Wire Lakes turnoff and the Gianelli Cabin Trailhead, and another trail heading east to the Buck Lakes and, eventually, to Huckleberry Lake. Swimming at Deer Lake is delightful, and fishing for nice-sized rainbow is good to great on both the lake and the inlet stream.

DAYS 3 and 4 (Deer Lake to Crabtree Camp Trailhead, 11.3 miles): Retrace your steps.

29 Pingree Lake

Trip Data: 11S 254940
4224516; 35.6 miles;
6/2 days

Topos: *Pinecrest, Cooper Peak*

Highlights: This trip visits some of Emigrant Wilderness's most beautiful lakes, which differ in character from granitic, dramatic, isolated Kole Lake, barely nestled in a mountain summit, to the densely forested, popular Pingree Lake. Incomparable beauty is found at every step.

HEADS UP! *The cross-country route between Karls and Pingree lakes is not difficult but requires navigational and scrambling skills and is not recommended for beginners.*

DAY 1 (Crabtree Camp Trailhead to Lilypad Lake, 5.1 miles): *(Recap: Trip 28, Day 1.)* Leaving the trailhead going south, hop Bell Creek and quickly come to a junction with the Chewing Gum Lake Trail (shown on the *Emigrant Wilderness* map but not on the 7.5' topo) to your left (north). Continue ahead (south) and curve east to a junction with a lateral trail to the right (south) to Pine Valley. Continue ahead (east) from this junction.

Pass the Emigrant Wilderness boundary and in 400 yards reach Camp Lake (7590'), where camping is poor. At a saddle just past Camp Lake, the trail to Bear Lake goes left (north); you go ahead (east).

The trail soon curves south to a ford of Lily Creek. Beyond the ford, switchbacks lead to a lengthy traverse through meadows, and you soon reach "Lilypad Lake" (7856'; 11S 250121 4227345), not named on the 7.5' topo or on the wilderness map and much larger than it appears on either map. There is good camping to the south, above the trail.

DAY 2 (Lilypad Lake to Deer Lake, 6.2 miles): *(Recap: Trip 28, Day 2.)* After a short climb east of Lilypad Lake, you reach an overlook where views include Piute Meadow. Keeping to the trees south of the west arm of Piute Meadow, the route passes a small campsite and presently fords Piute Creek. Only yards after Piute Creek, the unsigned Groundhog Meadow spur trail comes in from the right (south); you continue ahead, eastward.

Slog to tiny, 2-acre Piute Lake (7865'; good campsites on its north side). From Piute Lake onward (east) on this route, you can choose among many beautiful lakes and campsites.

From Piute Lake, ford West Fork Cherry Creek and then steeply ascend to an overlook above Gem Lake (8224'; limited camping). Just after rounding Gem Lake, ignore a lateral right (south) to Buck Meadow Creek. Your route continues straight ahead (east), and then climbs and skirts the north side of the meadow around Jewelry Lake (8399'; very poor camping but fair-to-good fishing).

From the east end of Jewelry Lake, it is a mile to the excellent campsites on the north side of Deer Lake (8482'; 11S 257676 4227795), where there is a junction with one trail north to the Wire Lakes turnoff and the Gianelli Cabin Trailhead, and with another trail heading east to the Buck Lakes. Fishing for nice-sized rainbow is good to great on both the lake and the inlet stream.

DAY 3 (Deer Lake to Pingree Lake, 6.5 miles, part cross-country): From the junction on Deer Lake's north shore, go east toward the Buck Lakes for about a half mile to another junction, where you turn right (south) toward Wood Lake and soon begin a descent.

You pass a small tarn on the right and cross several small streams(often dry at summer's end). Most of the descent is gentle, with several brief stretches of steep switchbacks. The final approach to Wood Lake (8270') is through a meadow, across which the heavily wooded lake is tantalizingly visible. The trail branches in this meadow: The left branch leads to good camping at Wood Lake, but you bear right (southwest). At first severely eroded, this trail crosses a low shoulder and then travels along the north shore of Wood Lake on a high, smooth granite slab with good views. The trail then drops, crosses the outlet stream, and goes downstream (west) a short distance to a junction with the Buck Meadow Creek Trail.

At this junction, you turn left (east), passing good camping at the west end of Wood Lake, and then travel along the south shore. Just east of the point where the shores compress the waters to a narrow neck, you reach the signed junction with the lateral south to Karls Lake. Turn right (south) at this junction and ascend a short, steep saddle. Next, you make a moderate descent over granite slabs (the trail is often indistinct) and re-enter a forest cover with a floor of corn lilies. After passing a packer camp, you find excellent camping along the very beautiful and irregular northwest shore of Karls Lake (8290'); there's even better camping at the narrows halfway along the lake's northwest side. There are many more granite islands than appear on the topo, and the entire lake is bordered with lodgepoles, also contrary to the topo.

From the northwest shore of Karls Lake, your route, now cross-country, soon becomes indistinct as you cross the scant quarter mile separating Karls Lake from the northernmost tip of Leighton Lake (8280'), an eerily beautiful wasteland of dead trees where there is no camping. In mid to late season, when the water level is low, the best route around Leighton

Lake is along the north side at the water's edge—you will have to leapfrog across dead trees. In early season, you will need to go a bit higher over huge granite boulders. There is no visible trail either way.

To leave the lake, go to its extreme western tip and then ascend west directly up the easy granite slabs. Be sure to look back into the lake basin during the climb to observe the cracks in these slabs, which are filled with seedling lodgepoles that are slowly breaking up the mountainside. Avoid the obvious lower saddle to the southwest and aim slightly north to the saddle just northeast of Kole Lake.

VIEWS

If you hanker for dramatic vistas, take a brief stroll up to the knob a half mile southwest of Kole Lake. There is nothing higher than this point west all the way to the Pacific Ocean, and you can also see the entire western end of Emigrant Wilderness, much of Yosemite to the south, and as far beyond as the atmosphere permits.

Kole Lake (8384') is unusual in that you ascend to the lake: It lies in a small hollow in a crest. Its shores are gently forested in lodgepole and carpeted with ferns and wildflowers. Granite slabs lead into the water, inviting you in for a swim. Wonderful, unused camping is available on all sides of the lake.

The 1.5-mile cross-country route from Kole Lake to Pingree Lake starts with a rapid descent down the granite slabs at the west end of Kole Lake and then levels out as it crosses gigantic slabs laced with streams. Stay to the north side of this flat, relatively close to the underside of the cliff to the north. The final part of the descent is over irregular but easy terrain. A use trail appears in the meadows bordering the east side of Pingree Lake (8162'; 11S 254940 4224516) and continues around the north side. Superb camping surrounds the lake. The shore of this large lake is very irregular, offering privacy for a swim, and the many granite islands tempt sunbathers.

DAYS 4–6 (Pingree Lake to Crabtree Camp Trailhead, 17.8 miles): Retrace your steps.

Gianelli Cabin Trailhead

8577'; 11S 247546 4231633

DESTINATION/ UTM COORDINATES	TRIP TYPE	BEST SEASON	PACE (HIKING/ LAYOVER DAYS)	TOTAL MILEAGE
30 Y Meadow Lake 11S 252587 3241363	Out & back	Mid or late	2/0 Leisurely	10
31 Wire Lakes 11S 257312 4229635	Out & back	Mid or late	4/1 Leisurely	24.8
32 Crabtree Camp Trailhead 11S 245407 4229620	Shuttle	Mid or late	4/1 Moderate, cross-country option	25.9
33 Kennedy Meadow 11S 292581 4194990	Shuttle	Mid or late	5/2 Leisurely	33.3

Information and Permits: Emigrant Wilderness is in the Stanislaus National Forest, and wilderness permits are required, but there are no quotas. For permit reservations, contact Stanislaus National Forest: Supervisor's Office, 19777 Greenley Road, Sonora, CA 95370; 209-532-3671; www.fs.fed.us/r5/stanislaus/visitor/emigrant.shtml. For on-demand permits, visit the Summit Ranger District, #1 Pinecrest Lake Road, Pinecrest, CA 95364; 209-965-3434. Bear canisters and stoves are strongly recommended. No campfires above 9000 feet, and no campfires within a half mile of Emigrant Lake. One-night camping limit per trip at the following lakes: Bear, Camp, Grouse, Powell, and Waterhouse.

Driving Directions: From the west, from the junction of highways 108 and 120 west of Sonora, go 33.5 miles northeast on Hwy. 108 to Cold Springs (east of Long Barn, west of the Pinecrest Y). Continue 1.2 miles east of Cold Springs and turn right on signed Crabtree Road. Or, from the east, drive west on Hwy. 108 over Sonora Pass to the Pinecrest Y. Continue about 2 miles to the signed Crabtree Road and turn left. Follow that paved road 6.8 miles (do not turn onto the road to the Dodge Ridge Ski Area) to a junction just before a pack station. Go straight ahead onto dirt road and drive 2.6 miles to a junction. Here, turn left and go about 4 miles to a T-junction with a dirt road to Dodge Ridge Ski Area. Turn right and go a short distance to the trailhead at the site of Gianelli Cabin.

30 Y Meadow Lake

Trip Data: 11S 252587 3241363; 10 miles; 2/0 days

Topos: *Pinecrest, Cooper Peak*

see map on p.122

Highlights: This beautiful route parallels a segment of the historic Emigrant Trail. En route to Y Meadow Lake, anglers can try their luck on two small but fairly productive lakes. Early-trip views from Burst Rock are panoramic.

HEADS UP! *Y Meadow Lake as such doesn't appear on the topo or the wilderness map; look for the lake above labeled "Y Meadow Dam."*

DAY 1 (Gianelli Cabin Trailhead to Y Meadow Lake, 5 miles): The trail begins northeastward in a meadow and soon ascends a steep slope covered with red fir and lodgepole and western white pine. After the first mile, the trail follows the mountain spine, and you can look down a thousand feet into the valley below, and perhaps see the remains of a shattered pioneer wagon. The trail tops the ridge at Burst Rock (9161'), a landmark for the old Emigrant Trail, and crosses the Emigrant Wilderness boundary; this vantage point offers excellent views to the north of Liberty Hill, Elephant Rock, the Dardanelles, Castle Rock, and the Three Chimneys. You can see as far as Mt. Lyell on the southeast border of Yosemite Park.

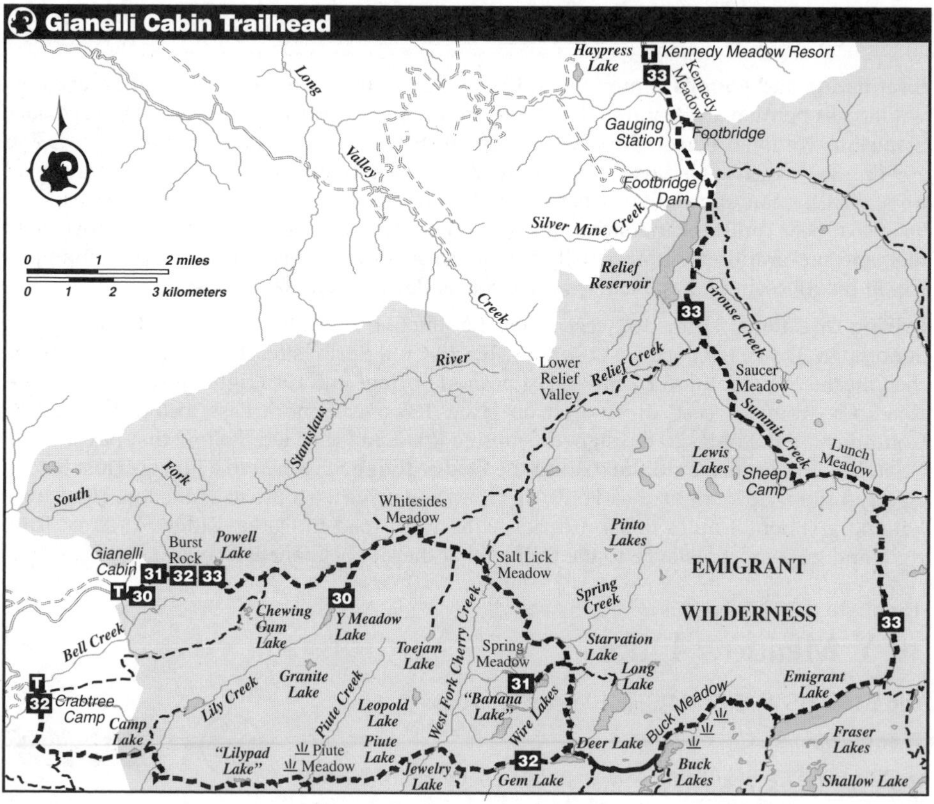

Gianelli Cabin Trailhead

Haypress Lake
Kennedy Meadow Resort
33
Kennedy Meadow
Gauging Station
Footbridge
Footbridge Dam
Silver Mine Creek
Relief Reservoir
33
Grouse Creek
Saucer Meadow
Summit Creek
Lewis Lakes
Lunch Meadow
Sheep Camp
Lower Relief Valley
Relief Creek
River
Stanislaus
Fork
South
Whitesides Meadow
Salt Lick Meadow
Pinto Lakes
EMIGRANT
Spring Creek
WILDERNESS
Gianelli Cabin
Burst Rock
Powell Lake
31 32 33
30
Chewing Gum Lake
Y Meadow Lake
30
Toejam Lake
Spring Meadow
Starvation Lake
Long Lake
Buck Meadow
Emigrant Lake
33
Bell Creek
Lily Creek
Granite Lake
Piute Creek
Leopold Lake
West Fork Cherry Creek
31
Spring Meadow
"Banana Lake"
Wire Lakes
Deer Lake
Buck Lakes
Fraser Lakes
32
Crabtree Camp
Camp Lake
"Lilypad Lake"
Piute Meadow
Piute Lake
Jewelry Lake
32
Gem Lake
Buck Lakes
Shallow Lake

Long Valley Creek

0   1   2 miles
0 1 2 3 kilometers

As the trail bears east along the ridge, you also have excellent views of the Stanislaus River watershed to the north and the Tuolumne River watershed to the south.

> **ABOUT GIANELLI CABIN**
>
> Gianelli Cabin is a hunting cabin dating back to 1905, according to Peter Browning's *Place Names of the Sierra Nevada*. Now, only part of the log cabin's base remains. As an Italian name, Gianelli is pronounced "jah-NEL-lee."

The trail descends gradually to a low saddle overlooking granitic Powell Lake (excellent camping). This small lake offers fishing for brook trout in early and late season, and the fine views to the northeast make this an attractive spot for a lunch break.

Your route then crosses a small ridge, descends through a forest of lodgepole, fir, and mountain hemlock, and arrives at the open stretches of meadowy Lake Valley, which offers a spectacular display of flowers even in late season. A faint fisherman's trail (0.7 mile) to Chewing Gum Lake turns right (south) through the meadow. Your trail continues ahead (generally east) from this junction.

From Lake Valley, it is 1.5 miles across another broad ridge to the turnoff to Y Meadow Lake. Here the route turns right (south) for a winding mile to the fair campsites at the north end of Y Meadow Lake (8602'; 11S 252587 4231363). The lake doesn't support fish due to fluctuating water levels; however, hikers comfortable with cross-country walking can head south 0.7 mile from Y Meadow Lake to the good fishing for brook at Granite Lake (poor-to-fair campsites).

DAY 2 (Y Meadow Lake to Gianelli Cabin Trailhead, 5 miles): Retrace your steps.

31 Wire Lakes

Trip Data: 11S 257312 4229635; 24.8 miles; 4/1 days

Topos: *Pinecrest, Cooper Peak*

Highlights: The Wire Lakes are a stepladder set of three memorable mountain lakes offering excellent angling and opportunities for secluded camping. Their location in the heart of the Emigrant Wilderness means you can dayhike to many other lakes.

DAY 1 (Gianelli Cabin Trailhead to Y Meadow Lake, 5 miles): *(Recap: Trip 30, Day 1.)* The trail begins northeastward in a meadow and soon ascends a steep slope. After the first mile, the trail follows the mountain spine. The trail tops the ridge at Burst Rock (9161') and crosses the Emigrant Wilderness boundary going generally east. The trail descends to a low saddle overlooking granitic Powell Lake and then crosses a small ridge, descends through forest, and arrives at Lake Valley. Where a faint fisherman's trail turns right (south) to Chewing Gum Lake, your trail continues ahead (generally east). Another 1.5 miles across another broad ridge brings you to the turnoff right (south) for 1 mile to Y Meadow Lake (8602'; 11S 252587 4231363).

DAY 2 (Y Meadow Lake to Upper Wire Lake, 7.4 miles): First, retrace your steps from Y Meadow Lake to the last trail junction. Here, your route turns right (northeast) toward very large Whitesides Meadow, where you may find grazing cattle. At the north end of this meadow, several aspens bear the etched names of pioneers who were buried here.

At a junction with the Eagle Pass Trail (left, west) your trail continues ahead (northeast), ascending a moderately timbered slope through astonishing wildflowers at

Whitesides Meadow's northeast end. On this ascent, the path meets a junction with a trail left (northeast) to Upper Relief Valley and Kennedy Meadow; you go ahead (east) as your trail begins a long curve generally southward. Soon your trail meets an unsigned path right (south) to Toejam Lake; stay on the main route (ahead/southeast) to another junction with a trail left (north) to Upper Relief Valley. Your trail turns right (south) here and presently dips to ford West Fork Cherry Creek (sometimes dry in late season) at Salt Lick Meadow (8520').

From here, the trail climbs to a tarn-dotted bench and then descends past several picturesque tarns southeast and then south to Spring Meadow. Tiny lakes sprinkle the green expanse of the meadow, and early- to midseason hikers will find lupine, paintbrush, and buttercup. Fishing for brook trout is fair to good along the tributary (Spring Creek) flowing through Post Corral Canyon.

A short mile farther southeast and south, you find a signed junction where you turn right (west and southwest) on a lateral and wind the remaining 0.4 mile along a ridge, past trees blasted by a lightning strike, to excellent campsites on the northwest side of Upper Wire Lake (8846'; 11S 257312 4229635). More isolated sites are on the east side, and there are equally good sites at "Banana Lake" (Middle Wire Lake), 0.3 miles southwest cross-country. Fishing on the Wire Lakes is good to excellent (with a midseason slowdown) for brook. The Wire Lakes make idyllic basecamps for exploring the many lakes nearby.

DAYS 3 and 4 (Wire Lakes to Gianelli Cabin Trailhead, 12.4 miles): Retrace your steps.

32 Crabtree Camp Trailhead

Trip Data: 11S 245407 4229620; 25.9 miles; 4/1 days

Topos: *Pinecrest, Cooper Peak*

Highlights: This route is popular with anglers, naturalists, photographers, and hikers alike. High, cold-water lakes and streams vie with deep fir forests and alpine meadows for visitors' attention, and the shortness of the shuttle for this trip almost makes it a loop.

Shuttle Directions: To access the take-out trailhead at Crabtree Camp from the west, from the junction of state highways 108 and 120 west of Sonora, go 33.5 miles northeast on Hwy. 108 to Cold Springs (east of Long Barn, west of the Pinecrest Y). Continue 1.2 miles east of Cold Springs and turn right on signed Crabtree Road. Or, from the east, drive west on Hwy. 108 over Sonora Pass to the Pinecrest Y. Continue about 2 miles more to the signed Crabtree Road and turn left. Follow this paved road 6.8 miles (do not turn onto the road to the Dodge Ridge Ski Area) to a junction just before a pack station. Go straight ahead onto dirt road for 2.6 miles to a junction. Go right and then ahead 0.7 miles to the trailhead parking lot beside Bell Creek.

Day 1 (Gianelli Cabin Trailhead to Y Meadow Lake, 5 miles): *(Recap: Trip 30, Day 1.)* The trail begins northeastward in a meadow and soon ascends a steep slope. After the first mile, the trail follows the mountain spine. The trail tops the ridge at Burst Rock (9161') and crosses the Emigrant Wilderness boundary going generally east. The trail descends to a low saddle overlooking granitic Powell Lake and then crosses a small ridge, descends through forest, and arrives at Lake Valley. Where a faint fisherman's trail turns right (south) to Chewing Gum Lake, your trail continues ahead (generally east). Another 1.5 miles across another broad ridge brings you to the turnoff right (south) for 1 mile to Y Meadow Lake (8602'; 11S 252587 4231363).

see map on p.122

HWY 108

Day 2 (Y Meadow Lake to Upper Wire Lake, 7.4 miles): *(Recap: Trip 31, Day 2.)* Return to the last trail junction and turn right (northeast) toward Whitesides Meadow, where you may find grazing cattle. At a junction with the Eagle Pass Trail (left, west), go ahead (northeast). Climb to a junction with a trail left (northeast) to Upper Relief Valley and Kennedy Meadow. Go ahead (east), curving generally southward. Soon your trail meets an unsigned path right (south) to Toejam Lake; go ahead (southeast) to another junction with a trail left (north) to Upper Relief Valley. Turn right (south) here and presently ford West Fork Cherry Creek at Salt Lick Meadow (8520').

From here, the trail climbs to a bench and then descends southeast and then south to Spring Meadow and then Post Corral Canyon. Farther southeast and south, you find a signed junction where you turn right (west and southwest) on a lateral 0.4 mile to excellent campsites on the northwest side of Upper Wire Lake (8846'; 11S 257312 4229635). Fishing on the Wire Lakes is good to excellent (with a mid-season slowdown) for brook.

DAY 3 (Upper Wire Lake to Piute Lake, 5.5 miles, optional cross-country route): From Upper Wire Lake, you can circle to Deer Lake by the longer trail route or descend through the Wire Lakes basin and go cross-country to the west end of Deer Lake.

The trail route: Retrace your steps to the junction with the main trail and turn right (south-southeast). Almost immediately, the route meets an unsigned lateral left (east) to Long Lake; your route continues ahead (south) toward Deer Lake. After a slight climb, the remaining distance to Deer Lake is a steady descent over a forested streamcourse that passes several small, unnamed lakes. On Deer Lake's north shore, you find a junction with a trail right (southeast) to the Buck Lakes and another left (southwest) to Jewelry Lake and the Crabtree Camp Trailhead.

The cross-country route: From Upper Wire Lake, head southwest to Banana Lake (Middle Wire Lake), where all semblance of trail vanishes. The easiest descent from here is to take the clear route through the meadowed area east of Banana Lake and then descend via the usually dry streamcourse to reach the Jewelry Lake/Deer Lake Trail about 0.3 mile west of Deer Lake.

With the routes rejoined, turn left (southwest) on the trail. The trail from Deer Lake to Jewelry Lake is a half-mile rocky descent westward to Jewelry Lake (poor camping; fair-to-good fishing for rainbow on the inlet's lagoons). Crossing the inlet stream, the route descends to warm little Gem Lake (8224'), where you ignore a lateral left (south) to Buck Meadow Creek and continue ahead, beginning a curve northwest. The trail descends steeply to a ford of West Fork Cherry Creek and then climbs to tiny Piute Lake (7873'; 11S 253781 4227559) with good campsites on its north side.

DAY 4 (Piute Lake to Crabtree Camp Trailhead, 8 miles): *(Recap in Reverse: Trip 28, Day 2, from Piute Lake through the trip's Day 1.)* After a long descent southwest and then west from Piute Lake, you avoid an unsigned lateral left (south) to Groundhog Meadow and continue ahead (west), soon fording Piute Creek to Piute Meadow. The trail stays in the trees on the meadow's south side before climbing to a viewpoint and then descending to Lilypad Lake (7856'; 11S 250121 4227345), perhaps your last chance for good camping but not quite 3 miles from Piute Lake.

Descend switchbacks to a ford of Lily Creek. Continue west to a saddle and a junction right (north) just before Camp Lake (7590'); continue ahead (west) on your main trail to Camp Lake (poor camping). Beyond Camp Lake, your trail presently avoids a lateral left

OPTION: CLOSING THE LOOP ON THE ROADS

Add a day, and you could close the loop by walking on the roads. Here you are at Crabtree Camp Trailhead, so it's left (west) 0.7 mile to a junction with the road to the Gianelli Cabin Trailhead, where you take a right (east and northeast) and head about 4 miles more to Gianelli Cabin. Hmm ... well, why not?

(south) to Pine Valley; continue ahead (west) here and soon curve north on a descent toward Crabtree Camp Trailhead. Just before the trailhead, you ford Bell Creek and bypass a spur right (east) to Chewing Gum Lake. In a few more steps northward, you're at the trailhead (7153'; 11S 245407 4229620), where your shuttle car or ride should be waiting.

33 Kennedy Meadow

Trip Data: 11S 292581 4194990; 33.3 miles; 5/2 days

Topos: *Pinecrest, Cooper Peak, Emigrant Lake, Sonora Pass*

see map on p.122

Highlights: This trip journeys through a cross-section of Emigrant Wilderness, touching some justly popular base-camping lakes, and from these points, you have access to the unusual and exciting surrounding country. Taken at a leisurely pace, this trip is one of the best possible weeklong excursions in the region, and—surprise!—it isn't a copy of the Kennedy Meadow to Gianelli Cabin trip coming up later in this book.

Shuttle Directions: From Hwy. 108, the turnoff for the take-out location, Kennedy Meadow, is 27 miles east of the Pinecrest Y (the turnoff to Pinecrest Lake, south of Strawberry) and 9.1 miles west of Sonora Pass. Turn south on the signed spur road to Kennedy Meadows. A half mile down the road there is signed public parking, where you can leave your car. One mile down the road is Kennedy Meadows Resort (lodgings, café, saloon, store, pack station) and the trailhead (6400'), where you could spend a night at the end of this trip.

DAY 1 (Gianelli Cabin Trailhead to Y Meadow Lake, 5 miles): *(Recap: Trip 30, Day 1.)* The trail begins northeastward in a meadow and soon ascends a steep slope. After the first mile, the trail follows the mountain spine. The trail tops the ridge at Burst Rock (9161') and crosses the Emigrant Wilderness boundary going generally east. The trail descends to a low saddle overlooking granitic Powell Lake and then crosses a small ridge, descends through forest, and arrives at Lake Valley. Where a faint fisherman's trail turns right (south) to Chewing Gum Lake, your trail continues ahead (generally east). Another 1.5 miles across another broad ridge brings you to the turnoff right (south) for 1 mile to Y Meadow Lake (8602'; 11S 252587 4231363).

DAY 2 (Y Meadow Lake to Upper Wire Lake, 7.4 miles): *(Recap: Trip 31, Day 2.)* Return to the last trail junction and turn right (northeast) toward Whitesides Meadow, where you may find grazing cattle. At a junction with the Eagle Pass Trail (left, west), go ahead (northeast). Climb to a junction with a trail left (northeast) to Upper Relief Valley and Kennedy Meadow. Go ahead (east), curving generally southward. Soon your trail meets an unsigned path right (south) to Toejam Lake; go ahead (southeast) to another junction with a trail left (north) to Upper Relief Valley. Turn right (south) here and presently ford West Fork Cherry Creek at Salt Lick Meadow (8520').

From here, the trail climbs to a bench and then descends southeast and then south to Spring Meadow and then Post Corral Canyon. Farther southeast and south, you find a signed junction where you turn right (west and southwest) on a lateral 0.4 mile to excellent campsites on the northwest side of Upper Wire Lake (8846'; 11S 257312 4229635). Fishing on the Wire Lakes is good to excellent (with a mid-season slowdown) for brook.

DAY 3 (Upper Wire Lake to Emigrant Lake, 7.5 miles): *(Partial Recap: Trip 32, Day 3, trail route, as far as Deer Lake.)* Retrace your steps to the junction with the main trail and turn right (south-southeast). Almost immediately, the route meets an unsigned lateral left (east) to Long Lake; your route continues ahead (south) toward Deer Lake. After a slight climb, the remaining distance to Deer Lake is a steady descent. On Deer Lake's north shore, you find a junction with a trail right (southeast) to the Buck Lakes and another left (southwest) to Jewelry Lake.

Leaving the Day 3 route of Trip 32, turn right toward the Buck Lakes and head east. At a lateral to Wood Lake (right, south), your route continues ahead (generally east), crosses over a low, rocky ridge with several tarns, and then descends steeply to join the Emigrant Lake/Cow Meadow Lake Trail on the west shore of Buck Lakes. At this junction, your route turns left (northeast) along the west side of Upper Buck Lake and follows Buck Meadow Creek as it crosses the long meadow at the lake's north end.

The route then veers east, fords Buck Meadow Creek, and crosses the steep, low ridge separating the Emigrant Lake and Buck Lakes basins. At Emigrant Lake, there is a junction with an unmaintained path right (initially west) to North Fork Cherry Creek. Your trail turns left (east-northeast) to trace Emigrant Lake's long north shore to several good campsites near the inlet (8827'; 11S 264854 4229109). At 230 acres, Emigrant Lake is the largest lake in this wilderness and is a longtime favorite of anglers because of the good-to-excellent rainbow fishing in its deep waters. Those who prefer stream fishing will find the lagoons near the inlet exciting, but the fish are smaller.

DAY 4 (Emigrant Lake to Summit Creek, 6.6 miles): *(Recap in Reverse: Trip 37, Day 2.)* Resume your trip east-northeast along Emigrant Lake's inlet. Just before a ford of the inlet, there's a junction: right (south) to Blackbird Lake and left (north) to Mosquito Pass. You turn north to Mosquito Pass (not named on the 7.5' topo), climbing along a tributary to the inlet stream, and presently ford to the stream's east side. Ascending generally north and upstream, you eventually reach a long, 9300-foot saddle with fields of granite and tiny meadows through which your trail winds. Presumably, the high point of this is 9377–foot Mosquito Pass. On the saddle's north side, you descend to ford Summit Creek and reach a junction at the east end of Lunch Meadow: right (east) to Emigrant Meadow Lake; left (west) to Kennedy Meadow.

Turn left and stroll west through Lunch Meadow along Summit Creek. The trail presently crosses a pumice slope from which it descends a little to curve around the hardened camping area called Sheep Camp. Near Sheep Camp, your trail bends north-northwest. Beyond Sheep Camp, at a little saddle, you start a descent of 400 rocky feet. At the bottom, the grade eases and you walk under red firs along Summit Creek, descending gradually to good camping along the creek (8200–8300'; 11S 261707 4235645). Some sites are closed due to overuse; look for nicer ones uphill of the trail. Fishing is poor.

DAY 5 (Summit Creek to Kennedy Meadow, 6.8 miles): *(Recap in Reverse: Trip 35, Day 1.)* Continue downstream along Summit Creek and drop into wet little Saucer Meadow. Past the meadow, the trail drops steadily and steeply through brush-covered volcanic rubble above the creek. Soon after the grade eases, you meet a lateral left (northwest, then southwest) to Lower Relief Valley; go ahead (north-northwest) here. Descend rocky switchbacks, ford Grouse Creek, and begin a scenic traverse high above Relief Reservoir.

Beyond the reservoir, you pass a PG&E dam-maintenance station and then meet a trail to Kennedy Lake (right, northeast). Going ahead (northwest) on the main trail, you soon cross a footbridge and descend, passing some seasonally striking cascades. The descent becomes steep and rocky for a time but soon eases as it curves along the base of a granite dome to a junction. Here, go left (west-southwest) to cross Middle Fork Stanislaus River on a footbridge, skirt the east side of Kennedy Meadow on what shortly becomes an old dirt road, cross a small ridge, and walk the road under dense forest to the guest parking lot at Kennedy Meadows Resort (6400'; 11S 292581 4194990), where this trip ends.

Your ride may be waiting for you here, or you may need to pick up your shuttle car by walking through the resort and along the paved road to it for a half mile to backpackers' parking on the east side of the road (distance not included).

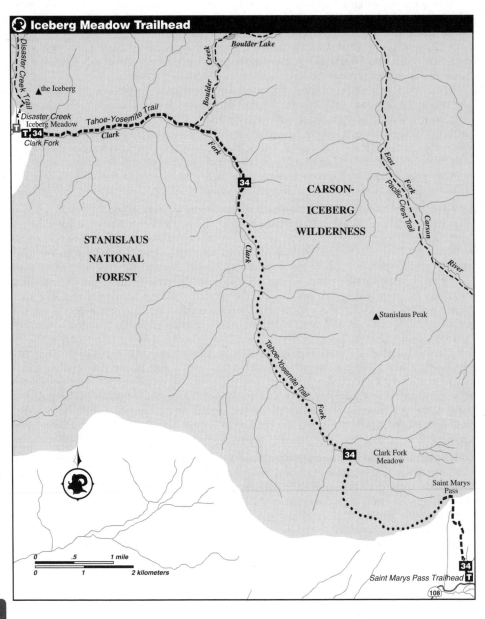

Iceberg Meadow Trailhead

Disaster Creek Trail
the Iceberg
Boulder Creek
Boulder Lake
Disaster Creek
Iceberg Meadow
Tahoe-Yosemite Trail
T 34
Clark Fork
Clark
34
East Fork
Pacific Crest Trail
CARSON-
ICEBERG
WILDERNESS
STANISLAUS
NATIONAL
FOREST
Clark
Fork
Carson
River
Stanislaus Peak
Tahoe-Yosemite Trail
Fork
34
Clark Fork
Meadow
Saint Marys
Pass
0   .5   1 mile
0   1   2 kilometers
34 T
Saint Marys Pass Trailhead
108

Iceberg Meadow Trailhead

6475'; 11S 259977 4255701

DESTINATION/ UTM COORDINATES	TRIP TYPE	BEST SEASON	PACE (HIKING/ LAYOVER DAYS)	TOTAL MILEAGE
34 Tahoe-Yosemite Trail Section 5: To Saint Marys Pass Trailhead 11S 268785 4246482	Shuttle	Mid to late	2/0 Strenuous, part cross-country	9.1 trail miles*

*Does not include the 3.7 road miles from the bridge over Arnot Creek at the beginning or the 9.6 road miles to Kennedy Meadow at the end.

Information and Permits: You must have a wilderness permit for overnight visits to this part of Carson-Iceberg Wilderness. TYT Section 5 is in Stanislaus National Forest: Summit Ranger District, #1 Pinecrest Lake Road, Pinecrest, CA 95364; 209-965-3434.

Driving Directions: The ill-signed turnoff from Hwy. 108 to paved Clark Fork Road lies 17.1 miles west of Sonora Pass, 20 miles east of the Pinecrest Y, and on the north side of the highway. Turn northeast here and follow this paved road for 9.2 miles to its end at Iceberg Meadow. Don't take any of the dirt roads that branch away from it. There's no parking lot; park off the road and on the shoulder as best you can. Through-hikers who are continuing from Section 4 should follow the trail directions below.

34 Tahoe-Yosemite Trail Section 5: To Saint Marys Pass Trailhead

Trip Data: 11S 268785 4246482; 9.1 trail miles, 2/0 days

Topos: *Disaster Peak, Sonora Pass*

Highlights: Your adventure begins as a stroll along lovely Clark Fork Stanislaus River, then turns into a cross-country scramble to the river's headwaters and beyond. From a view-rich granite rim high above the headwaters, you find an old trail down to Hwy. 108.

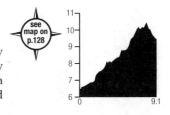

see map on p.128

HEADS UP! *If you begin your day at the end of Section 4, at the bridge where Clark Fork Road crosses Arnot Creek, turn east (face downstream above Arnot Creek and go to your left) on lightly traveled Clark Fork Road. Walk the road past Sand Flat Campground for 3.7 miles to the next section of foot trail at Iceberg Meadow, where the road ends. There is no footpath paralleling this segment. On the way, you bypass a trailhead for a northbound trail shortly before reaching Iceberg Meadow. This adds 3.7 miles to Day 1, below.*

Do not attempt this section unless you have good bouldering and navigation skills and the maps and compass or GPS unit to navigate with. The Carson-Iceberg Wilderness *map is wrong in this area: There is no real trail going all the way up to Clark Fork Meadow and Saint Marys Pass. With luck, you'll find some use trails and ducks, but don't count on it. Be prepared to correctly identify Sonora Peak in order to find Saint Marys Pass at the end of this section. Note also that the 7.5'* Disaster Peak *and* Sonora Peak *topos have 80-foot contour intervals instead of the usual 40-foot contour intervals.*

Shuttle Directions: The take-out trailhead at Saint Marys Pass is 1 mile west of Sonora Pass on Hwy. 108. Turn north onto this dirt road and follow it a short distance to the trailhead, where there's parking for a few cars.

DAY 1 (Iceberg Meadow Trailhead to Boulder Creek Ford, 4.7 miles): Whether you hiked the road or drove to this trailhead, at wet, flowery Iceberg Meadow beneath the towering lump of granite called the Iceberg, the TYT continues on the signed CLARK FORK TRAIL, which is on the right (south) side of the road as you face Iceberg Meadow. The duff trail is quite faint as you cross an unmapped trickle and soon curve between the meadow's fence and a creeklet. Heading east-northeast, you ford the creeklet and pass a trail sign just before zigzagging up into an area of large boulders where there's a nice viewpoint.

The trail then descends gradually to the north bank of Clark Fork Stanislaus River and continues east up the river, re-entering Carson-Iceberg Wilderness. The underfooting is alternately sand and duff beneath a moderate-to-dense cover of red and white firs and Jeffrey pines. The wet banks of tributaries host an abundant display of wildflowers, including columbine and monkeyflower. Alas, with the river on one side and steep slopes on the other side, the trail offers no legal campsites before it crosses Boulder Creek.

An easy 2.3 miles of hiking leads to an unsigned fork just before Boulder Creek flows into the river: left (northeast) up Boulder Creek to Boulder Lake, right (south) to Clark Fork Meadow. The left-hand route to Boulder Lake may seem the more heavily used. Nevertheless, you turn right on the TYT toward Clark Fork Meadow and ford Boulder Creek (steep banks; may be dangerous in early season). Leaving the ford, the route remains mostly within sight or sound of alder-and-willow-lined Clark Fork as it passes through a meadow that may be used for grazing and thus be full of cow pies and flies. Here a couple of poor campsites within sight of the trail and a couple of others in the alders nearer the river may lure campers.

From here, the trail curves south and ascends more and more steeply, climbing toward the highest point on the entire trail at Saint Marys Pass. Soon the grade becomes even steeper on rocky-dusty tread beside the cascading Clark Fork. An outcrop near a seasonal trickle offers a Spartan campsite beneath a juniper. Northbound hikers will experience their first views of the spectacular Dardanelles along this section of trail. Where the trail levels off, you find an unsigned fork and take the righthand branch. Beyond the junction, the trail passes a meadow near a stream boasting aspen, alder, willow, lodgepole, and cottonwood with some fair campsites, and a nighttime complement of foraging animals.

At a signed, almost streamside junction with the Seven Pines Trail, the right-hand fork crosses the Clark Fork, but the TYT continues ahead (south). The route grows increasingly faint through sloping meadows; the occasional duck helps you to stay on route, in spite of the appearance of multiple trails at times. Cows graze all over this slope, and some of the "trails" turn out to be merely cow paths. The goal in this section is to continue up the valley. The Carson-Iceberg Wilderness map is quite wrong here: There is no real trail coming down here from Saint Marys Pass.

Beyond the sloping meadows, the sandy trail veers east up an exposed, sage-dotted slope to the ford of a stream and then continues its ascent under a moderate forest cover of white and red firs, junipers, lodgepole pines, and western white pines. The route crosses seasonal tributary streams about every half mile, tributaries that drain the granite ridge that forms the Sierra Crest.

A long, gentle ascent leads to a ford of Clark Fork beside several fair-to-good campsites (8372'; 11S 265429 4250304). Just before these campsites, a trail branches left, but the TYT continues ahead.

DAY 2 (Clark Fork Ford to Saint Marys Pass Trailhead, 4.4 miles, part cross-country): After the ford, the ascent becomes moderate and then steep, winding among hemlocks, western white pines, and lodgepole pines, leaving the red firs behind. From here, the TYT is an ill-defined, unducked, very steep track that scrambles up slopes with granite outcroppings. The track leads to a small, lush meadow where you cross the stream and reach a campsite. Here, all semblance of a trail disappears, and the route continues southeast over boulders to Clark Fork Meadow. The "meadow" is now half forest and half grassland, almost encircled by steep walls of pine-and-hemlock-dotted granite. Above the granite, the upper basin is rimmed by reddish-brown and tan volcanic rocks, which are devoid of trees except for a few clumps of whitebark pine. A few poor campsites are spread around the meadow, which offers a superb display of mountain wildflowers in season. Clark Fork Meadow seems so remote that it's hard to imagine that there's a state highway just over the ridge. It's a good spot for a rest and for picking out Sonora Peak.

Hikers have created or found dozens of routes into (northbound) or out of (southbound) Clark Fork Meadow. The one described here is certainly not the only reasonable route, but it may be the easiest to follow. Beyond the head of the meadow, continue through forest, following a path of sorts near and north of the stream. Then, a few hundred feet after you cross a northeast-bank tributary, you find a split in the stream where it flows around either side of a little island after cascading down granite slabs. Cross to the east fork and turn directly uphill alongside the *other* fork, soon passing close under a granite cliff to the east of the route. (Warning: Don't follow ducks back to Clark Fork!)

For the first half mile, the occasionally ducked ascent is quite steep but mercifully shaded by moderate-to-dense hemlock forest. Where the slope decreases and the forest cover thins, begin to veer east onto a ridge dotted with whitebark pines. Remain on the ridge, resisting any temptation to drop into the region to the south, which is pleated with little gullies. The ridge gives way to granite terrain that bounds the Clark Fork drainage on the south; many of the outcroppings around here have a "billowy" appearance. From this vantage, Sonora Peak is undistinguished; a conical peak due north is far more striking. Over-the-shoulder views of the drainage you've ascended are quite astounding. An amazing display of seasonal alpine flowers huddles close to the windswept, decomposed granite "soil." If there were water here, hikers could find spectacular, albeit exposed, campsites.

Traverse high around the rim of this bowl, bypassing several false passes on the way east to Saint Marys Pass, a shallow saddle on the east of the first broad dome of reddish volcanic rock west of Sonora Peak. Saint Marys Pass (10,160+'), though bearing no sign with its name, is distinguished by a wilderness-related sign and a "star" of trails radiating from it. Only one of them heads downhill and south to the trailhead.

The trail south from Saint Marys Pass, though sometimes steep and loose, is easy to follow. It soon leads to an abandoned jeep road (shown as a trail on the topo map) that covers the last mile to Hwy. 108. The dirt road meets Hwy. 108 almost a mile west of Sonora Pass (9427'; 11S 268783 4246474 (field)).

IF YOU GET LOST

If you mistake a false pass for Saint Marys Pass and follow what turns out to be a use trail partway down one of the false passes west of it, as one of us did, all is not lost. The terrain is probably loose and strenuous but, with care, not all that dangerous. For one thing, you could climb back up and resume your walk toward Saint Marys Pass. Or, if you get too far down to climb back up and realize your error only when you find there's no real trail or jeep road, you can carefully work your way down to easier terrain and then work cross-country generally southeast (left-ish), angling toward the jeep road that descends from Saint Marys Pass. Turn right (south) when you meet it.

IF YOU'RE HIKING THE TYT SOUTH TO NORTH

Northbound hikers at Saint Marys Pass who are searching for where to begin the major descent to Clark Fork Meadow should make a lengthy westward traverse along the rim before veering north as soon as they have passed beyond the billowy granite outcroppings that line most of the route for the first mile or so from Saint Marys Pass. Here begins the little stream that flows down toward Clark Fork Meadow, and the northbound route follows the ridge that lies northeast of this stream's upper drainage basin. Then, near timberline, the use trail drops down to parallel the stream to Clark Fork Meadow.

CONTINUING TO TYT SECTION 6

You have just ended Section 5 of the TYT at the Saint Marys Pass Trailhead. The next trailhead, for Section 6 of the TYT, lies 9.6 road miles west and south at Kennedy Meadow (Kennedy Meadows Resort). There is no trail between these trailheads, only the highway and a spur road.

We strongly recommend that you get a ride between the Saint Marys Pass Trailhead and the trailhead at Kennedy Meadows Resort (or at least to the turnoff to the resort). Walking all the way down Hwy. 108 to the turnoff is dangerous: The highway is a steep, narrow, twisting road with inadequate shoulders.

If you have no choice but to continue on foot, or really *want* to continue on foot, we offer two choices: 1. Walk the 9.6 miles west and south down Hwy. 108 and then up the spur road to Kennedy Meadows Resort. 2. Walk 1 mile east and uphill to the PCT trailheads at Sonora Pass and follow the PCT southward for a while, bypassing the first two-and-a-half days of TYT Section 6. It would be a shame to miss those beautiful days on the TYT, but it would be an even bigger shame to get run over on Hwy. 108.

1. Optional route down Hwy. 108 and spur road to trailhead at Kennedy Meadow (9.6 miles): This is the longest stretch of roadside travel along the entire TYT. When you are walking on a road, try to walk facing oncoming traffic and assume that anyone operating a vehicle on that road is deaf, blind, and insane.

From the Saint Marys Pass Trailhead, turn right (west) on the highway, where a jagged crest of richly colored, dark volcanic rock on the south dominates the sparsely timbered high valley through which the road runs. Soon the highway makes a steep descent across the 9000-foot contour and then turns sharply right into a charming vale. Overnighters will find good campsites near Deadman Creek at several places in this high valley.

Beyond Chipmunk Flat, the road rises moderately as the creek descends, and soon the road is high above the cascading water. From a level stretch of road, a group of 10,000-foot peaks appears across the canyon of Middle Fork Stanislaus River. The road then descends gently under a sparse cover of young firs and Jeffrey pines, with a groundcover largely composed of manzanita and some sagebrush. Excellent views up the canyon of the Stanislaus reveal Granite Dome, which seems to stand athwart the canyon almost like a gigantic dam.

About 8.5 miles from where the roadside walk began, turn left (south) on a signed, paved road that passes two car-campgrounds as it rises gently for a mile past a backpackers' parking lot to Kennedy Meadows Resort (lodgings, café, store, saloon, pack station). At the far end of the resort, there is a parking lot where Section 6 of the TYT leaves "civilization," first as a closed dirt road and then as a footpath.

2. Optional Route up Hwy. 108 and south along the PCT: Take this alternative and rejoin the TYT's Section 6 partway through Day 3. Besides avoiding a long walk on Hwy. 108, this alternative avoids the loss of 3100 feet of hard-won elevation: Go left (east) from the turnoff to Saint Marys Pass Trailhead and walk along the highway for a mile to Sonora Pass and its PCT trailheads. Pick up the southbound PCT and then follow it south for 8.1 miles to a closed jeep road at a switchback. Here, you leave the PCT and follow that road south for 7.8 miles to meet the TYT at Grizzly Meadow.

Kennedy Meadow Trailhead

6400'; 11S 292581 4194990

DESTINATION/ UTM COORDINATES	TRIP TYPE	BEST SEASON	PACE (HIKING/ LAYOVER DAYS)	TOTAL MILEAGE
35 Summit Creek 11S 261707 4235645	Out & back	Early or mid	2/1 Leisurely	13.6
36 Emigrant Meadow Lake 11S 268152 4231050	Out & back	Mid or late	4/1 Leisurely	25.2
37 Emigrant Lake 11S 264854 4229109	Out & back	Mid or late	4/1 Leisurely	26.8
38 Cow Meadow Lake 11S 260404 4225352	Semiloop	Mid or late	7/2 Leisurely	46
39 Gianelli Cabin 11S 247573 4231605	Shuttle	Mid or late	7/3 Leisurely	43.1
40 Tahoe-Yosemite Trail Section 6: To Tuolumne Meadows 11S 292581 4194990	Shuttle	Mid or late	11/4 Moderate	71.3

Information and Permits: Emigrant Wilderness is in the Stanislaus National Forest, and wilderness permits are required, but there are no quotas. For permit reservations, contact Stanislaus National Forest: Supervisor's Office, 19777 Greenley Road, Sonora, CA 95370; 209-532-3671; www.fs.fed.us/r5/stanislaus/visitor/emigrant.shtml. For on-demand permits, visit the Summit Ranger District, #1 Pinecrest Lake Road, Pinecrest, CA 95364; 209-965-3434. Bear canisters and stoves are strongly recommended. No campfires above 9000 feet, and no campfires within a half mile of Emigrant Lake. One-night camping limit per trip at the following lakes: Bear, Camp, Grouse, Powell, and Waterhouse.

Driving Directions: The turnoff to Kennedy Meadow from Hwy. 108 is 27 miles east of the Pinecrest Y (the turnoff to Pinecrest Lake, south of Strawberry) and 9.1 miles west of Sonora Pass. Turn south on the signed spur road to Kennedy Meadow. A half mile down the road there is signed public parking, where you can leave your car. One mile down the road is Kennedy Meadows Resort (lodgings, café, saloon, store, pack station) and the trailhead (6400') where you can drop off passengers and packs and perhaps spend a night before starting your trip.

35 Summit Creek

Trip Data: 11S 261707 4235645; 13.6 miles; 2/1 days

Topos: *Sonora Pass, Emigrant Lake*

Highlights: A part of this route follows the historic Emigrant Trail used by pioneers crossing the Sierra between the areas around Bridgeport and Columbia. The scenery along the way is an absorbing study in glacial and volcanic terrain.

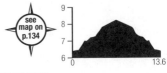

DAY 1 (Kennedy Meadow Trailhead to Summit Creek, 6.8 miles): Under a dense forest cover of Jeffrey pine, incense-cedar, sugar pine, juniper, and white fir, the trail crosses a small ridge to Kennedy Meadow itself and skirts the east side of the meadow. Beyond the meadow, the trail crosses Middle Fork Stanislaus River on a footbridge to reach a junction. Go left (southeast) along the base of a granite dome. The trail soon becomes steep and rocky and passes a series of cascades near the confluence of Kennedy and Summit creeks and more cascades as it crosses Summit Creek on a footbridge.

HWY 108

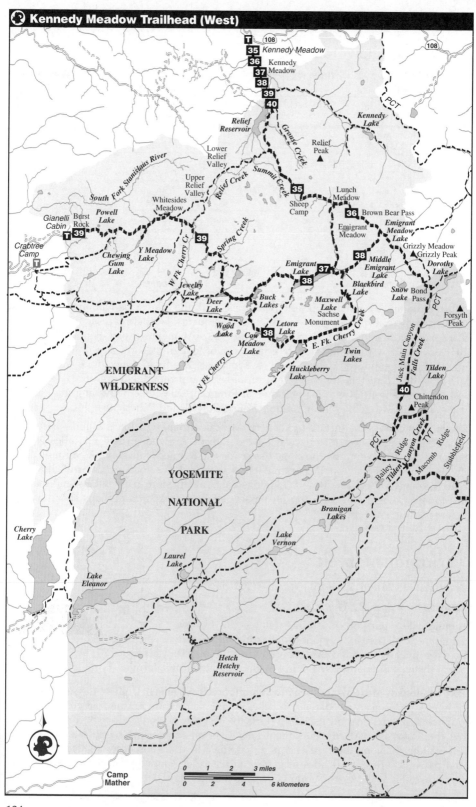

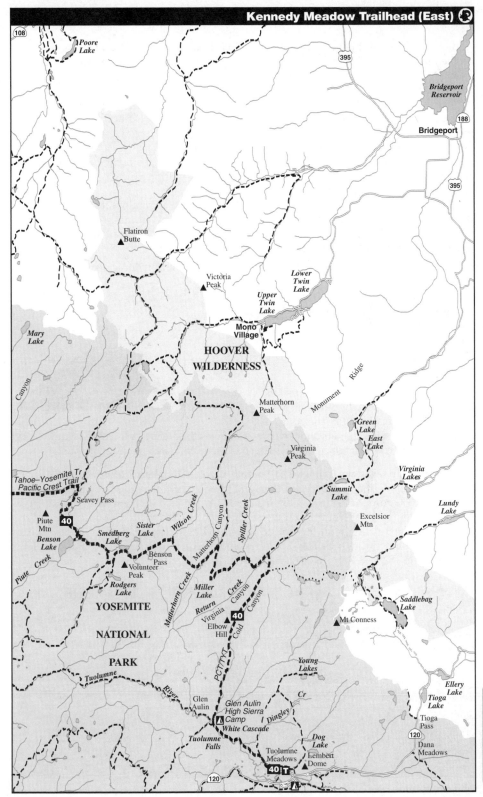

108

Poore
Lake

395

*Bridgeport
Reservoir*

188

Bridgeport

395

Flatiron
Butte

*Lower
Twin
Lake*

Victoria
Peak

*Upper
Twin
Lake*

*Mary
Lake*

Mono
Village

**HOOVER
WILDERNESS**

Canyon

Monument Ridge

Matterhorn
Peak

*Green
Lake*

*East
Lake*

Virginia
Peak

*Virginia
Lakes*

Tahoe–Yosemite Tr
Pacific Crest Trail

*Summit
Lake*

*Lundy
Lake*

Seavey Pass

Piute
Mtn

40

*Benson
Lake*

*Smedberg
Lake*

*Sister
Lake*

Wilson Creek

Matterhorn Canyon

Spiller Creek

Excelsior
Mtn

Benson
Pass

Volunteer
Peak

*Rodgers
Lake*

Piute Creek

*Saddlebag
Lake*

*Miller
Lake*

Return

Creek

Matterhorn Creek

Virginia

Canyon

Cold

Canyon

YOSEMITE

Elbow
Hill

40

Mt Conness

NATIONAL

*Young
Lakes*

PCT/TYT

PARK

Tuolumne

River

*Ellery
Lake*

Cr

*Tioga
Lake*

Glen
Aulin

Glen Aulin
High Sierra
Camp

Dingley

White Cascade

*Tuolumne
Falls*

Tuolumne
Meadows

*Dog
Lake*

Lembert
Dome

Tioga
Pass

120

Dana
Meadows

40

120

T

Beyond the footbridge is a false junction: Left is an abandoned track; go right to stay on the main trail to a junction with the Kennedy Lake Trail. Here, left (northeast) goes to Kennedy Lake; right (south) to Relief Reservoir. Go right, soon passing a PG&E dam-maintenance station, to an overlook of Relief Reservoir.

The trail contours high above the reservoir before reaching a shallow ford of Grouse Creek. Beyond here, the route ascends a series of rocky switchbacks and then veers southeast to pass a junction with the Lower Relief Valley Trail (left, northwest, then southwest) after 1 mile; continue ahead (south-southeast) at this junction.

Go left here to begin a steady, steep uphill climb to enter the brush-covered volcanic rubble above Summit Creek. The trail then drops into wet little Saucer Meadow, with one or two poor campsites on its edge.

With the multihued volcanic rock of Relief Peak on the left and white, glaciated granite on the right, the trail climbs along Summit Creek to several fair campsites between 8200 and 8300 feet (11S 261707 4235645). Some on the creek side of the trail are closed due to overuse; look for nicer ones uphill of the trail. Fishing is poor.

DAY 2 (Summit Creek to Kennedy Meadow Trailhead, 6.8 miles): Retrace your steps.

36 Emigrant Meadow Lake

Trip Data: 11S 268152 4231050;
25.2 miles; 4/1 days

Topos: *Sonora Pass, Emigrant Lake*

Highlights: Scenically, this route splits the terrain into two distinctly different parts. To the north, the basaltic and pumice slopes vividly disclose the volcanic overlay that gives the area its colorful reds and blacks. To the south, in contrast, glaciers have polished the granite into shining mirror slabs.

DAY 1 (Kennedy Meadow Trailhead to Summit Creek, 6.8 miles): *(Recap: Trip 35, Day 1.)* Begin hiking along the dirt road and then onto the foot trail that climbs to the false junction where you go right to stay on the main trail. At the next junction, with the Kennedy Lake Trail, you go right (south) to traverse above Relief Reservoir. Continue beyond the reservoir to the junction with the trail to Lower Relief Valley, where you go left (southsoutheast), climb through Saucer Meadow, and eventually reach the campsites along Summit Creek (8200–8300'; 11S 261707 4235645).

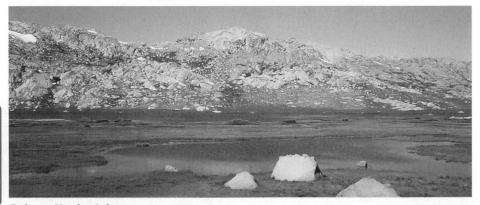

Emigrant Meadow Lake

DAY 2 (Summit Creek to Emigrant Meadow Lake, 5.8 miles): The trail continues up-canyon under red firs for a mile and then ascends 400 rocky feet to a little saddle beyond which is the hardened camping area called Sheep Camp. The main trail curves around Sheep Camp and then back to the creek, trending eastward past a meadow with a campsite at its east end. Next the trail crosses a pumice slope above huge, subalpine Lunch Meadow. At the meadow's east end there is a junction: left (ahead, east) to Emigrant Meadow Lake; right (south) across the creek to Emigrant Lake.

Go left, presently making the gradual but steady ascent, with Granite Dome and Relief Peak to the west, to Brown Bear Pass (9750'). The trail descends from the pass on a long traverse into the grassy, granite-walled basin containing Emigrant Meadow Lake (9407'; rainbow). As the trail swings around the top of the lake, it reaches a junction with a trail left (southeast) to Grizzly Meadow and Bond Pass on the TYT and right (south-southwest) to Middle Emigrant Lake.

The windy basin of Emigrant Meadow Lake offers sheltered camping among the boulders and battered trees on the saddle just south of the lake (11S 268152 4231050) and exposed sites on the rocky knolls northeast of the lake (11S 268350 4231929). Fishing is good for rainbow. This huge meadow was the traditional stopping place for emigrant trains on the first leg of their Sierra crossing.

DAYS 3–4 (Emigrant Meadow Lake to Kennedy Meadow Trailhead, 12.6 miles): Retrace your steps.

37 Emigrant Lake

Trip Data: 11S 264854 4229109; 26.8 miles; 4/1 days

Topos: *Sonora Pass, Emigrant Lake*

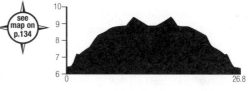

see map on p.134

Highlights: A longtime favorite with anglers, Emigrant Lake is often used as a base camp for short fishing trips to the numerous lakes that lie close by. Lush alpine meadows surrounding isolated snowmelt tarns contrast with vast slopes of red pumice and fields of polished granite.

DAY 1 (Kennedy Meadow Trailhead to Summit Creek, 6.8 miles): *(Recap: Trip 35, Day 1.)* Hike along the dirt road and then on the foot trail that climbs to the false junction where you go right to stay on the main trail. At the next junction, with the Kennedy Lake Trail, you go right (south) to traverse above Relief Reservoir. Continue beyond the reservoir to the junction with the trail to Lower Relief Valley, where you go left (south-southeast), climb through Saucer Meadow, and eventually reach the campsites along Summit Creek (8200–8300'; 11S 261707 4235645).

DAY 2 (Summit Creek to Emigrant Lake, 6.6 miles): *(Partial Recap: Trip 36, Day 2, from Summit Creek to junction in Lunch Meadow.)* Follow the trail along Summit Creek upstream and southeast, then climb 400 feet, curving around Sheep Camp, and from there going generally east along the creek to Lunch Meadow. At the meadow's east end there is a junction: left (ahead, east) to Emigrant Meadow Lake; right (south) across the creek to Emigrant Lake.

Leaving the Day 2 route of Trip 36, go right, ford the creek, and climb to a long, low, 9300-foot saddle, enjoying views of volcanic Relief Peak in the east and of granite Black Hawk Mountain in the west. Presumably, the high point of this saddle, at 9377 feet, is Mosquito Pass. The trail now winds through the long saddle with its fields of granite and tiny meadows. The valley on the other side of the saddle contains a tributary of North Fork

Cherry Creek (and of Emigrant Lake's inlet), over which there are views south to Michie and Haystack peaks.

The trail descends the east side of the tributary for some distance, passing a cross-country access to Mosquito Lake, before fording to the west side. Approaching Emigrant Lake, several use trails lead off to the right to tree-protected campsites well above the lake. The main trail avoids a trail left (south) to Blackbird Lake and continues ahead (generally northwest) to descend to the large meadow at the inlet of Emigrant Lake (8827'; 11S 264854 4229109; rainbow trout). There are good-to-excellent campsites at Emigrant Lake's nearby inlet, north side, and outlet.

DAYS 3–4 (Emigrant Lake to Kennedy Meadow Trailhead, 13.4 miles): Retrace your steps.

38 Cow Meadow Lake

Trip Data:
11S 260404
4225352;
46 miles;
7/2 days

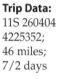

Topos:
Sonora Pass,
Emigrant Lake

Highlights: This is a fine choice for a mid-season fishing trip, as it circles the lake-dotted Cherry Creek watershed. A day's walk from your Cow Meadow Lake base camp permits anglers to sample almost 100 lakes. The route tours some of the finest scenery in Emigrant Wilderness, and the gentle terrain is ideal for beginning backpackers.

DAY 1 (Kennedy Meadow Trailhead to Summit Creek, 6.8 miles): *(Recap: Trip 35, Day 1.)* Hike along the dirt road and then on the foot trail that climbs to the false junction where you go right to stay on the main trail. At the next junction, with the Kennedy Lake Trail, you go right (south) to traverse above Relief Reservoir. Continue beyond the reservoir to the junction with the trail to Lower Relief Valley, where you go left (south-southeast), climb through Saucer Meadow, and eventually reach the campsites along Summit Creek (8200–8300'; 11S 261707 4235645).

DAY 2 (Summit Creek to Emigrant Lake, 6.6 miles): *(Partial Recap: Trip 36, Day 2, from Summit Creek to junction in Lunch Meadow.)* Follow the trail along Summit Creek upstream and southeast, then climb 400 feet, curving around Sheep Camp, and from there going generally east along the creek to Lunch Meadow. At the meadow's east end there is a junction: left (ahead, east) to Emigrant Meadow Lake; right (south) across the creek to Emigrant Lake.

(Partial Recap: Trip 37, Day 2, from junction in Lunch Meadow to Emigrant Lake.) Go right, ford the creek, and climb to a long, low, saddle.Wind through the saddle and into the valley on the other side along the east side of a tributary of North Fork Cherry Creek.

Ford the tributary's west side. Approaching Emigrant Lake, several use trails lead off to the right to tree-protected campsites well above the lake. At a junction with a trail left (south) to Blackbird Lake, continue ahead (generally northwest) to the large meadow at the inlet of Emigrant Lake (8827'; 11S 264854 4229109; rainbow trout; good camping on inlet, north side, and outlet).

DAY 3 (Emigrant Lake to Cow Meadow Lake, 7 miles): Follow the trail about 2 miles along the north side of Emigrant Lake to a junction at its northwest end: left (west) to Cow

Meadow Lake via North Fork Cherry Creek; right (west-northwest) to Cow Meadow Lake via Buck Meadow Creek.

Go right to cross a low, forested saddle and descend to ford Buck Meadow Creek. The trail turns south to traverse the long meadow north of Upper Buck Lake and then the west side of that lake (8313'; excellent camping around isthmus and east side, but no camping allowed on west shore) to a junction: right (southwest) to Deer Lake; left (south) to Lower Buck Lake. Go left to Lower Buck Lake.

At the next junction, the right fork leads south to the west side of Lower Buck Lake, and the left fork leads south and then east across an isthmus and to the east side of lower Buck Lake. Take the left fork, at first along the east side of Lower Buck Lake and then south to a saddle and to another junction: right (west) to Wood Lake; left (east) to Cow Meadow Lake.

Take the left fork and, under a lodgepole cover, descend steeply 600 feet to an unmarked, complex trail junction at North Fork Cherry Creek: left (north) on a faint, poorly maintained trail to Emigrant Lake; right (south) to the west side of Cow Meadow Lake; and ahead (west) to cross the creek. Go ahead to cross the creek and immediately veer southeast toward the north end of Cow Meadow Lake. The nearly level route reaches Cow Meadow Lake (7780'; 11S 260404 4225352; rainbows) and several excellent, well-used campsites.

DAY 4 (Cow Meadow Lake to Maxwell Lake, 7.5 miles): From the north end of Cow Meadow Lake, the trail climbs 560 feet to a signed junction: right, south-southwest, signed LOWER HUCKLEBERRY, to Huckleberry Lake; left, southeast, signed HUCKLEBERRY–ROUGH TRAIL.

Go left to the southwestern end of deep, serene Letora Lake (8351'; brook and rainbow). Leaving Letora Lake, the route angles south and then east, and descends a very rough trail to the northeast end of large Huckleberry Lake (7856'; brook and rainbow).

From the meadow at Huckleberry's northeast end, the trail heads upstream, passing a junction with the Lower Huckleberry Trail: right (south) to Lower Huckleberry; left (north) to East Fork Cherry Creek and Maxwell Lake. There are hardened campsites around this junction.

Take the left fork north, soon veering northeast and presently fording East Fork Cherry Creek. Now the trail ascends the creek's canyon. Views along this ascent include the large granite outcrop known as Sachse Monument (9405'). The trail passes an abandoned tungsten mine, joins a mining road, fords the creek, and continues ahead (north) at a lateral right (southeast) to Twin Lakes.

At the south end of Horse Meadow, the trail forks: left (northwest) to Maxwell Lake; ahead (north-northwest) to skirt Horse Meadow. Take the left fork up a timbered slope to Maxwell Lake (8662'; 11S 266169 4227269; brook trout). Choice campsites on the lake's north side have views of both the lake and Sachse Monument.

DAY 5 (Maxwell Lake to Emigrant Meadow Lake, 5.5 miles): From Maxwell Lake, the trail switchbacks generally northward up through moderate lodgepole cover and then winds through a long, rock-lined meadow past several beautiful lakelets to Blackbird Lake (9402'; excellent camping). At Blackbird's northwest tip, there's a junction: The main trail heads left (west) to Emigrant Lake, but your route, faint and hard to find, heads right, first north and then east around the top of the lake.

This unmaintained footpath ascends along the south side of North Fork Cherry Creek for about 1.5 miles before fording the creek. Beyond the ford, the trail is rutted into meadowy turf, overgrown from lack of maintenance. There are spectacular campsites along the creek.

The route grows steeper just south of Middle Emigrant Lake (9335; rainbow) and then levels out at the wet meadows at the foot of the lake. The path skirts the lake's west side, fords its inlet (difficult in footing and hard to see because of willows) and crosses a low, rocky saddle to Emigrant Meadow Lake's windy basin (9407'; rainbow). The best campsites are on this saddle (11S 268152 4231050); there are others on the north and south sides of Emigrant Meadow Lake.

DAY 6 (Emigrant Meadow Lake to Summit Creek, 5.8 miles): *(Recap in Reverse: Trip 36, Day 2.)* Depending on where you camped, follow the trail to the junction on Emigrant Meadow Lake's northeast edge and go left (northwest) over Brown Bear Pass and descend through Lunch Meadow and Sheep Camp down to the campsites along Summit Creek, 6.6 miles (8200–8300'; 11S 261707 4235645).

DAY 7 (Summit Creek to Kennedy Meadow Trailhead, 6.8 miles): *(Recap in Reverse: Trip 35, Day 1.)* Head down (north-northwest) along Summit Creek, through Saucer Meadow, ahead (right, south) at the Lower Relief Valley junction, ahead (left, south) at the Kennedy Lake Trail junction, past the false junction, and past Relief Reservoir to Kennedy Meadow Trailhead (6400'; 11S 261707 4235645).

39 Gianelli Cabin

Trip Data:
11S 247573
4231605;
43.1 miles;
7/3 days

see map on p.134

Topos: *Cooper Peak, Emigrant Lake, Sonora Pass, Pinecrest*

Highlights: After visiting the north side of Emigrant Wilderness, this trip turns south and traverses the beautiful, lake-dotted country of the Cherry Creek watershed. At Emigrant Meadow, the trail joins the old Emigrant Trail, and history buffs will have the opportunity to see this historic crossing as the pioneers did. Note, too, that this trip is not the same as the Gianelli Cabin Trailhead to Kennedy Meadow trip that appears earlier in the book.

Shuttle Directions: To get to Gianelli Cabin from Hwy. 108, drive to tiny Cold Springs (east of Long Barn and west of the Pinecrest Y). From there, head east 1.2 miles to a junction with paved Crabtree Road, and turn right. If coming from the east, drive west on Hwy. 108 past the Pinecrest Y and continue to this road junction, about 7.75 miles farther west, and turn left. Follow Crabtree Road 6.8 miles to a junction just before a pack station. Go straight ahead onto a dirt road and drive 2.6 miles to a junction. Turn left and go 4 miles to road's end at meadow containing the ruins of Gianelli Cabin.

DAY 1 (Kennedy Meadow Trailhead to Summit Creek, 6.8 miles): *(Recap: Trip 35, Day 1.)* Hike along the dirt road and then the foot trail that climbs to the false junction where you go right to stay on the main trail. At the next junction, with the Kennedy Lake Trail, you go right (south) to traverse above Relief Reservoir. Continue beyond the reservoir to the junction with the trail to Lower Relief Valley, where you go left (south-southeast), climb through Saucer Meadow, and eventually reach the campsites along Summit Creek (8200'–8300'; 11S 261707 4235645).

DAY 2 (Summit Creek to Emigrant Meadow Lake, 5.8 miles): *(Recap: Trip 36, Day 2.)* Walk up-canyon for a mile and then ascend 400 rocky feet to a saddle beyond, which is Sheep Camp. Follow the trail generally eastward to huge, subalpine Lunch Meadow. At the meadow's east end there is a junction: left (ahead, east) to Emigrant Meadow Lake; right (south) across the creek to Emigrant Lake.

HWY 108

Go left and presently climb to Brown Bear Pass (9750'). Then descend into the basin containing Emigrant Meadow Lake (9407'; rainbow) and a junction with a trail left (southeast) to Grizzly Meadow and Bond Pass on the TYT and right (south-southwest) to Middle Emigrant Lake.

DAY 3 (Emigrant Meadow Lake to Maxwell Lake, 5.5 miles): *(Recap in Reverse: Trip 38, Day 5.)* Pick up the trail south and then southwest along Emigrant Meadow Lake's east and south shore to cross a low ridge separating this lake's basin from that of Middle Emigrant Lake (9335T; rainbow trout). Make a difficult ford (dense willows, poor footing) of North Fork Cherry Creek (Middle Emigrant Lake's inlet and outlet) and then skirt the lake's west shore to its foot. Here the trail grows steeper on its way down to another ford. Now for about 1.5 miles to a junction at Blackbird Lake with a lateral left (south) past that lake. While the main trail goes ahead (west) toward Emigrant Lake, you turn left on the lateral to pass Blackbird Lake (9042'; excellent camping on all sides), wind through a long meadow, and descend switchbacks to the northeast end of Maxwell Lake (8662'; 11S 266169 4227269; good campsites on north side).

DAY 4 (Maxwell Lake to Cow Meadow Lake, 7.5 miles): *(Recap in Reverse: Trip 38, Day 4.)* The trail continues south-southeast to climb to the south end of Horse Meadow. At a junction here, a trail leads left (northeast) to Horse Meadow, but you continue ahead (east, then south) to meet East Fork Cherry Creek. As the trail curves west-southwest, you reach a junction with a trail left (southeast) to Twin Lakes and soon ford the creek. Staying near the creek, the trail briefly joins a mining road and passes an abandoned tungsten mine. After a long stroll west-southwest, the trail fords the creek again and passes through a forested area to a fork where left (south) goes to the south side of Huckleberry Lake (7856') and right (west) briefly grazes the lake's northeast shore. Go right to ascend west and then southwest on the very rough Huckleberry Trail, which curves north near an unnamed lake (8564') before climbing to Letora Lake (8351'). The trail quickly leaves Letora Lake behind on its way to a junction with the Lower Huckleberry Trail (left, south-southwest). You go right (generally northwest) and descend 560 feet on a sometimes blasted-out, sometimes cobbled trail to the east side of Cow Meadow Lake (7780'; 11S 260404 4225352).

DAY 5 (Cow Meadow Lake to Deer Lake, 3.5 miles): Leaving Cow Meadow Lake, the trail fords North Fork Cherry Creek and steps over an unmaintained trail that goes up and down the creek. Now the trail ascends steeply 600 feet amid a dense, predominantly lodgepole forest cover to a junction with a lateral to Wood Lake. Avoiding the lateral, you continue ahead to Lower Buck Lake (8305'). Fishing for rainbow is good on this lake and nearby Upper Buck Lake. Your trail crosses the isthmus separating Lower and Upper Buck lakes; fishing on both lakes for rainbow is good.

After crossing the isthmus, your route avoids a lateral left (south) to Lower Buck Lake as it curves left (north) to a junction with the Deer Lake Trail. Here, the route turns left (west) and climbs steeply for a half mile. Then it descends more gently for a mile past a junction with the Wood Lake Trail left (south) to that lake. Continue ahead (west) to the excellent campsites on the north side of Deer Lake (8450'; 11S 257803 4227867). This long lake has the same kind of subalpine meadow-fringing as Upper Buck Lake. The fine campsites, situated in small stands of lodgepole, look out across the lake's island-dotted surface. Fishing for rainbow is good to excellent.

DAY 6 (Deer Lake to Y Meadow Lake, 9 miles): From a trail junction at the middle of Deer Lake's north shore, turn right (north) and climb along an unnamed stream and past a series of inviting tarns. About 1.7 miles from Deer Lake, you meet first a lateral going right (east) to Long Lake, where you go ahead (north). Next you meet the Wire Lakes Trail going left (west).

(Recap in Reverse: Trip 31, Day 2.) Continue ahead (north) here and descend to the east end of Spring Meadow in Post Corral Canyon. The trail crosses Spring Creek and angles north and then northwest.

From Spring Meadow, the trail crosses a small ridge to Salt Lick Meadow, where it crosses tiny West Fork Cherry Creek (sometimes dry in late season) and soon curves west-northwest. Then the route ascends, passing the first of two trails leading right (northeast) to Upper Relief Valley and Kennedy Meadow. Continue ahead (west-northwest) and, 0.6 mile later, meet an unsigned trail leading left (south) to Toejam Lake. Going ahead here, you top a ridge and descend to Whitesides Meadow. At its head, you meet and continue ahead at a junction with the second trail right (northeast) to Upper Relief Valley.

Presently, you meet a trail west- and then northwest-bound (right) to Cooper Meadow and continue ahead again to the Y Meadow Lake Trail junction. Here, you turn left (south-west) and walk a winding 1 mile to the fair campsites at the north end of Y Meadow Lake (8600'; 11S 252574 4231353). Y Meadow Lake doesn't appear as such on the 7.5' topo; instead, look on the topo for "Y Meadow Dam" at the lake's south end.

DAY 7 (Y Meadow Lake to Gianelli Cabin, 5 miles): *(Recap in Reverse: Trip 30, Day 1.)* Return to the trail junction where you branched off to Y Meadow Lake and turn left (generally west) toward Gianelli Cabin. In about 1.5 miles, arrive in Lake Valley, where a faint angler's trail turns southwest toward Chewing Gum Lake. Your route ascends generally west, crosses a small ridge, and descends to a saddle overlooking Powell Lake.

Continue west along a ridge, topping out at Burst Rock (9161'). You continue westward on the ridge and presently descend to the ruins of Gianelli Cabin at the trailhead (8560'; 11S 247573 4231605).

40 Tahoe-Yosemite Trail Section 6: To Tuolumne Meadows

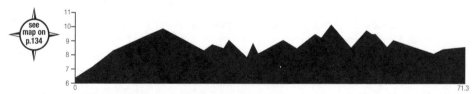

Trip Data: 11S 292581 4194990; 71.3 miles; 11/4 days

Topos: *Sonora Pass, Emigrant Lake, Tower Peak, Piute Mountain, Tiltill Mountain, Matterhorn Peak, Falls Ridge, Dunderberg Peak, Tioga Pass*

Highlights: The varied and incomparable scenery along this leg of the TYT—which travels from Kennedy Meadow to Tuolumne Meadows and offers emerald meadows, granitic and metamorphic peaks, jewellike lakes, bubbling creeks, panoramic views from ridges, and visits to deep canyons—more than justifies its length and sometimes taxing ups and downs.

HEADS UP! *Bear canisters are required in Yosemite National Park.*

Shuttle Directions: To access the take-out site at Tuolumne Meadows, head 7 miles west of Tioga Pass on Hwy. 120 (Tioga Road) in Yosemite National Park. It is walking distance east of Tuolumne Meadows Campground's entrance to prominent Lembert Dome on the southeast edge of expansive Tuolumne Meadows. Turn west onto a dirt road past the parking lot at Lembert Dome and find legal parking along that road, up to a gate across it (from which a spur road with more parking turns right to Tuolumne Stables). Your trip will end at that gate.

DAY 1 (Kennedy Meadow Trailhead to Summit Creek, 6.8 miles): *(Recap: Trip 35, Day 1.)* Hike along the dirt road and then onto the foot trail that climbs to the false junction where you go right to stay on the main trail. At the next junction, with the Kennedy Lake Trail, you go right (south) to traverse above Relief Reservoir. Continue beyond the reservoir to the junction with the trail to Lower Relief Valley, where you go left (south-southeast), climb through Saucer Meadow, and eventually reach the campsites along Summit Creek (8200–8300'; 11S 261707 4235645).

DAY 2 (Kennedy Meadow to Emigrant Meadow Lake, 5.8 miles): *(Recap: Trip 36, Day 2.)* Continue generally southeast up Summit Creek through Sheep Camp and Lunch Meadow. Go left (ahead, east) at the junction at Lunch Meadow's east end and, soon bearing southeast again, cross over Brown Bear Pass to Emigrant Meadow Lake (9407';11S 268152 4231050), where the better camping is on the saddle south of the lake.

DAY 3 (Emigrant Meadow Lake to Grace Meadow, 7.2 miles): Leave Emigrant Meadow Lake on the continuation of the trail you came in, soon reaching a junction with a spur left (north) to High Emigrant Lake. Go right here, continuing southeast and climbing to beautiful Grizzly Meadow, where Grizzly Peak stands solemn guard over two small lakes.

Shortly after the more easterly of the lakes passes out of view, a foot trail darts off to the right. You go ahead (south-southeast) on the main foot trail to meet an old, closed mining road in about 300 yards. Stay ahead (still south-southeast) on the road when another foot trail shortly darts off left (southeast) along the south slopes of Grizzly Peak.

For the next mile, the old road offers tantalizing views over East Fork Cherry Creek to the peaks of northern Yosemite. Where the road then forks, the right fork leads west to some old mining claims, while your route continues ahead (southeast) to lovely Summit Meadow and, in a half mile, to another fork. The right fork goes southwest to Snow Lake, while the TYT turns left (east) and ascends, presently curving south, 300 feet up a moderate slope dotted with lodgepole and hemlock. At an unsigned junction with a track that goes right (southwest), the TYT goes left (south) on trail again and soon reaches Bond Pass, a low saddle (9800') between Emigrant Wilderness and Yosemite National Park. From here to Tuolumne Meadows, firearms, hunting, and pets are prohibited.

You step across the pass and into the park, descending southeast and in quarter mile meeting the alternate route coming in from the left (northeast). Continue ahead (southeast) and in another quarter mile meet the PCT coming in on the left (northeast) from Dorothy Lake.

Turn right (south-southwest) on the combined PCT/TYT and continue your descent into the upper end of lush, damp, and stunning Jack Main Canyon, where the trail roughly parallels Falls Creek (trout). Early-morning travelers are likely to spot deer still grazing as well as signs of black bears, particularly during gooseberry season. This next stretch of trail is an idyllic series of tiny meadows interspersed with dense forest, all alongside murmuring Falls Creek. To the east, somber Forsyth Peak and black-and-white Keyes Peak cap the canyon walls.

Today's goal is long, rolling Grace Meadow (8800–8640'; 11S 270738 4224679—approximately in the meadow's center along the trail). As easy as Jack Main Canyon is on the eye, it is tough on the seeker of a campsite. With camping prohibited on meadows and with the forest often very dense and damp, it can be hard to find a legal, flat, dry campsite in Jack Main Canyon. Good luck.

DAY 4 (Grace Meadow to Tilden Lake, 5.2 miles): From Grace Meadow, the nearly level PCT/TYT leads 5 miles through numerous meadows. Much of the trail is lined with huckleberries, and during early summer, lavender shooting stars bloom in abundance along parts of the route. Chittenden Peak and its northern satellite serve as impressive reference points for gauging your progress toward the junction where the TYT turns east to Tilden Lake.

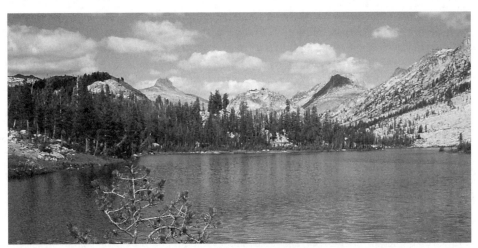

Tilden Lake, Day 4's destination, and Saurian Crest (background left)

Nearing the junction, you see and hear the roar of the impressive falls on Tilden Creek, rushing to join Falls Creek. In a little more than a half mile beyond the confluence of Tilden and Falls creeks, the TYT and the PCT part company. Go left (east) on the TYT, ford Falls Creek (difficult in early season) in 80 yards near a possible campsite, and parallel the creek upstream for a half mile. Under the steep, black-streaked south face of Chittenden Peak, the TYT begins climbing rough switchbacks for 700 feet to the basin holding long, sublime Tilden Lake (8900'; 11S 271071 4219974 for southwest shore). Many well-used campsites line the southeast and southwest shores. Views of Saurian Crest to the north are breathtaking.

DAY 5 (Tilden Lake to Rancheria Creek, 8.5 miles): The trail curves around the narrow, southwest toe of Tilden Lake, skirting a teardrop-shaped bay on its way to a pronounced, crescent-shaped bay on the lake's southeastern shore. Here, the trail may fade out completely; when Tilden Lake is high, the meadow around the crescent-shaped bay may be under a sheet of water, as is the trail through it. Veer south through this meadow and into a shallow draw to pick up the trail again. It soon passes over a tiny ridge and into the upper end of the canyon through which Tilden Canyon Creek flows out of lakelets dwarfed by the size of nearby, but now invisible, Tilden Lake. The TYT gently descends this canyon, passing poor campsites near the canyon's lower end.

The TYT curves west around the base of Peak 9362T and switchbacks down to a junction where it rejoins the PCT 3 miles from Tilden Lake. Turn left (south) on the combined PCT/TYT; right (west) on the PCT goes to Wilma Lake. From here on, the TYT follows the PCT on the way to Tuolumne Meadows.

The PCT/TYT soon reaches another junction where it turns left (southeast) across Tilden Canyon Creek to begin a gradual and then steeply switchbacking climb of Macomb Ridge.

HWY 108

> **CROSSING THE WASHBOARD**
>
> This is the first ridge of several northeast-southwest ridge-and-canyon systems you will tackle as the PCT/TYT pushes its way generally eastward against the "grain" of what's often called "northern Yosemite's washboard country." Ascend a ridge, drop into the next canyon, almost immediately ascend the next ridge, drop into the next canyon…until the mind reels and feet ache. Even so, the magnificent scenery of northern Yosemite is adequate reward for all your effort.

You may think you've topped Macomb Ridge when you happily descend a quarter mile to a meadow, but—surprise!—you still have one more short, steep ascent to top Macomb Ridge. From the top, you make a long descent into Stubblefield Canyon, first contouring northeast through low chaparral on the mountainside and then dropping down a rocky, steep, cobblestoned trail to the canyon's floor and stream. You can search out campsites under red firs in Stubblefield Canyon if you're ready to stop.

The PCT/TYT fords the stream (difficult in early season) and soon climbs on short, steep switchbacks up the unnamed ridge between Stubblefield and Kerrick canyons. Halfway up, a spring provides a chance to refill your water bottles or hydration packs. East of the gap atop this ridge, there's a small lake that may provide a campsite.

From the ridgetop, the PCT/TYT makes a long, somewhat exposed descent into Kerrick Canyon near the ford of Rancheria Creek (7940'; 11S 274209 4213969) as the route swings eastward. On this side of the creek (the north side), there are pleasant, well-used campsites.

DAY 6 (Rancheria Creek to Benson Lake, 7.3 miles): Fording Rancheria Creek here may be difficult in early season, but your route picks up on the creek's south bank. At a junction on the other side, a trail leads right (south-southwest) to Bear Valley, while the PCT/TYT goes ahead (east) upstream on a winding, undulating, often ascending traverse of Kerrick Canyon's south wall. As it passes below the heavily fractured north face of Piute Mountain, the trail is sometimes high above the creek, sometimes on its banks. Many little tributaries to Rancheria Creek break this leg into lush gardens of monkeyflower, tiger lily, shooting star, bush lupine, corn lily, columbine, and goldenrod.

At the next junction, the left fork continues up-canyon (west-northwest) toward Arndt Lake and Kerrick Meadow, while the PCT/TYT turns right (south-southwest) to climb steeply in search of Seavey Pass. Two gaps that aren't Seavey Pass precede the signed pass, which is 30 feet lower than the second gap before it. Ponds in this area offer the occasional camping opportunity.

From Seavey Pass, the PCT/TYT drops past a stately, rock-bound tarn before plummeting steeply over eroded trail alongside a riotous, unnamed stream that feeds the Benson Lake alluvial fan. It's rocky, weary going, alleviated only by the fine scenery: Volunteer Peak across Piute Creek and a splashing waterfall springing from the ridge of Piute Mountain.

Where the trail finally levels out on the valley floor, it crosses sandy, alluvial sediments and sees some marked changes in the flora. Although the route seems sandy and arid at first, it soon becomes tangled in bracken fern, overflow streamlets, and dense forest that sometimes make the trail difficult to follow through the overgrowth and boggy conditions.

At a signed junction just before the ford of Piute Creek, a spur trail branches right (southwest) 0.3 mile to popular, well-used Benson Lake (7581'; 11S 278374 4211043), famed for its large beach and pleasant swimming. There are sandy campsites on the lake's northeast shore, but they can be very buggy in mosquito season. The spur winds along the northwest bank of Piute Creek through corn lily, bracken, tiger lily, and swamp onion, to the beach. Fishing in Benson Lake is good for rainbow and eastern brook trout. This area, however, is down in a "hole" from which every way out is up!

DAY 7 (Benson Lake to Smedberg Lake, 4.5 miles): Return to the main trail and turn right (southeast). Soon the PCT/TYT fords Piute Creek (difficult in early season) and starts a 1900-foot ascent over the next 3 miles. The first pitch takes hikers beneath giant firs to a brush saddle, then descends 0.3 mile to a ford of Smedberg Lake's outlet creek (difficult in early season). The next leg switchbacks up over metamorphic rock to another, easier stream crossing. The following leg is a steady, moderate 1-mile ascent to the simplest of these three stream fords, followed by switchbacks southward up to a lovely, meadowed area and a junction with a trail to Murdock Lake: right (southwest) to Murdock Lake; left (west) on the PCT/TYT toward Smedberg Lake.

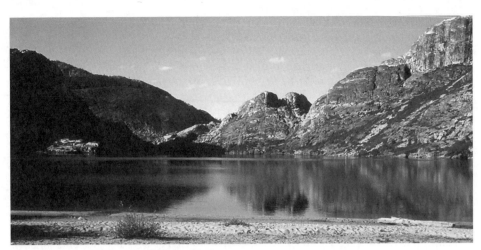

Benson Lake from its large, inviting beach

In a quarter mile more, the PCT/TYT meets a trail right (south) to Rodgers Lake, a half mile away and offering better camping than you'll find at sometimes crowded Smedberg Lake. The PCT/TYT goes left (northeast) here to curve around Volunteer Peak, plunge down a narrow canyon, climb up a ridge, and—finally—descend to the south shore of lovely Smedberg Lake (9219'; 11S 281748 4210078) and its campsites.

DAY 8 (Smedberg Lake to Matterhorn Canyon, 6.5 miles): Beyond the oasis of Smedberg Lake, the PCT/TYT resumes its steep, rocky, upward course to Benson Pass (10,139'), passing through a high meadow where there may be campsites if there is still water, and making its last climb over a heavily eroded surface and through sparse whitebark pine and hemlock. From Benson Pass, views to the northeast are excellent; on the pass's eastern flanks, weathered and blanched whitebark pines grow directly out of the ochre scree in tight clusters about 25 feet to 50 feet apart.

From Benson Pass, the PCT/TYT drops steeply, then gently, then steeply again to splashing Wilson Creek (campsites), crosses this stream, and winds down through an increasingly dense forest cover of mostly lodgepole pines. After fording Wilson Creek for the third time, the trail plunges steeply 500 feet down through lodgepole and hemlock to the floor of deep Matterhorn Canyon. Matterhorn Canyon's creek is a meandering stream flowing alternately through willowed meadows and stands of mixed lodgepole and western white pine. The trail turns north and follows the stream for 1 mile to several good campsites and to swimming holes just upstream in granite potholes. Or ford the creek to more good campsites a little downstream (8480' at the ford; 11S 288137 4210225). Fishing for eastern brook and rainbow trout is good.

DAY 9 (Matterhorn Canyon to Virginia Canyon, 5.8 miles): The PCT/TYT fords the creek (difficult in early season) and meets the Matterhorn Canyon Trail (left, north-northeast) in about 80 yards. Travelers on the PCT/TYT turn right (south) up the imposing, steep, forested canyon wall. About two dozen steep switchbacks gain the 1100 feet necessary to reach a saddle where hikers can see the striking peaks to the north.

PEAK IDENTIFICATION

On the left of gaping Matterhorn Canyon are Doghead and Quarry peaks and, farther away, some of the peaks of noted Sawtooth Ridge. The great white hulk just to the right of the canyon is multi-summited Whorl Mountain, and to its right are the dark gray Twin Peaks Ridge, pointed and rusty-colored Virginia Peak, and pointed and light gray Stanton Peak.

From this saddle, the PCT/TYT descends gently south for more than a half mile to the meadow just north of scenic but campsite-less Miller Lake, hemmed in by white granite walls on the east and a wet meadow elsewhere. Here, the route makes a hairpin turn northeastward on a gentle ascent past several handsome ponds where a hiker anxious to stop might find a campsite. Beyond two gaps on this ascent, the trail descends slightly to a meadowed bench and then rises slowly up a narrow canyon on deep, decomposed-granite soil to a forested pass.

> **HISTORICAL NOTE**
>
> This pass was the original route between Spiller Creek and Matterhorn canyons, discovered by Lt. Nathaniel McClure of the 4th US Cavalry in 1894, during the time when the Cavalry were the guardians of the new national park. The National Park Service was formed in 1916.

Now the route descends numerous switchbacks through a moderate-to-dense forest of lodgepole and western white pine, mountain hemlock, and red fir, which give blessed shade to the northbound hiker climbing this steep slope. There are fine views of Shepherd Crest and the Mt. Conness complex of peaks on this steady descent. Just beyond the ford of Spiller Creek (campsites nearby), an unsigned trail starts up Spiller Creek's canyon.

The PCT/TYT bears right (southeast) and then northeast as it rounds the nose of the ridge separating Spiller Creek's canyon from Virginia Canyon, a relatively easy transition compared to the ridge-canyon transitions since the trail left Tilden Creek's canyon far to the west. The "northern Yosemite washboard" is at last losing its ferocity.

On Virginia Canyon's floor, you meet the trail up-canyon (left, north-northeast) toward the park's northeastern boundary at Summit Lake. Just beyond is a ford of the canyon's creek, Return Creek, a ford that can be difficult throughout the season; a crossing a quarter mile upstream may be easier. There are fair campsites upstream here on the west side and better campsites beyond the ford on the east bank (8560' near the ford; 11S 291514 4209335).

DAY 10 (Virginia Canyon to Glen Aulin, 8 miles): From the last trail junction, you bear right (northeast) on the PCT/TYT to ford Return Creek (or detour a quarter mile upstream to the easier ford, then follow a use trail downstream on the creek's east side). On the other side of this ford, there are some adequate campsites, and beyond them the trail hooks south to make a gentle descent along cascading Return Creek to the ford of smaller McCabe Creek. This may be the last water before Glen Aulin in late season.

Next, the trail climbs on moderately steep switchbacks to a junction with the trail left (northeast) up McCabe Creek to McCabe Lakes; you go right (southwest) into Cold Canyon for a long, gentle descent, at first through patches of moderate-to-dense forest abounding in birdlife (chickadees, juncos, warblers, flycatchers, woodpeckers, bluebirds, robins, evening grosbeaks). In Cold Canyon, when there's water, you may also be able to camp in the occasional dry, forested patch.

Continuing the descent of Cold Canyon, the trail passes through cool, moist forest and into long, broad meadows that are usually dry by late season. However, about 0.75 mile beyond the last junction, there may be water in late season close under Point 9182T. And at a stream fork shortly beyond a *very* large boulder on your west, you may find water in late season. Then the trail climbs over a saddle in a low, forested ridge, and gently descends for about a half mile. Over the next mile, always near Cold Canyon's creek (mostly dry in late season), the level, rutted path passes a few possible campsites.

From here, the trail leaves the creek and descends a series of easy switchbacks about halfway to the Tuolumne River. There's a campsite where the trail touches the creek again.

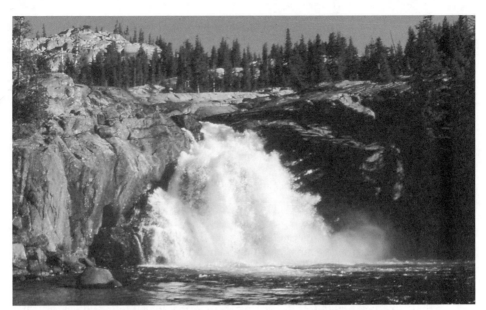

White Cascade, next to Glen Aulin High Sierra Camp

On the final, rocky downhill to the river, you catch glimpses of Tuolumne Falls and the White Cascade, and their roar carries all the way across the canyon.

Within sight of Glen Aulin High Sierra Camp, you reach a junction with the Tuolumne River Trail right (northwest) through the Grand Canyon of the Tuolumne. Good campsites are unfortunately rare along the Tuolumne there. In 15 yards, you come to a spur trail that goes left to cross Conness Creek on a footbridge to Glen Aulin High Sierra Camp (7910'; 11S 287493 4198572), where you may find meager supplies at its tiny store, campsites in its adjacent backpackers' campground (small sites close together in the rocks; potable water from a tap), and hot meals by reservation if the camp has places available (check and pay at the store).

Camping along the PCT/TYT is prohibited between Glen Aulin and the TYT's end at Tuolumne Meadows.

DAY 11 (Glen Aulin to Tuolumne Meadows, 5.7 miles): Return to the PCT/TYT and head briefly ahead southwest to cross the Tuolumne River just below the roar and foam of stunning White Cascade. The trail, sometimes hard to follow here, climbs along the river to a junction with the trail right (west) to McGee and May lakes. Staying on the PCT/TYT, you go left (southeast) here and continue climbing upriver, passing a fine viewpoint of crashing Tuolumne Falls. In the right lighting, you can get a superb photograph of the falls here.

Beyond, you ascend past a series of sparkling rapids separated by large pools and wide sheets of clear water spread out on slightly inclined granite slabs—one of the most beautiful stretches of the whole TYT. Soon the trail crosses the river for the last time, again on a footbridge, and climbs a little way above the gorge the river has cut here. Across the stream you'll spot basaltic "Little Devils Postpile," the only volcanic formation anywhere around here. The trail shortly descends to large, polished, granite slabs near the river and follows a sometimes ducked route across them for a mile or so.

When the tread resumes, you soon come right to the river's edge at an extremely scenic, wide bend far across which rise granite domes and peaks; beyond, you shortly cross the three branches of Dingley Creek (may be dry by late season). The trail gradually leaves the river behind for a while as the river turns south and the trail continues southeast to meet the trail to Young Lakes (left, north). You go ahead (still southeast) on the PCT/TYT to touch the northwest edge of Tuolumne Meadows before crossing the three branches of Delaney Creek, whose last branch is the only one that is a significant crossing and where there may still be water by late season.

Just beyond that ford, a spur trail takes off left (north) for Tuolumne Stables, while you veer right to ascend a long, dry, sandy ridge. From the tiny, reed-filled ponds atop this ridge, the trail drops gently down through meadowed pockets and stands of lodgepole pine to pass near Parsons Memorial Lodge and above rusty-red Soda Springs in a wooden enclosure. This very last leg is an alternate route of the JMT.

Now the PCT/TYT picks up a closed dirt road bearing east above the north edge of Tuolumne Meadows and follows it past interpretive displays to a locked gate (8590'; 11S 292581 4194990) with a road leading ahead to Hwy. 120, the Tioga Road (the right fork at this gate leads to the stables). The TYT ends here.

Go ahead toward Lembert Dome's abrupt southwest face to find your pick-up ride or your shuttle car. The Cathedral Range across the meadow provides inspiring scenery, as you finish your 186-mile journey from Meeks Bay to Tuolumne Meadows.

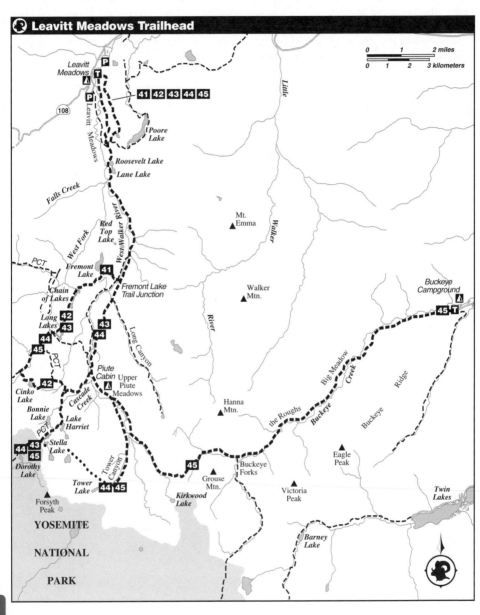

Leavitt Meadows Trailhead

Leavitt Meadows
41 42 43 44 45
Poore Lake
Roosevelt Lake
Lane Lake
Falls Creek
West Walker River
West Fork
Red Top Lake
Mt. Emma
Walker
PCT
Fremont Lake
41
Chain of Lakes
Fremont Lake Trail Junction
Long Lakes
42
43
43
44
Walker Mtn.
Buckeye Campground
45
T
45
PCT
Piute Cabin
Upper Piute Meadows
River
Long Canyon
Cinko Lake
42
Cascade Creek
Bonnie Lake
Lake Harriet
Hanna Mtn.
Big Meadow Creek
Buckeye
Buckeye Ridge
the Roughs
Stella Lake
PCT
44
43
45
Dorothy Lake
Tower Canyon
45
Buckeye Forks
Eagle Peak
Tower Lake
44
45
Grouse Mtn.
Kirkwood Lake
Victoria Peak
Twin Lakes
Forsyth Peak

YOSEMITE

NATIONAL

PARK

Barney Lake

HWY 108

Leavitt Meadows Trailhead

7123'; 11S 276948 4245965

DESTINATION/ UTM COORDINATES	TRIP TYPE	BEST SEASON	PACE (HIKING/ LAYOVER DAYS)	TOTAL MILEAGE
41 Fremont Lake 11S 276852 4236745	Semiloop	Mid or late	2/0 Moderate	19.5
42 Cinko Lake 11S 273454 4231779	Out & back	Mid or late	4/0 Moderate	28
43 Dorothy Lake 11S 272782 4228362	Semiloop	Mid or late	4/1 Moderate	34
44 Tower Lake 11S 276629 4226741	Semiloop	Mid or late	5/2 Moderate, part cross-country	40
45 Buckeye Forks 11S 283366 4227850	Shuttle	Early or mid	5/2 Moderate, part cross-country	41.4

Information and Permits: The proposed Hoover Wilderness Additions are managed by Humboldt-Toiyabe National Forest (Bridgeport Ranger District). While not yet official wilderness, permits are still required. Contact the Bridgeport Ranger District: HCR 1 Box 1000, Bridgeport, CA 93517; 760-932-7070; www.fs.fed.us/r4/htnf. Note that the trip to Dorothy Lake enters Yosemite National Park; once you step across the park's boundary, all of the park's rules and restrictions apply. Also note that the USDA/USFS *Hoover Wilderness* map is much more accurate about trails in this area than are the 7.5' topos.

Driving Directions: Just 7.8 miles east of Sonora Pass on Hwy. 108, there's a backpackers' parking lot on the east side of the road (Hwy. 108 runs north-south through here), about 200 yards south of Leavitt Meadows Campground. Overnighters must park here (water; toilet) and walk the 200 yards to the campground, which is also on the east side of the road. From there, work your way down to the lower campground road, along which this trailhead lies, just before a steel bridge over West Walker River. Only day-use parking is permitted here.

41 Fremont Lake

Trip Data: 11S 276852 4236745; 19.5 miles; 2/0 days

Topos: *Pickel Meadow, Tower Peak*

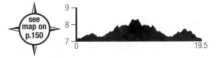

Highlights: You visit several lovely lakes on this beautiful route. An ideal weekend for the beginner, this trip offers off-trail excursions to other lakes for the more advanced backpacker.

DAY 1 (Leavitt Meadows Trailhead to Fremont Lake, 9 miles): Walk across the bridge over West Walker River. Avoid a use trail right around an outcrop and instead follow the main trail as it ascends briefly and in a quarter mile reaches a junction where you turn right (west) onto the West Walker River Trail—not on the topos but on the wilderness map. Descend a sagebrush-covered arid slope toward West Walker River. Just before its banks, the trail meets a snarl of use trails as well as its own continuation. Go left as the sandy West Walker River Trail, very exposed here, curves south and ascends gradually along the lower slopes of the ridge east of Leavitt Meadows.

The river meanders through this huge meadow, and you can see a trail from the pack station heading across the meadow toward your route. Continue ahead (south) at any junctions, including the one with the trail from the pack station. Far up the river canyon, Forsyth Peak stands majestically on the border of Yosemite.

MOUNTAIN MAHOGANY

Close beside the trail, you may observe many tall specimens of an almost tree-sized shrub called mountain mahogany. Despite the leaves' dry, tough appearance, the local mule deer love to eat them. The plant is particularly striking in the early fall, when the styles (part of the flowers) are white, silky, 3-inch plumes growing by the hundreds on each bush.

Around 1.5 miles, the trail enters sparse forest and ascends to a little saddle. Then, at about 1.75 miles, you meet a signed junction with a trail left (east) to Secret and Poore lakes. You go ahead (south) here. Note this junction: On the semilooping return trip, you will take the north fork to Secret Lake. For now, continue south to algae-bottomed Roosevelt Lake, ringed with a sparse fringe of Jeffrey pines. There are some undistinguished campsites on the west side of the lake, and sometimes fishing is good for brook trout.

The trail leads next over a granite shoulder and down to the outlet of Lane Lake, nearly a twin of Roosevelt and only a few yards from it. This outlet usually dries up by midsummer, but the dead lodgepole pines southwest of the ford are testimony to flooding earlier in the season. From the ford, the rocky-dusty trail ascends briefly southeast and then levels off as it passes several lovely aspen groves, some with lush grass floors even into late season.

More than a mile from Lane Lake, you descend to the willow-lined banks of the river, crossing a small but vigorous tributary, and in 0.125 mile reach the main stream's east bank. You ascend gently near the river for a quarter mile through a cool forest of mixed conifers, aspens, and cottonwoods, and then veer away on a steeper ascent that fords another tributary. Now you climb steeply to a saddle with junipers and Jeffrey pines, which offers fine views up the West Walker Valley to Forsyth Peak and the Sierra Crest.

Descending over a sandy trail, you pass the signed turnoff right to Hidden and Red Top lakes and continue ahead, ascending along the east bank of a narrow section of West Walker River.

ALONG THE RIVER HERE

This rocky stretch of trail alongside the river gives access to many pleasant, granite-bottomed potholes. Here the river tumbles along in a series of small falls and cascades that have carved a narrows through the white granite that typifies the middle of the West Walker River Valley. The upper walls are of barren, metavolcanic rock that ranges the color spectrum from black to reds and yellows.

At a wide spot, the trail splits, and signs direct stock users to go right and cross the river. You continue ahead (south) on the east bank; the trails will rejoin later. Where the river valley opens onto a forested flat buzzing with mosquitoes in early season, there's a signed junction, the east-side Fremont Lake Trail junction (7928'; 11S 277808 4236251), directing you right (west) some 150 yards to a wide spot where you can ford the river (very dangerous in early season; a serious wade at any time).

Across the river and on its west bank, the trail curves briefly downstream through lodgepoles and past some well-used campsites to a junction with the stock-users' trail. The joined trails immediately reach another signed Fremont Lake Trail junction. Turn left (northwest) here and soon begin climbing dusty, gradual-to-moderate switchbacks that eventually lead to a saddle topped with juniper and Jeffrey pine. This saddle offers views south to Tower Peak.

From the saddle, your trail descends gently to a signed junction with the trail left (south-southwest) to Chain of Lakes. Go ahead (northwest) here and, in 100 yards, reach Fremont Lake, ringed by moderate-to-dense lodgepole and juniper. Around the south end of the lake in the timber are fair campsites (8243′; 11S 276852 4236745), and fishing for rainbow and eastern brook is good.

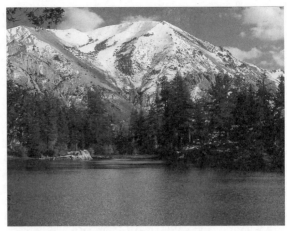

Secret Lake is one of Day 2's scenic delights.

DAY 2 (Fremont Lake to Leavitt Meadows Trailhead, 10.5 miles): Retrace your steps of Day 1 to the signed junction with the trail to Secret Lake. For a trip that is 1.5 miles shorter, you could continue retracing Day 1 for an out-and-back trip, but you'll miss Secret Lake and some fine scenery.

To begin the loop part of this trip, turn right (north-northeast) toward Secret Lake, almost immediately reaching a junction with a trail continuing northeast to Poore Lake. You turn left (north-northwest) to curve above Secret Lake—lovely but no secret. Surrounded by trees, Secret Lake has several overused campsites. Beyond the lake, the rocky trail ascends and then follows the crest. Expansive views in all directions invite you to linger; many of the trees you pass are stunted and hauntingly shaped by wind. Beyond a flat covered with sagebrush and mountain mahogany, the trail drops steeply through a wooded pocket, across a little meadow, down sagebrush slopes, and past a line of aspens. After the aspens, the trail hooks sharply west across a meadow, in the middle of which you may notice faint use trails right and north to Millie Lake (definitely not worth your trouble). Continue west across the iris-dotted meadow, bob over a low ridge, and reach another use trail, this one on your left. Ignore it and continue northwest to close the loop part of this trip.

From here, turn right and retrace your steps to the trailhead, campground, and, finally, the backpackers' parking lot.

42 Cinko Lake

Trip Data: 11S 273454 4231779; 28 miles; 4/0 days

Topos: *Pickel Meadow, Tower Peak*

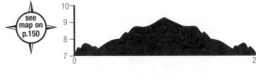

Highlights: This interesting route traces West Fork West Walker River to its headwater cirque beneath the Sierra Crest, passing through three life zones as it goes. Of the several trips in this drainage, this offers one of the best exposures to the geological, topographical, and biological features of this country.

DAY 1 (Leavitt Meadows Trailhead to Fremont Lake, 9 miles): *(Recap: Trip 41, Day 1.)* Cross the bridge over West Walker River and follow the main trail a quarter mile to a junction where you turn right (west) onto the West Walker River Trail—not on the topos but on the wilderness map. Descend to a snarl of use trails as well as your trail's continuation. Go left with the West Walker River Trail, which curves south and ascends gradually along the lower slopes of the ridge east of Leavitt Meadows. Continue ahead (south) at any junctions, including the one with the trail that crosses the meadow from the pack station. At about 1.75 miles, you meet a signed junction with a trail left to Secret and Poore lakes. Go ahead (south) to Roosevelt Lake, cross a low shoulder, and reach Lane Lake. Beyond, the trail eventually descends to the river's east bank and wanders south along it. At the signed turnoff right to Hidden and Red Top lakes, go ahead (south) and presently reach a wide spot where stock users go right to cross the river. Go ahead (south) to the signed east-side Fremont Lake Trail junction (7928'; 11S 277808 4236251) where you go right (west) to ford the river (very dangerous in early season; a serious wade at any time). Across the river, the trail curves briefly downstream to join the stock-users' trail. The trail immediately turns left (northwest) on the signed Fremont Lake Trail and switchbacks to a saddle. Descend to a signed junction with the trail left (south-southwest) to Chain of Lakes. Go ahead (northwest) and, in 100 yards, reach Fremont Lake with campsites at its south end (8243'; 11S 276852 4236745).

DAY 2 (Fremont Lake to Cinko Lake, 5 miles): Return to the last junction and turn right (south-southwest) toward Chain of Lakes on an ascent that steepens as it crosses open, granite-sand slopes with little shade. The first of three large granite domes that tower over the east side of Chain of Lakes comes into view, and the trail crosses to the north of it. Then, on a gently descending path through an increasingly dense forest cover, you pass a signed trail left (northwest) to Walker Meadows. Go right (south-southwest), step across the Chain of Lakes' outlet, and arrive at the Chain of Lakes—mostly tiny, green, lily-padded lakes. The trail leaves the last and largest of the Chain of Lakes and ascends gently past a small, unnamed lake north of Lower Long Lake. A few yards beyond, the trail veers right (west and then south) around the north side of Lower Long Lake (campsites).

> **SANDPIPERS**
>
> The rock in the center of the lake is a favorite midday resting place for the sandpipers that live here. Anglers seeking the pan-sized rainbow here will enjoy watching the sandpiper's low, skimming flight.

More campsites are found a few yards farther up the trail at Upper Long Lake. The trail jogs around the northwest end of Upper Long Lake, fords its intermittent outlet stream, and meets a lateral going left (southeast) to West Walker River and Lower Piute Meadows. Your route turns right (northwest) past a picturesque tarn to West Fork West Walker River and a signed junction with the PCT and a lateral that almost parallels the northbound PCT—it's actually a former PCT route—northwest toward Walker Meadow. If you turned right (northwest) on the PCT, you'd cross a bridge to a campsite on the river's west side.

But you don't cross, and you don't pick up the lateral. Instead, go left (southwest) on the PCT for a short way along West Fork West Walker River's east side to a fork. Here you leave the PCT by taking the right fork southwest along the tumbling "river" (the PCT goes left and south-southwest). Good campsites dot both sides of the West Fork near the junction. Occasional droopy-topped hemlocks appear along the pleasant ascent from the campsites, and many wildflowers bloom here, including shooting star, penstemon, bush lupine, aster, columbine, goldenrod, heather, Mariposa lily, wallflower, woolly sunflower, and fleabane. This gentle-to-moderate climb continues along the southeast side of the stream to the foot of a large, white granite dome. Here, the trail fords to the northwest side of the creek.

> **GEOLOGY LESSON**
>
> Contrasts between the dark volcanic rock and the white granite underlayment of this part of the Sierra are nowhere more marked than in this valley, and the viewer is assailed with dark battlements of multihued basalt and sheer escarpments of glacially smoothed batholithic granite. William H. Brewer, head of the Brewer Survey party that passed near here in July 1863, took note of the volcanic surroundings, saying, "…in the higher Sierra, along our line of travel, all our highest points were capped with lava, often worn into strange and fantastic forms: rounded hills of granite, capped by rugged masses of lava, sometimes looking like old castles with their towers and buttresses and walls, sometimes like old churches with their pinnacles, all on a gigantic scale, and then again shooting up in curious forms that defy description."

This ascent takes you to timberline, where the trees become stunted and include occasional, altitude-loving whitebark pines. At a signed junction, your route takes the left fork southeast along a clear trail to Cinko Lake. You ford West Fork West Walker River and pass a charming meadow with a tiny tarn. Then the trail makes a brief, moderate ascent to the intermittent north outlet of arrowhead-shaped Cinko Lake (there is another outlet on the south side of the lake). The trail emerges at the lake's edge (9212'; 11S 273454 4231779), next to the north outlet, where there are several good campsites. Fishing for rainbow and eastern brook may be good.

DAYS 3–4 (Cinko Lake to Leavitt Meadows Trailhead, 14 miles): Retrace your steps to the trailhead, 14 miles.

43 Dorothy Lake

Trip Data: 11S 272782 4228362; 34 miles; 4/1 days

Topos: *Pickel Meadow, Tower Peak*

Highlights: Touring the headwaters of the West Fork West Walker River and the headwaters of Cascade Creek and Falls Creek would be an ambitious undertaking in any one trip, but this trip boasts more. Near Dorothy Lake, the culmination of the trip, you'll see the unusual Forsyth Peak "rock glacier."

DAY 1 (Leavitt Meadows Trailhead to Fremont Lake, 9 miles): *(Recap: Trip 41, Day 1.)* Cross the bridge over West Walker River and follow the main trail a quarter mile to a junction where you turn right (west) onto the West Walker River Trail—not on the topos but on the wilderness map. Descend to a snarl of use trails as well as your trail's continuation. Go left with the West Walker River Trail, which curves south and ascends gradually along the lower slopes of the ridge east of Leavitt Meadows. Continue ahead (south) at any junctions, including the one with the trail that crosses the meadow from the pack station. At about 1.75 miles, you meet a signed junction with a trail left to Secret and Poore lakes. Go ahead (south) to Roosevelt Lake, cross a low shoulder, and reach Lane Lake. Beyond, the trail eventually descends to the river's east bank and wanders south along it. At the signed turnoff right to Hidden and Red Top lakes, go ahead (south) and presently reach a wide spot where stock users go right to cross the river. Go ahead (south) to the signed east-side Fremont Lake Trail junction (7928'; 11S 277808 4236251) where you go right (west) to ford the river (very dangerous in early season; a serious wade at any time). Across the river, the trail curves briefly downstream to join the stock-users' trail. The trail immediately turns left (northwest) on the signed Fremont Lake Trail and switch-backs to a saddle. Descend to a signed junction with the trail left (south-southwest) to Chain of Lakes. Go ahead (northwest) and, in 100 yards, reach Fremont Lake with campsites at its south end (8243′; 11S 276852 4236745).

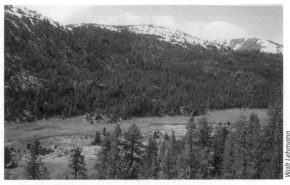

Walt Lehmann

DAY 2 (Fremont Lake to Dorothy Lake, 9 miles): *(Partial Recap: Trip 42, Day 2.)* Return to the Chain of Lakes Trail junction and turn right (south-southwest) toward

Leavitt Meadows

Chain of Lakes on an ascent that steepens as it crosses open slopes. Then descend to a junction with a signed trail left (northwest) to Walker Meadows. Go right (south-southwest) to the Chain of Lakes. Beyond the last and largest of the Chain of Lakes, ascend past a small lake and shortly veer right (west and then south) around the north side of Lower Long Lake (campsites; more campsites at Upper Long Lake). The trail jogs around the northwest end of Upper Long Lake, fords its intermittent outlet stream, and meets a lateral to West Walker River. Turn right (northwest) to West Fork West Walker River and a signed junction with the PCT and a lateral that almost parallels the northbound PCT. Go left (southwest) on the southbound PCT along the river's east side to a fork. Leave the PCT by taking the right fork southwest along the "river" (good campsites nearby). Climb along the southeast side of the stream before fording to the northwest side of the creek. Continue ascending to a signed junction; take the left fork southeast to Cinko Lake. Ford West Fork West Walker River and soon climb to the intermittent north outlet of Cinko Lake. The trail emerges next to the lake's north outlet (9212′; 11S 273454 4231779; campsites).

Leaving the Day 2 route of Trip 42, follow the trail along Cinko's north shore. From the southeast side of Cinko Lake, the trail winds down a lodgepole-and-hemlock-clothed hillside to an unnamed stream. Then it climbs slightly, veering east away from the stream, and makes a short, steep descent to a beautiful lakelet. About 0.125 mile past the lake, you briefly touch the stream again before veering away. In another 0.125 mile, the trail crosses this persistent tributary on a wooden bridge and soon passes three tarns on the right. Continuing levelly through a tarn-filled saddle here, the trail curves northeast to meet the PCT again, and you turn right (southeast) on the PCT toward Dorothy Lake, ascending through a thinning forest cover of lodgepole, hemlock, and whitebark pine. Shortly, you cross a deep, narrow stream on a rickety bridge.

The PCT continues southeast and then south to a junction with a trail left (northwest) down nearby Cascade Creek to West Fork Walker River. You turn right (generally south) to stay on the PCT here; the west side of this trip's loop ends here, and it's now out and back to Dorothy Lake. Soon you ford Cascade Creek near a large, east-bank campsite, climb away from the creek to ascend near Lake Harriet's noisy outlet, and presently ford that outlet. After this ford, the trail ascends more steeply, winds along island-dotted Harriet's west shore (campsites better on the east shore), and becomes rocky after passing the lake. Briefly ascend tight switchbacks before leveling out through a meadowy section to ford the stream joining Stella and Bonnie lakes. After another moderate, rocky ascent, the trail levels past the grassy north arm of Stella Lake. (At the northeast end of this arm, a ducked cross-country route to Lake Ruth and Lake Helen departs from your route.)

The long, low saddle on which Stella Lake sits ends at Dorothy Lake Pass (9528′), where there is an excellent view of Dorothy Lake to the southwest. To the southeast are V-notched views of Tower Peak, and to the south, the granite grenadiers of Forsyth Peak.

This is the boundary with Yosemite National Park. From the pass, the trail descends steadily into the park over a rocky slope full of pikas and marmots. As the trail skirts the north side of this beautiful lake, which is the source of Falls Creek, it winds through lush grass and willow with patches of shooting star, elephant heads, goldenrod, paintbrush, whorled penstemon, pussypaws, and false Solomon's seal.

HISTORY LESSON

This stretch of the north shore was not so lush when the first recorded explorer of this lake walked here. Lt. N.F. McClure, of the 4th Cavalry, came this way in 1894, noting, "Grazing here was poor, and there had evidently been thousands of sheep about."

The trail passes three windy campsites along the north shore before arriving at the good campsites at the west end of the lake (9397'; 11S 272782 4228362). Fishing for rainbow and occasional eastern brook is good except during a midsummer slowdown. This lake makes an excellent base-camp location for exploring and fishing the nearby lakes in the upper Cascade Creek basin, and for viewing the Forsyth Peak "rock glacier."

"ROCK GLACIER"

This phenomenon can be viewed from the unnamed lake south of Dorothy Lake. Seen from here, it is a prominent "river" of rock flowing in a long, northwest-curving arc. This arc begins on the northeast face of Forsyth Peak, then curves down the easternmost ravine, and points its moving head toward Dorothy Lake. Composed of coarse rock that tumbled from Forsyth Peak's fractured face, it hides an underlayment of silt, sand, and fine gravel, and it depends upon ice caught between larger boulders for its mobility.

DAY 3 (Dorothy Lake to Fremont Lake Trail Junction, 8 miles): First, retrace the steps of the previous hiking day, now northeast on the PCT, as far as the PCT's junction with the trail to Cinko Lake and the trail down Cascade Creek. Turn right (northeast) here to begin the east side of the loop part of this trip by descending switchbacks on the north side of tumbling Cascade Creek, past Cascade Falls. Near the bottom of this descent, the forest, now including stately red firs, becomes thicker. As the trail nears West Walker River, the descent levels, and then the route fords the river near an old corral.

Beyond the ford, you reach a junction with the West Walker River Trail; turn left (north and downstream) on it. You shortly ford a tributary and then meet the lateral left (northwest) to the Long Lakes and the PCT. You continue ahead (north) on the river's east side and ascend a little before dropping to and skirting the east side of large Lower Piute Meadows. Next, the sand-and-duff trail crosses a saddle and descends to ford Long Canyon's creek and reach a junction with a trail right (southeast) up Long Canyon to Beartrap Lake. Go ahead (north-northeast) here and in about a quarter mile beyond the creek meet the east-side Fremont Lake Trail junction (7928'; 11S 277808 4236251) where, on Day 1 of this trip, you turned left and northwest to ford West Walker River and rejoin the stock trail at the Fremont Lake Trail junction. The loop part of this trip ends here.

To end your day, you can either take the left fork across the river (again) to the west-side campsites passed on Day 1, or you can continue ahead and downstream on the river's east side to other good campsites. Fishing in the deeper holes of this section of the river is good for rainbow.

DAY 4 (Fremont Lake Trail Junction to Leavitt Meadows Trailhead, 8 miles): From the Fremont Lake Trail junction on the east side of West Walker River, retrace the rest of Day 1 of this trip.

44 Tower Lake

Trip Data: 11S 276629
4226741; 40 miles;
5/2 days

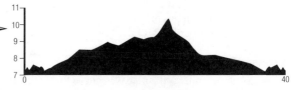

Topos: *Pickel Meadow,*
Tower Peak

Highlights: Combine the pleasures of the preceding trip to Dorothy Lake with a beautiful cross-country segment. Its strenuousness guarantees solitude to those who take it—and they'll also enjoy views of the alpine crest seldom seen by anyone except cross-country travelers.

HEADS UP! The cross-country segment of this trip is for experienced backpackers only.

DAY 1 (Leavitt Meadows Trailhead to Fremont Lake, 9 miles): *(Recap: Trip 41, Day 1.)* Cross the bridge over West Walker River and follow the main trail a quarter mile to a junction where you turn right (west) onto the West Walker River Trail—not on the topos but on the wilderness map. Descend to a snarl of use trails as well as your trail's continuation. Go left with the West Walker River Trail, which curves south and ascends gradually along the lower slopes of the ridge east of Leavitt Meadows. Continue ahead (south) at any junctions, including the one with the trail that crosses the meadow from the pack station. At about 1.75 miles, you meet a signed junction with a trail left to Secret and Poore lakes. Go ahead (south) to Roosevelt Lake, cross a low shoulder, and reach Lane Lake. Beyond, the trail eventually descends to the river's east bank and wanders south along it. At the signed turnoff right to Hidden and Red Top lakes, go ahead (south) and presently reach a wide spot where stock users go right to cross the river. Go ahead (south) to the signed east-side Fremont Lake Trail junction (7928'; 11S 277808 4236251) where you go right (west) to ford the river (very dangerous in early season; a serious wade at any time). Across the river, the trail curves briefly downstream to join the stock-users' trail. The trail immediately turns left (northwest) on the signed Fremont Lake Trail and switchbacks to a saddle. Descend to a signed junction with the trail left (south-southwest) to Chain of Lakes. Go ahead (northwest) and, in 100 yards, reach Fremont Lake with campsites at its south end (8243'; 11S 276852 4236745).

DAY 2 (Fremont Lake to Dorothy Lake, 9 miles): *(Partial Recap: Trip 42, Day 2.)* Return to the Chain of Lakes Trail junction and turn right (south-southwest) toward Chain of Lakes on an ascent that steepens as it crosses open slopes. Then descend to a junction with a signed trail left (northwest) to Walker Meadows. Go right (south-southwest), step across the Chain of Lakes' outlet, and arrive at the Chain of Lakes. Beyond the last and largest of the Chain of Lakes, ascend past a small, unnamed lake and a few yards past it, veer right (west and then south) around the north side of Lower Long Lake (campsites; more campsites at Upper Long Lake). The trail jogs around the northwest end of Upper Long Lake, fords its intermittent outlet stream, and meets a lateral to West Walker River. Turn right (northwest) past a picturesque tarn to West Fork West Walker River and a signed junction with the PCT and a lateral that almost parallels the northbound PCT. Go left (southwest) on the southbound PCT for a short way along the river's east side to a fork. Leave the PCT by taking the right fork southwest along the "river" (good campsites nearby). Climb along the southeast side of the stream before fording to the northwest side of the creek. Continue ascending to a signed junction; take the left fork southeast to Cinko Lake. Ford West Fork West Walker River and soon climb to the intermittent north outlet of Cinko Lake. The trail emerges next to the lake's north outlet (9212'; 11S 273454 4231779; campsites).

Leaving the Day 2 route of Trip 42, follow the trail along Cinko's north shore. From the southeast side of Cinko Lake, the trail winds down to an unnamed stream. Then it veers east away from the stream and descends to a lakelet. About 0.125 mile past the lake, you briefly touch the stream again before veering away. In another 0.125 mile, the trail crosses this persistent tributary on a wooden bridge and soon passes three tarns on the right. Continuing levelly through a tarn-filled saddle here, the trail curves northeast to meet the PCT again; turn right (southeast) on the PCT toward Dorothy Lake, shortly crossing a stream on a rickety bridge.

The PCT continues southeast and then south to a junction with a trail left (northwest) down nearby Cascade Creek to West Fork Walker River. You turn right (generally south) to stay on the PCT here; the west side of this trip's loop ends here, and it's now out and back to Dorothy Lake. Soon you ford Cascade Creek, climb away, and presently ford Lake Harriet's outlet. Beyond, the trail ascends more steeply, winds along Harriet's west shore and ascends tight switchbacks before leveling out to ford the stream joining Stella and Bonnie lakes. After another ascent, the trail levels past the north arm of Stella Lake. (At the northeast end of this arm, a ducked cross-country route to Lake Ruth and Lake Helen departs from your route.)

The trail presently reaches Dorothy Lake Pass (9528') and descends along the lake's north side to campsites on its west side (9397'; 11S 272782 4228362).

DAY 3 (Dorothy Lake to Tower Lake, 5 miles, part cross-country): From the Dorothy Lake campsites, return on the PCT to Stella Lake, where there are multiple choices for going generally southeast to lakes Ruth and Helen and Tower Lake. One of them is a ducked cross-country route that rounds the northeast end of Stella Lake and then climbs over a rock-and-grass ledge system along the east side of the intermittent stream joining Stella Lake and Lake Ruth to arrive at the outlet end of Lake Ruth (excellent campsites). Continuing to Lake Helen, the route skirts the east side of the lake for a short distance and then ascends a long, gentle swale to the southeast. Several small tarns mark the crossover point to the Lake Helen drainage (good campsites on the north side). Your route, keeping to the south side of Lake Helen, fords the tiny but noisy southwest inlet and then crosses the rocky slope directly south of the lake. At the southeast inlet, the route fords and ascends moderately southeast to a lovely grass bench. The remaining ascent to the obvious saddle in the southeast crosses steeper sections; possible routes may be better on the left (north) side of the cirque wall. This steep pitch brings you to a saddle offering incomparable views.

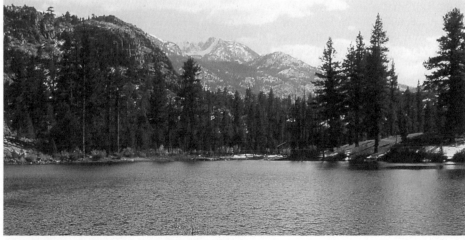

Day 1 of all Leavitt Meadows trips passes Lane Lake.

THE VIEWS FROM HERE

Included in the views are, from north to west, Wells Peak, White Mountain, Sonora Peak, Stanislaus Peak, Leavitt Peak, Kennedy Peak, Relief Peak, and Forsyth Peak. To the east and southeast the view encompasses, from east to south, Flatiron Butte, Walker Peak, Buckeye Ridge, the Kirkwood Creek drainage, Grouse Mountain, Hunewill Peak, Hawksbeak Peak, Kettle Peak, Cirque Mountain, and Tower Peak. You can also see most of the lakes of the Cascade Creek drainage, as well as Tower Lake at the foot of Tower Peak. Tower Peak is not the tallest, but it is the most spectacular peak of Yosemite's North Boundary Country, and it has served as a landmark for over a century.

Descending from the saddle on the southeast side, you cross rock and scree to a rocky bench, and from there a grass-and-ledge system to a lakelet just north of Tower Lake. The route then rounds the south nose of a granite ridge to Tower Lake's willowed outlet and fords to the fair campsites centered in the only stand of timber found here on the east side of the outlet (9540'; 11S 276629 4226741). Fishing for golden trout is fair to good, and there are also good campsites a half mile down the outlet stream.

DAY 4 (Tower Lake to Fremont Lake Trail Junction, 9 miles): Also on the east side of Tower Lake's outlet, you find an eastbound trail. Take this trail as it descends over a rocky slope close to the north side of the outlet stream.

THE VIEWS FROM HERE

This descent offers a view of a dramatic avalanche chute that slices the slope on the northeast side of Kirkwood Creek's canyon. Over your shoulder, back toward Tower Peak, the view is dominated by the northern extension of Tower Peak. This classic white-granite pinnacle soon obliterates views of Tower Peak itself, and it stands as mute testimony to the obdurate granite's resistance to glacial erosion.

The rocky descent soon reaches timberline and then fords the outlet stream where Tower Lake's outlet meets the tiny stream draining the glacier to the south. From here, the trail and the stream bear generally north, and you now descend on the outlet's east side as it becomes the named West Walker River and flows through Tower Canyon.

Presently, you ford a nameless tributary and beyond the ford, curve northward as you wind down through a dense forest of lodgepole and hemlock. Then the trail fords West Walker River to its west side and climbs above narrows bracketed by almost vertical granite walls, between which the stream is a plummeting ribbon well below. Ahead, you can see the West Walker River valley through the trees. A short, easy descent on duff trail soon brings you down to beautiful Upper Piute Meadows. Skirt the huge meadow on its west side. Leaving its north end, the sandy trail passes a turnoff to Piute Cabin, a Forest Service trail-maintenance station, fords the river, meets a junction with the trail coming in sharply on your right from the south, a trail which has just descended Kirkwood Creek's canyon. From here, the trail veers away from the river on a gentle descent.

MOO?

The cattle seen in some years in Upper Piute Meadows are part of the Forest Service's "multiple use" administrative concept. Cowflops have been reported as far away as the head of Thompson Canyon—and it may be logically assumed that they were a result of allowing grazing here.

After jogging around a marshy section, the trail again nears the river and soon reaches a junction with the trail left and southwest up Cascade Creek.

(Partial Recap: Trip 43, Day 3, from the junction with the West Walker River Trail.) From the junction, go ahead (downstream and generally north): You shortly ford a tributary and then meet the lateral left (northwest) to the Long Lakes and the PCT. You continue ahead, curving north-northeast, on the river's east side and presently skirt the east side of large Lower Piute Meadows. Beyond, the trail crosses a saddle, descends to ford Long Canyon's creek, and reaches a junction with a trail right (southeast) up Long Canyon to Beartrap Lake. Go ahead (north-northeast) here and in about a quarter mile beyond the creek meet the east-side Fremont Lake Trail junction (7928'; 11S 277808 4236251) where, on Day 1 of this trip, you turned left and northwest to ford West Walker River and rejoin the stock trail at the Fremont Lake Trail junction. The loop part of this trip ends here.

To end your day, you can either take the left fork across the river (again) to the west-side campsites passed on Day 1, or you can continue ahead and downstream on the river's east side to other good campsites. Fishing in the deeper holes of this section of the river is good for rainbow.

DAY 5 (Fremont Lake Trail Junction to Leavitt Meadows, 8 miles): From the Fremont Lake Trail junction on the east side of West Walker River, retrace the rest of Day 1 of this trip.

45 Buckeye Forks

Trip Data: 11S 283366 4227850; 41.4 miles; 5/2 days

Topos: *Pickel Meadow, Tower Peak, Buckeye Ridge*

see map on p.150

Highlights: Using two major eastside drainages, this trip circumnavigates Walker Mountain and Flatiron Ridge, and is about evenly split between high country and lower, forested areas. It's a great choice for novices with a couple of shorter trips behind them, who are looking for a longer trip with some of the challenge of cross-country travel.

HEADS UP! The cross-country segment of this trip is for experienced backpackers only.

Shuttle Directions: To access the take-out location at the Buckeye Campground from Hwy. 395 in Bridgeport, turn toward the Sierra on Twin Lakes Road near the town's north end and follow that road for 7 miles (avoid a turnoff left to Hunewill Guest Ranch) to a junction signed BUCKEYE CAMPGROUND. Turn right on the dirt road here and pass Doc and Al's Resort as you go 4 more miles to a T-junction with the dirt road just beyond Buckeye Creek. Turn left here and go 1.1 miles, passing through a USFS campground, to the end of the road. Alternatively, you could drive 3.8 miles north of Bridgeport on Hwy. 395 and then turn left on signed, dirt Buckeye Road; drive 6 miles, avoiding a dirt road on the right as you negotiate a hairpin turn, through the campground to the road's end.

DAY 1 (Leavitt Meadows Trailhead to Fremont Lake, 9 miles): *(Recap: Trip 41, Day 1.)* Cross the bridge over West Walker River and follow the main trail a quarter mile to a junction where you turn right (west) onto the West Walker River Trail—not on the topos but on the wilderness map. Descend to a snarl of use trails as well as your trail's continuation. Go left with the West Walker River Trail, which curves south and ascends gradually along the lower slopes of the ridge east of Leavitt Meadows. Continue ahead (south) at any junctions, including the one with the trail that crosses the meadow from the pack station. At about 1.75 miles, you meet a signed junction with a trail left to Secret and Poore lakes. Go ahead (south) to Roosevelt Lake, cross a low shoulder, and reach Lane Lake. Beyond, the trail eventually descends to the river's east bank and wanders south along it. At the signed turnoff right to Hidden and Red Top lakes, go ahead (south) and presently reach a wide spot where stock users go right to cross the river. Go ahead (south) to the signed east-side Fremont Lake Trail junction (7928'; 11S 277808 4236251) where you go right (west) to ford the river (very dangerous in early season; a serious wade at any time). Across the river, the trail curves briefly downstream to join the stock-users' trail. The trail immediately turns left (northwest) on the signed Fremont Lake Trail and switchbacks to a saddle. Descend to a signed junction with the trail left (south-southwest) to Chain of Lakes. Go ahead (northwest) and, in 100 yards, reach Fremont Lake with campsites at its south end (8243'; 11S 276852 4236745).

DAY 2 (Fremont Lake to Dorothy Lake, 9 miles): *(Partial Recap: Trip 42, Day 2.)* Return to the Chain of Lakes Trail junction and turn right (south-southwest) toward Chain of Lakes on an ascent that steepens as it crosses open slopes. Then descend to a junction with a signed trail left (northwest) to Walker Meadows. Go right (south-southwest), step across the Chain of Lakes' outlet, and arrive at the Chain of Lakes. Beyond the last and largest of the Chain of Lakes, ascend past a small, unnamed lake and a few yards past it, veer right (west and then south) around the north side of Lower Long Lake (campsites; more campsites at Upper Long Lake). The trail jogs around the northwest end of Upper Long Lake, fords its intermittent outlet stream, and meets a lateral to West Walker River. Turn right (northwest) past a picturesque tarn to West Fork West Walker River and a signed junction with the PCT and a lateral that almost parallels the northbound PCT. Go left (southwest) on the southbound PCT for a short way along the river's east side to a fork. Leave the PCT by taking the right fork southwest along the "river" (good campsites nearby). Climb along the southeast side of the stream before fording to the northwest side of the creek. Continue ascending to a signed junction; take the left fork southeast to Cinko Lake. Ford West Fork West Walker River and soon climb to the intermittent north outlet of Cinko Lake. The trail emerges next to the lake's north outlet (9212'; 11S 273454 4231779; campsites).

Leaving the Day 2 route of Trip 42, follow the trail along Cinko's north shore. *(Partial Recap: Trip 43, Day 2, from Cinko Lake to Dorothy Lake.)* From the southeast side of Cinko Lake, the trail winds down to an unnamed stream. Then it veers east away from the stream and descends to a lakelet. About 0.125 mile past the lake, you briefly touch the stream again before veering away. In another 0.125 mile, the trail crosses this persistent tributary on a wooden bridge and soon passes three tarns on the right. Continuing levelly through a tarn-filled saddle here, the trail curves northeast to meet the PCT again; turn right (southeast) on the PCT toward Dorothy Lake, shortly crossing a stream on a rickety bridge.

The PCT continues southeast and then south to a junction with a trail left (northwest) down nearby Cascade Creek to West Fork Walker River. You turn right (generally south) to stay on the PCT here; the west side of this trip's loop ends here, and it's now out and back to Dorothy Lake. Soon you ford Cascade Creek, climb away, and presently ford Lake Harriet's outlet. Beyond, the trail ascends more steeply, winds along Harriet's west shore and ascends tight switchbacks before leveling out to ford the stream joining Stella and Bonnie lakes. After another ascent, the trail levels past the north arm of Stella Lake. (At the northeast end of this arm, a ducked cross-country route to Lake Ruth and Lake Helen departs from your route.)

The trail presently reaches Dorothy Lake Pass (9528') and descends along the lake's north side to campsites on its west side (9397'; 11S 272782 4228362).

DAY 3 (Dorothy Lake to Tower Lake, 5 miles, part cross-country): *(Recap: Trip 44, Day 3.)* From the Dorothy Lake campsites, return on the PCT to Stella Lake, where there are multiple choices for going generally southeast to lakes Ruth and Helen and Tower Lake. One of them is a ducked cross-country route that rounds the northeast end of Stella Lake and then climbs over a rock-and-grass ledge system along the east side of the intermittent stream joining Stella Lake and Lake Ruth to arrive at the outlet end of Lake Ruth (excellent campsites). Continuing to Lake Helen, the route skirts the east side of the lake for a short distance and then ascends a long swale to the southeast. Several small tarns mark the crossover point to the Lake Helen drainage. Your route, keeping to the south side of Lake Helen, fords the tiny but noisy southwest inlet and then crosses the slope directly south of the lake. At the southeast inlet, the route fords and ascends moderately southeast to a bench. The remaining ascent to the obvious saddle in the southeast crosses steeper sections; possible routes may be better on the left (north) side of the cirque wall to a saddle.

Descending from the saddle on the southeast side, you cross rock and scree to a rocky bench, and from there a grass-and-ledge system to a lakelet just north of Tower Lake. The route then rounds the south nose of a granite ridge to Tower Lake's outlet and fords to the fair campsites centered in the only stand of timber found here on the east side of the outlet (9540'; 11S 276629 4226741).

DAY 4 (Tower Lake to Buckeye Forks, 9 miles): *(Partial Recap: Trip 44, Day 4, from Tower Lake to Upper Piute Meadows and the junction with Kirkwood Creek canyon's trail.)* Also on the east side of Tower Lake's outlet, you find an eastbound trail. Take this trail as it descends close to the north side of the outlet stream to a confluence with a stream from the glacier to the south. From here, bear generally north and descend on the outlet's east side as it becomes the named West Walker River and flows through Tower Canyon. Still descending, ford a nameless tributary and curve northward to ford West Walker River to its west side and climb above the narrows. A short descent brings you down to Upper Piute Meadows. Skirt the huge meadow on its west side, avoid the turnoff to Piute Cabin, ford the river, and reach a junction with a trail coming in sharply on your right from the south, a trail which has just descended Kirkwood Creek's canyon.

Leaving the Day 4 route of Trip 44, turn right (southeast) onto the Kirkwood Creek trail and ascend moderately through dense lodgepoles, passing below a spectacular avalanche chute. The ascent steepens as the trail turns east and then northeast along cascading Kirkwood Creek, which here offers some inviting pools. After a steep rise, you reach the saddle (9908') on the divide between the West Walker River and Buckeye Creek drainages; there are fine views of Hawksbeak Peak to the south and red and black volcanic slopes to the north.

The trail next descends moderately northeastward under sparse-to-moderate forest cover on duff and rock to the headwaters of North Fork Buckeye Creek, fording the streams a few times before curving east on the named creek's north shore. Camping may be found along the stream from here on. Then, in a final steep descent, the trail drops to Buckeye Forks (8423'; 11S 283366 4227850) where, near an old cabin, it meets the trail descending from Buckeye Pass to the south. There are good campsites near the old cabin, and fishing in Buckeye Creek is good for rainbow and eastern brook.

BUCKEYE FORKS CABIN

The old snow-survey cabin here—possibly the oldest US Snow Survey shelter—is of log-tenon construction and is believed to have been built in 1928. When built, the cabin was surrounded by open meadow; the ubiquitous lodgepole and willow have since overgrown the meadow. This dense growth is undoubtedly due to the nearby colony of beavers, which has repeatedly flooded this section between Buckeye Forks and the Roughs. The consequent buildup of sediments and the high-water table supported forest growth. However, what the beaver giveth, it also taketh away. If this dense forest were flooded again, these healthy trees would drown. That happened downstream, where the bleached, white, ghost snags are skeletal reminders of the beaver's role in the evolutionary web. After humans, beavers have the greatest single impact on the natural environment.

DAY 5 (Buckeye Forks to Buckeye Roadend, 9.4 miles): From the cabin, the trail continues to descend steadily over alternating duff, sand, and rock past beaver-gnawed and -felled aspen.

FLORA AND FAUNA

In spite of the beavers' appetite for aspen, the forest along the creek is dense, and it serves as a foraging grounds for all manner of birdlife, including flickers, chickadees, juncos, robins, Williamson's sapsuckers, hummingbirds, and nuthatches.

As the canyon narrows between high, glacially polished granite walls, the trail curves northeast and enters the Roughs. Here, the sometimes swampy trail winds along the left bank of Buckeye Creek, overshadowed by sheer, rounded granite to the north and polished spires to the south. Good campsites can be found in the Roughs. You presently make a steep ascent over black metasedimentary shale to a juniper-topped saddle and the boundary of Hoover Wilderness. Just beyond the saddle, views down Buckeye Canyon are spectacular: The lush grasslands of Big Meadow provide a soft counterpoint to the ruggedness of Flatiron and Buckeye ridges.

A few hundred steep yards down from the saddle, you ford a vigorous creek and then descend over a rocky, exposed slope on a long traverse. This steady descent is the last of the precipitous terrain, and the remainder of the walk is over long, gradual slopes covered with sagebrush, mountain mahogany, bitterbrush, and mule ears. Occasional clumps of aspen occur where the trail crosses a tributary or where it veers close to Buckeye Creek, and they provide welcome shade on a hot afternoon. In these well-watered sections, you'll see colorful clumps of monkeyflower, goldenrod, lupine, shooting star, paintbrush, and penstemon. Eventually, you reach Big Meadow, a charming 2-mile-long grassland full of Belding ground squirrels and morning-feeding deer.

BACK IN 1870...

At one time, around 1870, this meadow rang with the sounds of axes and the whirring of a sawmill blade. Here, the Upper Hunewill mill operated to provide mining timber. Near the fence at the bottom of the meadow, the observant passerby can make out the signs of an abortive effort to construct a flume to carry water from Buckeye Creek to Bodie.

You pass through a gate in a fence at the bottom of the meadow and immediately head right, downhill, to ford Buckeye Creek (difficult in early season). From the creek, the trail leads up a small ridge and then undulates over several more ridges, generally within sight of the stream. Beyond a viewpoint for seeing a beaver dam, the trail traverses a hillside clothed in head-high aspen trees and flowers (in season), including scarlet gilia. After crossing two little rills, you can look through the trees and down to another large meadow, which you skirt on a level trail under aspen, juniper, red fir, and lodgepole pine trees. About a half mile farther, you cross an unmapped stream that flows late into summer. Soon the trail becomes an abandoned, two-track road, and you stroll through a sagebrush field squeezed between the lodgepole pines that border the creek and a large stand of aspen trees on the nose of a ridge that protrudes onto the canyon bottom.

The next section of trail passes through alternating green meadows and gray sagebrush fields, with constant good views of the towering north and south walls of Buckeye Canyon. Past one last, fairly large meadow, you come to a fence with both a hikers' gate and a stock gate. Here you begin the last mile of this five-day journey under Jeffrey and ponderosa pines, red firs, and quaking aspens. This last mile is a gentle downhill stroll that ends at the parking lot at Buckeye Campground's west end (7230'; 11S 294180 4234456).

STATE HIGHWAY 120 TRIPS

No trans-Sierra highway offers as many delightful trailheads as does Hwy. 120, largely because it crosses through Yosemite National Park. It's no surprise, then, that the scenery along trips from Hwy. 120 is simply spectacular. From west to east, we present trips from these trailheads: Hetch Hetchy, White Wolf, Tenaya Lake, Cathedral Lakes, Elizabeth Lake (Tuolumne Meadows Campground), Lembert Dome, Lyell Canyon-PCT/JMT, Mono Pass, and Saddlebag Lake. All are in Yosemite except for the last.

Each trailhead is unique: Hetch Hetchy, the lowest, is best in early season when its waterfalls are at their fullest. White Wolf, the westernmost of the high trailheads along 120, is a gateway to the Grand Canyon of the Tuolumne River. Tenaya Lake offers quick access to the scenic backcountry around Sunrise Mountain. Cathedral Lakes is a very popular way to pick up the northernmost section of the JMT to those lakes and beyond to enjoy some lovely meadow and forest scenery. Elizabeth Lake leads to that lake and, better yet, to a beautiful cross-country jaunt to a lake in the heart of the Cathedral Range. Lembert Dome is the door to a busy section of the PCT as well as to three secluded lakes far from the PCT's traffic. Lyell Canyon-PCT/JMT serves not only those bustling trails but also trails leading to what many consider Yosemite's most spectacular and wild backcountry. From Mono Pass, backpackers can turn away from that pass and exit Yosemite via a lightly used route into a splendid lakes basin in Ansel Adams Wilderness. Saddlebag Lake, lying just east of Yosemite, offers an easy way into a charming little lakes basin as well as to cross-country adventures from that basin into Yosemite.

It's no wonder that aspiring backpackers from all over the world flock to 120!

TRAILHEADS: Hetch Hetchy
White Wolf
Tenaya Lake
Cathedral Lakes
Elizabeth Lake
Lembert Dome
Lyell Canyon-PCT/JMT
Mono Pass
Saddlebag Lake

HWY 120

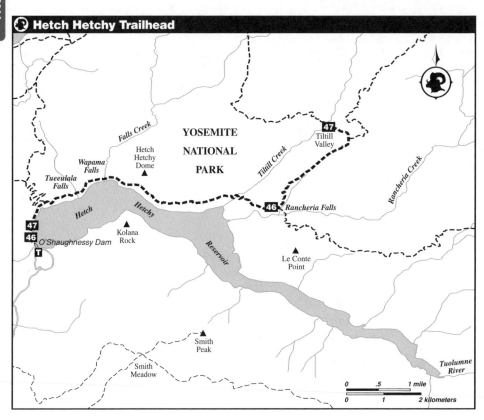

Hetch Hetchy Trailhead

YOSEMITE
NATIONAL
PARK

Falls Creek

Hetch
Hetchy
Dome

Wapama
Falls

Tueeulala
Falls

Tiltill Creek

Tiltill
Valley

47

Rancheria Creek

46   Rancheria Falls

Hetch   Hetchy

47
46   O'Shaughnessy Dam
1

Kolana
Rock

Reservoir

Le Conte
Point

Smith
Peak

Tuolumne
River

Smith
Meadow

0   .5   1 mile
0   1   2 kilometers

Hetch Hetchy Trailhead

3813'; UTM 11S 255088 4203527

DESTINATION/ UTM COORDINATES	TRIP TYPE	BEST SEASON	PACE (HIKING/ LAYOVER DAYS)	TOTAL MILEAGE
46 Rancheria Creek 11S 261587 4204361	Out & back	Early	2/0 Leisurely	13
47 Tiltill Valley 11S 263106 4206554	Out & back	Early	4/0 Leisurely	18.6

Information and Permits: These trips enter Yosemite National Park: Yosemite Permits, PO Box 545, Yosemite National Park, CA 95389; 209-372-0740; www.nps.gov/yose/wilderness/permits.htm. Bear canisters are required; pets and firearms are prohibited.

Driving Directions: Your first goal is to get to Evergreen Lodge. Eastbound, take Hwy. 120 (Tioga Road) east toward Yosemite's Big Oak Flat entrance station, to the junction with Evergreen Road, just outside the park and just north of the entrance station. Turn right and follow Evergreen Road east and then north about 6.6 miles to Evergreen Lodge. Westbound, take Hwy. 120 to Evergreen Road, just before Yosemite's Big Oak Flat entrance station, and turn left. Follow Evergreen Road about 6.6 miles to Evergreen Lodge.

From the lodge, continue on Evergreen Road north to its junction with the Hetch Hetchy Road by Camp Mather (private). Bear right on Hetch Hetchy Road and into Yosemite National Park. Follow the narrow, winding road to its end at a large roadend loop with parking at its north end, by O'Shaughnessy Dam, 9.5 miles from Evergreen Lodge.

46 Rancheria Creek

Trip Data: 11S 261587 4204361; 13 miles; 2/0 days

Topos: *Hetch Hetchy Reservoir*, Hetch Hetchy Reservoir, Lake Eleanor

Highlights: Eager opening-day anglers will find good fishing along Rancheria Creek. Beautiful 25-foot Rancheria Falls tumbles into large, inviting pools—a great end to a fine trip.

DAY 1 (Hetch Hetchy Trailhead to Rancheria Creek, 6.5 miles): From the trailhead at the south end of the dam (3813'), cross this 600-foot-long piece of concrete and immediately plunge into a quarter-mile-long, poorly lit tunnel. Although 8 miles of the Grand Canyon of the Tuolumne River were put under a reservoir for the sake of San Francisco's water supply, the actual intake for the aqueduct is 17 miles downstream in a relatively ordinary part of the canyon.

The first 0.7 mile of the route is on the now closed, badly deteriorated service road to Lake Eleanor (part of San Francisco's water project). Upon leaving the tunnel, the road winds along the hillside above Hetch Hetchy's high-water mark. Views across the water include, from the left, seasonal Tueeulala (twee-LAH-lah) Falls, Wapama Falls, Hetch Hetchy Dome, and Kolana Rock. Soon the road begins a gentle, shaded ascent through canyon live oak, incense-cedar, Douglas fir, California bay, California grape, big leaf maple, and poison oak.

At a junction, turn right (northeast) onto the signed trail to Rancheria Creek (the left fork climbs eventually to Laurel Lake). Now there are Digger pines and live oaks for shade. The trail winds along a sunny bench where glacial polish and glacial erratics remind you that at times during the Pleistocene Epoch glaciers up to 60 miles long—the longest in the Sierra—flowed down this canyon.

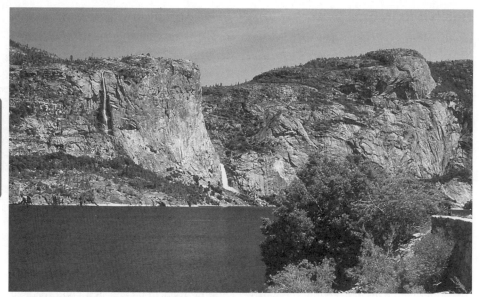

Hetch Hetchy Reservoir (foreground); Tueeulala Falls (left); Wapama Falls (center)

After crossing Tueeulala Falls's creek, you descend some 100 feet of granite stairs to the bridges over Falls Creek. During high runoff, the bridges may be under water. In early season, vast, crashing Wapama Falls will cover these bridges with spray.

Beyond the creek, the fly-infested trail climbs an impressive granite dome onto a meadowy ledge system where you have an airy view of the water below. In spring, wildflowers dot the meadows here and you can see monkeyflower, paintbrush, and Sierra onion. This hike usually boasts a great variety of wildlife, and animals commonly seen include alligator lizard, Steller jay, and California ground squirrel.

Past the ledges, the trail makes a long descent and crosses Tiltill Creek on a bridge. Here, the creek tumbles down its gorge 60 feet below you. From here you climb onto the low ridge separating Tiltill Creek and Rancheria Creek. About 0.75 mile beyond the bridge, the trail enters a shaded flat where you reach a junction where the main trail forks left (north) toward Tiltill and Pate valleys, and where you turn right (south-southeast) onto a spur trail to streamside campsites a quarter mile below Rancheria Falls (4520'; 11S 261587 4204361). The falls drop 25 feet into deep, swirling pools. Fishing in Rancheria Creek is poor to good for rainbow trout.

DAY 2 (Rancheria Creek to Hetch Hetchy Trailhead, 6.5 miles): Retrace your steps.

47 Tiltill Valley

Trip Data: 11S 263106 4206554;
18.6 miles; 4/0 days

Topos: *Hetch Hetchy Reservoir*, Lake Eleanor,
Hetch Hetchy Reservoir

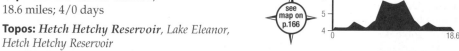

Highlights: This route tours the northern edge of Hetch Hetchy Reservoir. Across the lake, the views of Kolana Rock and the sheer granite walls of the Grand Canyon of the Tuolumne are majestic, contrasting pleasantly with the intimate serenity of Tiltill Valley.

DAY 1 (Hetch Hetchy Trailhead to Rancheria Creek, 6.5 miles): *(Recap: Trip 46, Day 1.)* Follow the road and then trail along Hetch Hetchy Reservoir, and at a junction, go ahead (generally east); the left fork goes north to Laurel Lake. Your trail takes you over Falls and Tiltill creeks. At a junction about 0.75 mile from the bridge over Tiltill Creek, turn right (south-southeast) down the spur trail to camping (4520'; 11S 261587 4204361) on Rancheria Creek.

DAY 2 (Rancheria Creek to Tiltill Valley, 2.8 miles): Return up the spur trail to the junction with the main trail. Turn right (north) and begin climbing the main trail, soon reaching the next junction, where the trail to Tiltill Valley goes left (switchbacking northward) to continue the climb, and the Pate Valley Trail goes right (generally east). Go left here. The trail to Tiltill Valley climbs steeply for a full 1200 feet up to a timber-bottomed saddle. As the trail descends on the north side of the saddle, it traverses a pine forest with a sprinkling of incense cedar and black oak.

This duff trail emerges at the east end of Tiltill Valley, a long meadow that, in early spring, is usually quite wet and boggy at the east end. You may not even notice a tributary of Tiltill Creek that's shown on the topo, as well as a "ford" of it. Lodgepole pine fringes the meadow, and the valley is flanked by polished outcroppings of granite and by brush-covered slopes. Just beyond the "tributary ford," you may spot a junction where one fork goes ahead (north) to Lake Vernon and the other goes right (east) on a rarely used route to Tiltill Meadow and eventually to the PCT.

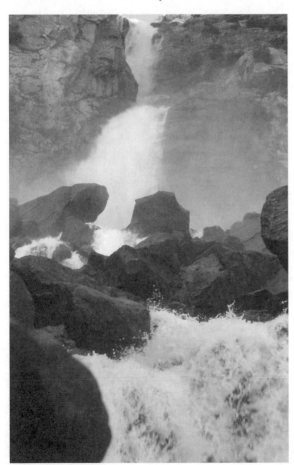

Go ahead across the meadow toward the base of Tiltill Valley's towering north wall, curve west, and find the excellent campsites just south of the Tiltill Creek ford (5600'; 11S 263106 4206554). These camping places, located in an isolated stand of lodgepole and sugar pine, afford excellent views in both directions down the meadows. Campers have an uninterrupted vantage point from which to watch the large variety of wildlife that make this meadow their home. Fishing for rainbow in Tiltill Creek is excellent in early season.

DAYS 3–4 (Tiltill Valley to Hetch Hetchy Trailhead, 9.3 miles): Retrace your steps.

Wapama Falls

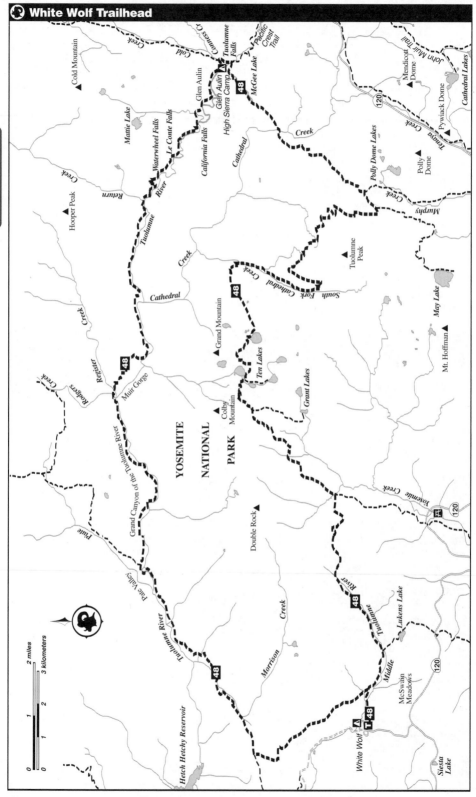

HWY 120

White Wolf Trailhead
7875'; 11S 267002 4194683

DESTINATION/ UTM COORDINATES	TRIP TYPE	BEST SEASON	PACE (HIKING/ LAYOVER DAYS)	TOTAL MILEAGE
48 Grand Canyon of the Tuolumne 11S 278985 4201207	Loop	Early to late	6/1 Moderate	50

Information and Permits: These trips enter Yosemite National Park: Yosemite Permits, PO Box 545, Yosemite National Park, CA 95389; 209-372-0740; www.nps.gov/yose/wilderness/permits.htm. Bear canisters are required; pets and firearms are prohibited.

Driving Directions: Just 32.3 miles west of Tioga Pass on Hwy. 120 is the signed turnoff to White Wolf Lodge and Campground, on the north side of the road. Follow this spur road 1.1 miles to parking opposite White Wolf Lodge, just before the campground entrance.

48 Grand Canyon of the Tuolumne

Trip Data: 11S 278985 4201207; 50 miles; 6/1 days

see map on p.170

Topos: *Hetch Hetchy Reservoir, Tuolumne Meadows, Tamarack Flat, Hetch Hetchy Reservoir, Ten Lakes, Falls Ridge, Tenaya Lake*

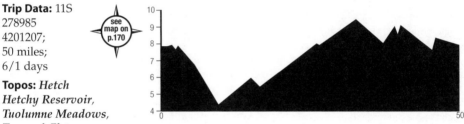

Highlights: In taking this trip, you'll experience firsthand what the mighty Tuolumne River has created over tens of millions of years. The trip's highest and lowest points are more than 5600 vertical feet apart! If you have only a couple of days, an out-and-back trip based on Day 1 of this trip, as far as Morrison Creek, makes an easy weekender with a fine view of the canyon.

HEADS UP! *Bears are serious problems along this route. If the preceding winter was a heavy one, this trip may be hazardous in early season because of high water and hazardous at any time if needed bridges have been swept away by high runoff. By late season in a dry year, the pond at the end of Day 4 may be dry.*

DAY 1 (White Wolf Trailhead to Pate Valley, 9.5 miles): Just opposite White Wolf Lodge, the trail begins by skirting the south side of White Wolf Campground. Avoid the many use trails from the campground and head generally east on a gradual ascent through lodgepole pines. After crossing seasonal Middle Tuolumne River, you reach a signed junction: ahead (east) to Lukens Lake; left (northwest) on your route. It's here that you begin the loop part of this trip.

Turning left, you continue almost levelly to eventually cross a nearly imperceptible ridge. Now descending, the trail follows a lush creek to a beautiful, forest-fringed meadow. After skirting this meadow, the route climbs gently for an easy mile to a more open, distinctive ridgetop. Here, you stand on the crest of a moraine that was deposited by a glacier that once flowed down the Grand Canyon of the Tuolumne.

From here, you begin descending a slope that eventually leads to the bottom of the canyon. On the way, you avoid a lateral left (west) to Harden Lake and continue ahead (north-northeast). At first you cannot see the canyon, as the trail crosses several more lateral-moraine crests. As you lose altitude, the forest cover changes rapidly: Lodgepole pine and red fir soon give way to western white pine, Sierra juniper, and Jeffrey pine.

As the grade steepens and the forest cover thins, you get your first views across the canyon. Where the trail crosses some glacially polished bedrock, you can take a break and consider that ice once filled this canyon to this height—and more—during the ice ages of the Pleistocene Epoch. Continuing into denser forest again, you meet incense cedar, white fir, and quaking aspen, which indicates a locally high water table. After many switchbacks, the route meets a signed junction with another trail west to Harden Lake.

Turn right (east-northeast) and continue descending along a forested slope where you catch views of broad Rancheria Mountain across the canyon to the north. Along this section, you meet more lower-elevation trees, including black oak, sugar pine, and, near an unmarked creek, some alder. Soon you can hear Morrison Creek to the right as you cross a densely forested bench, where a plank bridge helps keep your feet dry. A little beyond, the forest cover opens, and just south of a bedrock granite ridge, there are good campsites near the creek—your goal if you're doing a weekender out-and-back trip to Morrison Creek.

Leaving the Morrison Creek campsites, you soon begin the final plunge to the bottom of the Grand Canyon of the Tuolumne, still more than 2000 feet below. At first, the trail descends steeply on switchbacks beside Morrison Creek, through white fir, incense cedar, sugar pine, and dogwood. After dropping about 500 feet, the trail veers north and views open up dramatically.

At 5700 feet, you cross a bench where you can stop for serious views of this phenomenal canyon, including Hetch Hetchy. You can camp here as long as Morrison Creek flows nearby (usually through midsummer). As you descend, the flora continues to change rapidly and includes canyon live oak and, where you cross now seasonal Morrison Creek, incense-cedars and black oaks.

The last 1500 feet to the bottom are mostly across exposed slopes where the very steep trail is often cobblestoned with wedge-shaped rocks intricately fitted together to form a staircase of various-sized steps. Along this breathtaking descent you can see and hear the Tuolumne River far below. At 5000 feet, the trail crosses an unmapped seasonal creek channel which is also an avalanche chute in the winter. Five hundred feet lower, you cross another mapped seasonal creek. Both of these creeks can be dangerous torrents when runoff is high. At 4400 feet, the grade levels briefly, and you pass a moraine-dammed pond

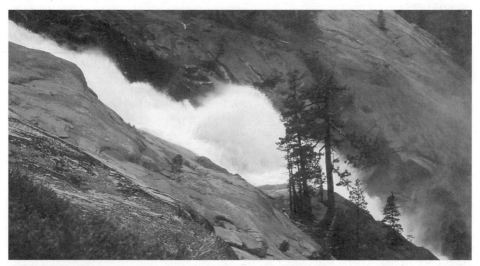

In early season, Waterwheel Falls stops Day 3's travelers in their tracks.

before entering tall forest again. Another 200-foot descent brings you to the canyon floor at Pate Valley, where there are campsites near the river (4225; 11S 269819 4200488).

If you'd like to camp in grander forest away from the burned area, continue up-canyon, and in 1 to 1.5 gentle miles, before the first bridge over the river, you'll find several excellent campsites in a cathedral forest of tall incense-cedars, white firs, and ponderosa pines.

DAY 2 (Pate Valley to Tuolumne Canyon, 7 miles): Today's journey takes you deep into the Grand Canyon of the Tuolumne—the less-traveled stretch from Pate Valley to Waterwheel Falls. Not only is this the least-traveled section upriver, it's also through the narrowest and deepest part of the canyon.

Assuming you didn't go upriver to forested campsites at the end of Day 1, the level trail continues upriver over 1.5 miles to cross one and then another channel of the river via bridges; the short section between these two bridges can flood in a very wet year. Once on the north side of the river, which you'll stay on until Glen Aulin, you enter another burned area and come to a junction with the Pleasant Valley Trail (left). Turning right (generally east) onto the trail leading upriver, you pass through a brief, narrow, marshy part of the valley.

> **WHY THE MARSH?**
> Perhaps bedrock, acting like an underground dam, has forced groundwater near the surface here to produce a lush, muddy area. Though it's too wet for trees, many species of water-loving flowers and shrubs thrive here, including cow parsnip and rushes.

Beyond, the trail returns to the river for a while, and you cross a short section of cobblestones set in cement to withstand flooding. You may need to wade this section, which may be dangerous in early season after a wet winter. If you find it unsafe, turn back.

More gentle ascending brings you to another older, burned area where the fire was hot enough to burn large trees as well as the ground cover. Just beyond this area, you come to some fantastically large and deep pools in the bedrock—a fine swimming and fishing spot. From here, the canyon narrows, and the trail stays close to the river for a mile that includes some spots where you may have to wade during high water.

This beautiful, shady stretch of canyon gives way to a wider, sunnier valley that is very deep. Partway through this valley, the trail climbs away from the river, up an open slope. Near the climb's start is a stately campsite just downstream from a large pool at the base of some wide slabs in the river. You'll find a number of reptiles in the canyon's drier areas, like these open slopes. The most common is the blue-bellied Western fence lizard, though there are a variety of snakes in the canyon, including a few rattlesnakes.

After nearly 2 miles, the canyon again narrows as you approach Muir Gorge. Named after a man who eagerly sought out inaccessible places, Muir Gorge is the only part of the canyon whose walls are too steep for a trail, so you're obliged to climb around it. Beyond two live-oak-shaded campsites, the trail begins climbing well above the river, and at one point you can look straight up the dark chasm of Muir Gorge.

The trail crosses Rodgers Canyon's creek on a bridge and then adjacent Register Creek on another bridge. The route then briefly heads up the side canyon of Register Creek before climbing south over a low, shady ridge. After a short descent, you switchback steeply up for 500 feet to a granite ridge. It is well worth a short detour to peer down into mysterious Muir Gorge.

The descent back to the river is mostly shady, and the canyon again widens above Muir Gorge. Where granite slabs come down to the river, the trail can be wet in early season, though climbing above high water is easy. In another quarter mile, you come to a seasonal stream channel in white gravel. Between the trail and the river there's an excellent campsite (about 5500'; near 11S 278985 4201207).

DAY 3 (Tuolumne Canyon to McGee Lake, 9.5 miles): Like the first day, this day is a long one, and if you break it up into two days, you could take more time to be near the water-falls upriver. The ascent is gentle for about a mile until the canyon again narrows, and you approach close under the looming south wall above. Nearing the base of this cliff, you pass some seasonally flooded campsites before beginning a steeper section of the canyon. The last Douglas fir and bay laurel fall behind as you climb alongside the river for about a mile.

When the canyon again widens, you're in dense forest on a flat away from the river. Another half mile brings you into the open, close to the river, and you pass some low falls that barely hint at the awesome features to come. Soon you bridge Return Creek and quick-ly begin climbing again. Waterwheel Falls loom above, and, in early season, these falls are at their best: thunderous and spectacular as protrusions in the granite throw wheeling sprays of water far out into the air. Don't be in a hurry, because these falls are best viewed from below, and on a hot day, you'll appreciate their cooling spray as you begin to climb the steep switchbacks up and around the falls. Waterwheel Falls are in dayhiking range on Hwy. 120 for sturdy hikers, and your solitude will temporarily end here.

The trail returns to the river just above the brink of the falls and climbs behind a low bedrock ridge for about a quarter mile to an open, juniper-dotted slope. Beyond, the trail again steepens as you climb past a short lateral trail to Le Conte Falls, which are well worth getting close, but not too close, to. Leaving behind the last cedars and sugar pines, the trail becomes increasingly steep and sunny until you come close under the massive south but-tress of Wildcat Point.

The grade eases before you reach California Falls. A relatively short climb brings you near the top of these, the third and lowest of the three major falls below Glen Aulin. Glen Aulin itself, through which you soon pass, has suffered from fire, and the many dead-and-ready-to-topple trees make it dangerous for camping.

CYCLES OF NATURE

Where the trail swings close to the river, there is one unburned area. Nature continues her cycles here, as fire is a regular player in the ecology of Sierra forests. You can see the timely succession of plant and animal species. Aspen is quick to grow back because, unlike conifers, it can resprout from the crown of its roots; therefore, aspen is an early-successional plant species, while firs, which need shade to grow, are late-successional trees.

After more than a mile of level ground, you leave Glen Aulin proper while skirting between a granite slope and the river and then climb briefly to a junction with the PCT/TYT. Turn right (south) on the PCT/TYT and almost immediately meet a spur trail left (east) that crosses Conness Creek on a bridge to Glen Aulin High Sierra Camp. There's a backpackers' campground with piped water and bear boxes next to the camp, and you may be able to reserve a meal at the camp's dining room (check at the office, which also has a small store). If someone in your party needs help, this is the place to stop and get it as long as the camp is open.

Staying on the PCT/TYT, you cross the Tuolumne River on a bridge in a few more yards. White Cascade plummets into a large pool just east of the bridge, and occasionally the trail just beyond the bridge is flooded but easily negotiable. Leaving the river, you climb, sometimes on slabs where the trail is hard to follow, to a junction where the PCT/TYT turns left (southeast) and you turn right (southwest) onto the signed May Lake Trail. Now in forest, the grade is easy, and soon you come to the northeast end of peaceful McGee Lake. The more secluded campsites at this lake are at its southwest end (8112'; 11S 286107 4197620). McGee Lake has outlets at either end and thus drains into both the Tuolumne River and Cathedral Creek.

DAY 4 (McGee Lake to Tuolumne Peak Ridge, 6.5 miles): From the northwest end of McGee Lake, the trail descends southwest to cross the southwest outlet of McGee Lake and then Cathedral Creek. Though a seasonal stream, Cathedral Creek can be a wet ford in early season. From Cathedral Creek, you begin climbing, steeply at first and then more gently, as you bear south-southwest and cross a low ridge. Continuing south-southwest, the mostly shady trail ascends gently for more than a mile to a junction with the Murphy Creek Trail (left, south), 2.5 miles from Cathedral Creek.

MURPHY CREEK TRAIL AND POLLY DOME LAKES

From this trip's route, this trail descends for about 3 miles generally south along Murphy Creek and past the swampy Polly Dome Lakes to the signed trailhead on Hwy. 120 across from Tenaya Lake. If someone in your party needs to bail out, this is probably the first good place to do so since Day 1. There is camping on the west side of the largest Polly Dome Lake (Lake 8714), under Polly Dome's north face, about a half mile cross-country southeast when you leave the Murphy Creek Trail at a trailside pond on your left as you descend.

Turning right (west and then southwest) away from the Murphy Creek Trail, the trail goes another level half mile to a junction with the trail to May Lake, where you again turn right (southwest). After heading southwest for another quarter mile, the route bends north and begins climbing the lower eastern slopes of Tuolumne Peak. At first, the ascent is gentle and the views are minimal, but as you gain altitude, both the grade and the views increase until you reach the northeast ridge of Tuolumne Peak at a first and then a second high point. Just below to the west is a small pond, and a short descent brings you to it (9822'; 11S 282285 4195642).

ENJOYING THE VIEWS

This ridgetop marks the highest point of the trip, at almost 9900 feet. To the east, beyond Tuolumne Meadows, rises the Sierra Crest; to the south of the meadows stands the ice-sculpted Cathedral Range; to the north, the Grand Canyon of the Tuolumne lies hidden behind Falls Ridge; and to the northeast is the massive, white southwest face of Mt. Conness.

Even more impressive views can be found by climbing partway up Tuolumne Peak. Centrally located in almost the middle of Yosemite National Park, and higher than any other point around here except Mt. Hoffman, Tuolumne Peak offers some of the most comprehensive views in the entire park.

DAY 5 (Tuolumne Peak Ridge to Ten Lakes, 6.5 miles): This area north of Tuolumne Peak is probably the least-traveled part of this loop, and if your speed and energy permit, you may want to linger here.

Leaving the pond heading west and then northwest, the winding trail climbs up and down for more than a mile to an overlook above South Fork Cathedral Creek's canyon. The trail then switchbacks down to the west, contours south, and switchbacks west again, into the canyon.

Turning north, you descend along the east side of the creek for 2 miles to a seasonally wet ford and continue heading north briefly before turning west to climb out of the creek's canyon. As you switchback up this open slope, you can see down into the deep canyon of Cathedral Creek and beyond to the north side of the much deeper Grand Canyon of the Tuolumne. Where the slope eases, the trail enters forest again. After a mile, the trail begins heading down, and soon you reach the northeast shore of the easternmost and largest of the Ten Lakes, Lake 9398 (9424'; 11S 279163 4197756). Good campsites can be found on the north and west sides of the lake.

(Note that the next and final day is a very long one, and you may wish to continue to the lower Ten Lakes as described for Day 6 before stopping.)

DAY 6 (Ten Lakes to White Wolf Trailhead, 11 miles): Today, the last day, is a very long and demanding one. Heading northwest from the easternmost of the Ten Lakes, the route is nearly level for a half mile before turning southwest to descend to the south shore of the large, most popular, western Ten Lake (campsites; last reliable water before a creek crossing past Half Moon Meadow).

Just west of this lake, the trail meets a lateral left (south) to the higher, southwestern Ten Lakes (quieter campsites). Your trail continues ahead (northwest) and then crosses their outlet. Soon you begin a switchbacking climb 600 feet to the broad ridge on the west side of Ten Lakes Basin. As you cross the top of this gently sloping upland at Ten Lakes Pass, you have extensive views in most directions, providing you with a final overview of the Tuolumne River drainage.

Descending southwest, the grade is at first gentle as you go right (west) at a junction with the Grant Lakes Trail on the left (south). Soon, however, the trail becomes steep and switchbacking until you reach the north side of Half Moon Meadow. The trail skirts the meadow's north side before continuing to descend southwest, crossing a creek about 0.75 mile from Half Moon Meadow's north side; this creek, a tributary of Yosemite Creek, may provide the first water since Ten Lakes in late season. Continue the generally southwestern descent; the grade eases briefly as the trail makes a short northwest jog, and then you resume your descent for another 1.5 miles. Just beyond a small creek (another Yosemite Creek tributary; may be dry by late season), you leave the Ten Lakes Trail and turn right (generally west) toward White Wolf.

> **VISITING TEN LAKES AND GRANT LAKES FROM HWY. 120**
>
> If you go ahead (south) here on the Ten Lakes Trail, you'll descend into the valley of Yosemite Creek for about 2.25 often exposed miles, sometimes steeply and always far from the creek, before leveling out as you approach a small, unsigned, dirt parking lot on the north side of Hwy. 120. On the other side of the highway is the paved turnout and signed trailhead for the Yosemite Creek Trail. Both lots are just west of the highway bridge over Yosemite Creek. You can make a trip from Hwy. 120 to extremely popular Ten Lakes by reversing the directions in this sidebar as far as the junction with the trail to White Wolf and then reversing the Day 6, Ten Lakes to White Wolf, description above. The main lake of the Ten Lakes (Lake 8947) is unbelievably overused. You'll find quieter camping at Lake 9021, southwest of Lake 8947, or the easternmost lake, Lake 9398, the destination of Day 5 of the loop trip. Or visit slightly less popular Grant Lakes by taking the Grant Lakes lateral at Ten Lakes Pass for about a mile south and down to lower Grant Lake.

Heading for White Wolf and ascending gently to moderately, the trail climbs 1.5 miles to a forested ridge. Here you enter the drainage of the Middle Tuolumne River and begin the last descent. Heading down through a quiet forest of lodgepole pine and red fir, the trail soon crosses the headwaters of the Middle Tuolumne River and then follows it southwest along a very gentle slope.

After 2 miles near the river, you meet the popular Lukens Lake Trail coming in on the left. Go ahead (west) for a nearly level mile to meet the trail to Pate Valley on your right (northwest) to close the loop. It's now just an easy mile back to the road and civilization at White Wolf Trailhead (7875'; 11S 267002 4194683).

Tenaya Lake Trailhead

8150'; 11S 282465 4189314

T

DESTINATION/ UTM COORDINATES	TRIP TYPE	BEST SEASON	PACE (HIKING/ LAYOVER DAYS)	TOTAL MILEAGE
49 Sunrise High Sierra Camp 11S 285820 4185899	Out & back	Mid or late	2/1 Leisurely	11.4
50 Yosemite Valley– Happy Isles Trailhead 11S 274550 4179235	Shuttle	Mid or late	2/1 Moderate	17.3

HWY 120

Information and Permits: These trips enter Yosemite National Park: Yosemite Permits, PO Box 545, Yosemite National Park, CA 95389; 209-372-0740; www.nps.gov/yose/wilderness/permits.htm. Bear canisters are required; pets and firearms are prohibited.

Driving Directions: Just 15.8 miles west of Hwy. 120's Tioga Pass and just past the west end of Tenaya Lake, there is a signed trailhead on the south side of the road at a turnout with a small parking lot and a toilet. The trail starts at a closed, gated road.

49 Sunrise High Sierra Camp

Trip Data: 11S 285820 4185899; 11.4 miles; 2/1 days

Topos: *Tenaya Lake*

Highlights: This trip follows very popular trails, but the breathtaking scenery you enjoy along the route more than makes up for the lack of solitude.

see map on p.178

HEADS UP! The 7.5' Tenaya Lake *topo shows a campground between this trailhead and Tenaya Lake's southwest shore. This campground is closed.*

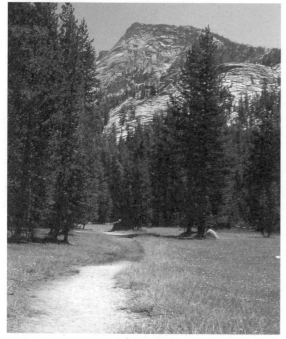

Tenaya Peak as seen early in the trip

DAY 1 (Tenaya Lake Trailhead to Sunrise High Sierra Camp, 5.7 miles): Walk about 150 feet down the road east to a marked trail on your right, turn right (northeast) briefly to the edge of a flowery meadow, and find a trail junction: right (southwest) to May Lake; left (east) to Sunrise Lakes. Go left on this trail, the Forsyth Trail, soon crossing Tenaya Lake's outlet and curving right (south) at a sign. At 0.2 mile, you reach a junction where you go right (south-southwest) toward Sunrise High Sierra Camp, briefly paralleling the outlet before veering left in an area of slabs. Beyond, you begin a rocky, gradual-to-moderate climb to a spot offering views of Sunrise Mountain, Clouds Rest, and several granite domes.

From the viewpoint, the trail descends into a bouldery wash,

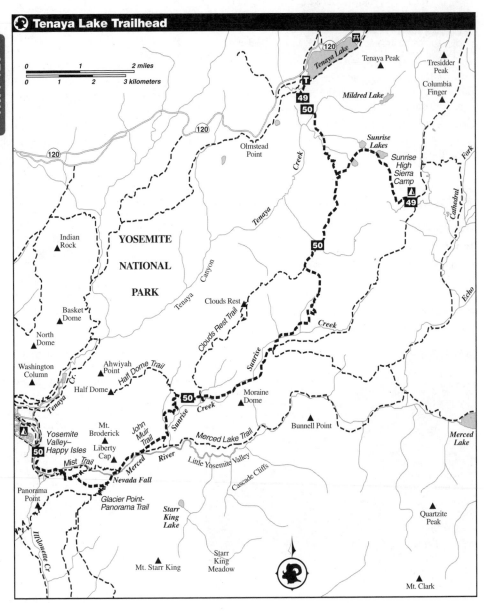

Tenaya Lake Trailhead

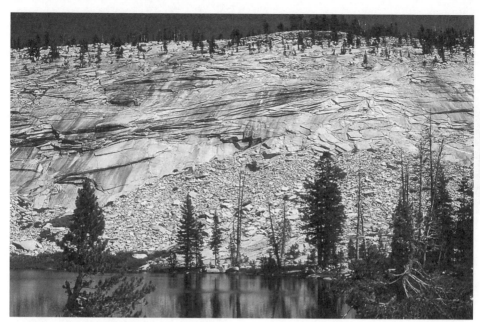

Exfoliating dome above Lower Sunrise Lake

tops a low rise, and crosses the multi-stranded outlet of Mildred Lake at nearly 1.25 miles. Now the path begins a moderate-to-steep ascent in forest, fording several more streams (may be dry by late season) before beginning a steep, exposed, view-rich, switchbacking slog up Sunrise Mountain.

ABOUT THE SCENERY

To the south, notice the long, gradual slope falling from Clouds Rest. This slope is a 4500-foot drop, one of the largest continuous rock slopes in the world.

Roughly southwest of this climb is Tenaya Canyon. The Indian name for Tenaya Creek, *Py-wi-ack* ("Stream of the Shining Rocks"), is apt, for this canyon exhibits the largest exposed granite area in Yosemite, and its shining surfaces are barren except for sporadic clumps of hardy conifers that have found root in broken talus pockets.

As spectacular as the view is, be sure to enjoy the dozens of wildflower species that seasonally grow on the slopes you're climbing, among them pussypaws, penstemon, paintbrush, lupine, streptanthus, aster, larkspur, brodiaea, and buttercup.

Eventually, mountain hemlocks close in around the trail, restricting views but offering welcome shade. Finally the switchbacks end, and the trail levels on a welcome saddle as it arrives at a signed junction (9224'; 11S 283538 4186577) with the trail to Sunrise High Sierra Camp.

Turning left (east), you leave the Forsyth Trail and stroll on a nearly level path under a sparse forest cover of pine and fir until the trail dips for about a quarter mile to the first Sunrise Lake.

After passing the west side of the lake on a trail fringed with red mountain heather, you cross the outlet and ascend gradually northeast. Then the trail levels off and wanders roughly north through a sparse lodgepole forest. The second Sunrise Lake comes into view on the left, but you veer east and climb away from it, paralleling its inlet some distance from the cascading water. The few trees here are not enough to block the views of granite domes all around. Then the trail skirts the south side of the meadow-fringed highest Sunrise Lake and begins a gradual ascent by crossing the lake's inlet stream.

Continuing southeast, you cross a little saddle and descend gradually almost straight south from the upper lake. After passing most of the hogback lying east of you, you swing northeast and switchback down to a bench overlooking spacious Long Meadow (may be dry late in the year). There are fair campsites here. It's possible to reserve a meal at adjacent Sunrise High Sierra Camp; do this at its office/store.

DAY 2 (Sunrise High Sierra Camp to Tenaya Lake Trailhead, 5.7 miles): Retrace your steps.

50 Yosemite Valley–Happy Isles Trailhead

Trip Data: 11S 274550 4179235; 17.3 miles; 2/1 days

Topos: *Yosemite, Tenaya Lake, Merced Peak, Half Dome*

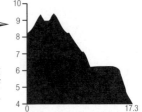

Highlights: Along an elevation change of more than 5000 feet (mostly downhill), this route covers most of Yosemite's life zones and adds to the scenery of the preceding trip, Tenaya Lake to Sunrise High Sierra Camp, the beauty of the Merced River with its quiet, winding stretches, slides, cascades, and earth-shaking waterfalls.

Shuttle Directions: You cannot drive to the take-out Happy Isles Trailhead, but you can leave a car in Curry Village and take a shuttle to and from there. Whether you drive from the west or the east, get to the junction of highways 140 and 120 in Yosemite Valley. On what is now the Yosemite Valley Road, drive east and deeper into the valley—a somewhat confusing effort, as parts of this road are one way, and you must follow signs toward your prearranged pick-up point, or, if you are leaving a car, toward overnight parking near Curry Village. Note that private cars cannot drive the Yosemite Valley Road east beyond the big parking lot at Curry Village. Weary hikers will probably want to ride the free shuttlebus from the Happy Isles bus stop to their pick-up point or to Curry Village parking. Or they can walk 1 mile more generally west on paved trail to Curry Village parking.

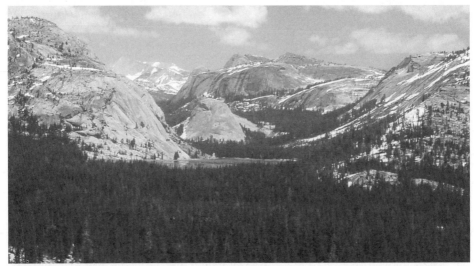

Left to right in middle ground: massive Polly Dome; tiny Pywiak Dome with Tenaya Lake visible below the trees at Pywiak's foot; the northwest slope of Tenaya Peak

DAY 1 (Tenaya Lake Trailhead to Sunrise Creek, 8.7 miles): *(Partial Recap: Trip 49, Day 1, from Tenaya Lake Trailhead to the signed junction on the saddle on Sunrise Mountain with the trail to Sunrise High Sierra Camp.)* From the trailhead, walk about 150 feet down the road to a marked trail on your right, turn right (northeast), and at a junction go left (east) to Sunrise Lakes on the Forsyth Trail. Cross Tenaya Lake's outlet, curve south at a sign, and reach a junction where you go right (south-southwest) toward Sunrise High Sierra Camp. Beyond, you begin a rocky, gradual-to-moderate climb, descend into a wash, top a rise, and cross Mildred Lake's outlet. Ascend, crossing a few seasonal streams, before beginning a steep, exposed, view-rich, switchbacking slog up Sunrise Mountain. Finally, the switchbacks end, and the trail levels on a saddle as it arrives at the signed junction with the trail to Sunrise High Sierra Camp (9224'; 11S 283538 4186577).

Leaving the Day 1 route of Trip 49, stay on the Forsyth Trail and go right to begin a generally southward, 320-foot, switchbacking descent. At the bottom of the descent, the trail rises over a talus-swollen little ridge and drops beside a pleasant-looking lakelet. Continuing south, the trail ascends a lightly forested hillside to three unnamed streams that you cross in quick succession (campsites near the second). This slope is boggy until mid season, and the plentiful groundwater nourishes rank gardens of wildflowers throughout the summer. Leveling off beyond the streams, your trail meets the spur trail right (southwest) to the summit of Clouds Rest.

VISITING CLOUDS REST
Hikers with plenty of energy may take this short lateral west (2.5 miles) to this lofty prominence. Views from Clouds Rest are among the most spectacular in the Sierra, including a 4500-foot continuous granite slope stretching all the way down to Tenaya Creek and rising on the other side—the largest exposed granite area in the Park.

At the Clouds Rest junction, your route turns left (southeast) and meanders over sandy, level terrain for a half mile, detouring around many fallen trees, before it starts its plunge toward Sunrise Creek. This switchbacking descent is a little tough on the knees but repays you: The green fir and pine forest is a classic of its kind, and occasional views down into the Merced River Canyon are sweeping in their range.

Finally the trail approaches a stream, parallels it for almost a half mile, fords it, and then fords Sunrise Creek (8032'; 11S 281761 4182005) to the fair campsites upstream some 200 yards on the south side of Sunrise Creek. Fishing for small rainbow and brook is poor to fair.

DAY 2 (Sunrise Creek to Yosemite Valley-Happy Isles Trailhead, 8.6 miles): Return to the trail and turn left (west-southwest) on it to continue your trip. In less than 0.2 mile, after the trail swings southward, you reach a junction with the JMT and go ahead (south) on the JMT. After less than another 0.2 mile, the JMT meets the trail left (east) to Merced Lake; you go right (west), staying on the JMT. The JMT here is bounded on the north by the Pinnacles (the south face of Clouds Rest) and on the south by Moraine Dome.

MORAINE DOME
François Matthes, in an interesting "detective story" written in the form of a geological essay, discusses Moraine Dome extensively. He deduced, using three examples, that the moraines around the dome were the product of at least two glacial ages—a notion contrary to the thinking of the time. The morainal till of the last glacial age characterizes the underfooting of the descent into Little Yosemite Valley.

A mile past the last junction, ford Sunrise Creek in a red fir forest whose stillness is broken only by the sounds of the creek and the occasional Steller's jay. In another mile, you ford Sunrise Creek again (campsites), shortly ford a tributary (more campsites), and then meet the trail coming down from Clouds Rest at a T-junction (still more campsites). You may temporarily mistake the broad, well-worn use trails to the campsites here for the main trail. At this junction, go left (southwest) on the JMT.

In less than a half mile from there, you meet the signed lateral right (northwest) to Half Dome (about 4 miles round trip). At this junction, turn left (briefly southeast) on the shady JMT, beginning switchbacks down through a changing forest cover. After the trail levels out, it forks; you go right (southwest) into the west end of Little Yosemite Valley. (The left, south, fork would take you to improved campsites in Little Yosemite Valley along Sunrise Creek and the Merced River.) A summer ranger may be on duty nearby.

The fork you've taken is a JMT shortcut angling across Little Yosemite Valley, and your trail soon meets the main route through Little Yosemite Valley to Merced Lake. From this junction, you turn right (west), shortly ascend out of Little Yosemite Valley, and then descend near the Merced River for about a half mile toward Nevada Fall. A few hundred yards before the roaring fall, the JMT meets the famous Mist Trail. Both descend toward Yosemite Valley, but this trip stays on the JMT by going left (south along the river) from this junction, near which there are some pit toilets. Along the river, slabs and pools beckon, but stay out of the rushing water or you'll be swept over 594-foot Nevada Fall to your death. Lookout points on the river's north side offer close-ups of the fall.

MIST TRAIL

The Mist Trail drops very steeply on tight, slippery switchbacks to the foot of Nevada Fall, flattens out briefly, fords the Merced River on a footbridge, passes a junction with the lower end of the Clark Trail (left and uphill to the JMT), passes the Emerald Pool, and then climbs a steep slab to the top of Vernal Fall. The trail then descends along, and is usually soaked by spray from, Vernal Fall. Not only is the descent itself very steep, but the rock "steps" you must descend are high, wet, and slippery. You will almost certainly get drenched here. After the Mist Trail levels out below Vernal Fall, it rejoins the JMT. We don't recommend the Mist Trail for backpackers, but it's a dayhikers' challenge and delight.

Continuing this journey, the JMT crosses above Nevada Fall on a footbridge to the river's south side and presently meets a couple of junctions with the Panorama Trail, which started at Glacier Point and ends here. At both junctions, go ahead (west) on the JMT to begin long, mostly paved switchbacks that are steep—but not nearly as steep as the Mist Trail. Over-the-shoulder views back to Nevada Fall are splendid, and views down the Merced River canyon to Liberty Cap and Sierra Point are excellent, too. At Clark Point, the upper end of the previously mentioned Clark Trail (on the right), enjoy the view and then continue down the JMT by going ahead (generally west).

After a long descent on switchbacks, the JMT levels out and meets a signed HORSE TRAIL coming in from the left. Avoid that and go ahead (west) on the JMT; the Mist Trail shortly joins the JMT from the right. The JMT then curves north to the Merced's south bank and crosses the river on a footbridge that offers a superb view of 317-foot Vernal Fall. On the south side of the river, before you cross the bridge, there are a drinking fountain on the right and restrooms on the left.

Once across the bridge and on the river's north side, the trail climbs a little before descending steeply again. On this final descent, you may glimpse Illilouette Fall high in Illilouette Gorge across the river as you pass the gorge's mouth. The JMT presently passes above the Happy Isles (two rocky islets in the Merced) and then a gauging station and the remains of a bridge to the Happy Isles. At last, the trail levels out near its end, where it meets the road that curves through Yosemite Valley's floor (4023′; 11S 274550 4179235).

There's a bridge across the Merced to your left; cross it to the Happy Isles bus stop, where you can pick up a free Valley shuttlebus to numerous Valley destinations where you may have arranged for a stay or for someone to pick you up—or you can ride it to Curry Village parking. If you have a car waiting for you and have some energy left, you can follow the paved path northwest beyond the bus stop for a mile to the overnight parking lot near Curry Village (distance not included in this trip).

HWY 120

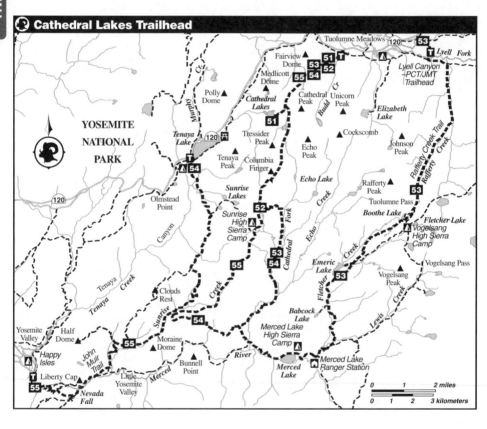

Cathedral Lakes Trailhead

Cathedral Lakes Trailhead

8576'; 11S 290424 4194431

DESTINATION/ UTM COORDINATES	TRIP TYPE	BEST SEASON	PACE (HIKING/ LAYOVER DAYS)	TOTAL MILEAGE
51 Upper Cathedral Lake 11S 290424 4194431	Out & back	Mid or late	2/0 Leisurely	7.4
52 Sunrise High Sierra Camp 11S 285820 4185899	Out & back	Mid or late	4/1 Leisurely	16.8
53 Lyell Canyon- PCT/JMT Trailhead 11S 294306 4194865	Shuttle or loop	Mid or late	5/1 Leisurely-moderate	34 (shuttle) or 36.2 (loop)
54 Tenaya Lake 11S 282465 4189314	Shuttle	Mid or late	4/1 Leisurely	25.4
55 Yosemite Valley- Happy Isles Trailhead 11S 274550 4179235	Shuttle	Mid or late	3/0 Moderate	22.4

Information and Permits: These trips enter Yosemite National Park: Yosemite Permits, PO Box 545, Yosemite National Park, CA 95389; 209-372-0740; www.nps.gov/yose/wilderness/permits.htm. Bear canisters are required; pets and firearms are prohibited.

Driving Directions: Just 8.3 miles southwest of Tioga Pass on Hwy. 120, in Tuolumne Meadows, and a short distance west of the Tuolumne Meadows Visitor Center, there is a broad, bare area with bear-resistant food lockers on the south side of the road. The bare area, once a parking lot, is now blocked off by boulders so that you can't get a car into it. This means that you must find parking somewhere off the asphalt and on the shoulders of Hwy. 120; this on-shoulder parking can be very crowded in the summer. You must leave any food and other smelly items in the lockers rather than in your car. The trail starts from the far end of the bare area.

51 Upper Cathedral Lake

Trip Data: 11S 290424 4194431; 7.4 miles; 2/0 days

Topos: *Tenaya Lake*

Highlights: We admit it: The Cathedral Lakes can be crowded, especially during the day. But the scenery is classic Yosemite: a

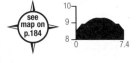

basin of gray-white granite holding an azure lake whose serene waters reflect the unmistakable, elegant spire of Cathedral Peak. Lower Cathedral Lake is as lovely as Upper Cathedral Lake, but as of this writing, Lower Cathedral Lake is closed to camping. No matter which lake is open to camping when you go, this trip is ideal for beginners. It's also a fine dayhike.

HEADS UP! *While this trip is written for Upper Cathedral Lake, it's possible the Park Service will decide to close Upper Cathedral Lake to camping and allow camping at Lower Cathedral Lake for a while before switching again. We include directions for Lower Cathedral Lake, too. Fires are not permitted in Cathedral Basin.*

DAY 1 (Cathedral Lakes Trailhead to Upper Cathedral Lake, 3.7 miles): From the ex-parking lot, head generally southwest on a gently ascending, overused trail that is very dusty except after rain. In just a few steps from the trailhead, the JMT joins your route at a step-across junction; continue ahead, southwest. Now the track begins to climb more steeply. Along the way, you glimpse two of Tuolumne Meadows' famed granite domes, Fairview and Medlicott. After 0.75 mile of ascent under a welcome forest cover, the trail levels off and descends to a small meadow that is boggy in early season. From here you can see the dramatically shaped tops of Unicorn Peak and the Cockscomb; the apparent granite dome in the south is in reality the north ridge of Cathedral Peak, whose steeples are out of sight over the "dome's" horizon.

The trail cruises gently through more little meadows set in hemlock forest and then dips near a stream. After a little more walking, you discover one of the sources of that stream—a robust spring on a shady set of switchbacks. Beyond this climb, the tread levels off on the west slope of Cathedral Peak and makes a long, gentle, sparsely forested descent on sandy underfooting to a junction with the spur trail to Lower Cathedral Lake: ahead (southeast) to Upper Cathedral Lake; right (south) to Lower Cathedral Lake.

TO LOWER CATHEDRAL LAKE

If Upper Cathedral Lake is closed to camping and you must go to Lower Cathedral Lake, turn right (south) at this junction and curve downhill through a meadow to cross a creek. Continue steeply downhill now on rocky track that's booby-trapped with tree roots. Ford streams several times in the extensive meadow you must cross to get to the granite slabs ringing Lower Cathedral Lake (9292'; 11S 286891 4191277); look for campsites here.

Continue ahead toward Upper Cathedral Lake on an easy climb for a little more than a half mile, soon entering Cathedral Basin. Nearing this day's goal, the trail dips slightly into the shallow bowl that holds the lake (9602'; 11S 287650 4190823); the sandy trail stays a little above and east of the lake. Rugged Tressider Peak lies southwest of the lake, while the delicate steeples of Cathedral Peak rise to the northeast. Look for campsites well away from the water.

TO BE OR NOT TO BE GLACIATED

The rounded, polished tops of the domes seen earlier prove that the domes were completely covered by ice, while the jagged summits of Cathedral and Tressider peaks prove that they stood a few hundred feet above the grinding ice and hence were not rounded and smoothed by it.

DAY 2 (Upper Cathedral Lake to Cathedral Lakes Trailhead, 3.7 miles): Retrace your steps.

52 Sunrise High Sierra Camp

Trip Data: 11S 285820 4185899; 16.8 miles; 4/1 days

Topos: *Tenaya Lake*

see map on p.184

Highlights: This leg of the JMT, also known as the Sunrise Trail, is a justly famous and popular route on its own. From much of the route, hikers enjoy superlative views of whole subranges in the distance as well as of spectacular peaks nearby.

DAY 1 (Cathedral Lakes Trailhead to Upper Cathedral Lake, 3.7 miles): *(Recap: Trip 51, Day 1.)* From the ex-parking lot, head generally southwest; in a few steps, the JMT joins your route at a step-across junction: Continue ahead (southwest) to begin to climb more steeply. After 0.75 mile of ascent, the trail levels off and descends to a small meadow.

The trail undulates through meadow and hemlock forest and then dips near a stream. You presently meet a robust spring on a shady set of switchbacks. Beyond this climb, the tread levels off on Cathedral Peak's west slope and descends to a junction with the spur trail to Lower Cathedral Lake: ahead (southeast) to Upper Cathedral Lake; right (south) to

Lower Cathedral Lake. (If camping is closed at Upper Cathedral Lake, head to Lower Cathedral Lake instead by going right here and descend to that lake: 9292'; 11S 286891 4191277.)

Continue ahead toward Upper Cathedral Lake and in a little over a half mile dip slightly into the bowl that holds the lake (9602'; 11S 287650 4190823). Camp well away from water.

DAY 2 (Upper Cathedral Lake to Sunrise High Sierra Camp, 4.7 miles): Regain the JMT/Sunrise Trail and follow it up and south to Cathedral Pass, where the excellent views include Cathedral Peak, Tressider Peak, Echo Peaks, Matthes Crest, the Clark Range farther south, and Matterhorn Peak far to the north. Beyond the pass is a long, beautiful swale, the headwaters of Echo Creek, where the mid-season flower show is alone worth the trip.

The JMT/Sunrise Trail continues climbing gradually along Tressider Peak's east flank to the actual high point of this trail, a marvelous viewpoint overlooking most of southern Yosemite National Park. The inspiring panorama includes the peaks around Vogelsang High Sierra Camp in the southeast, the whole Clark Range in the south, and the peaks on the Park border in both directions farther away.

Beyond this point, the trail switchbacks quickly down to the head of the upper lobe of Long Meadow, levels off, and leads down a gradually sloping valley dotted with little lodgepole pines to the head of the second, lower lobe of l-o-n-g Long Meadow (may be dry by late season). At a junction with the trail left (east) to Echo Creek, continue ahead (south).

Follow the trail on its meadowy descent to the fair campsites along the stream near Sunrise High Sierra Camp (9333'; 11S 285820 4185899). The High Sierra Camp is near the south end of the meadow, almost out of sight on a bench above and west of the trail. There are other well-used campsites south of the High Sierra Camp on the bench west of the meadow. The view east across Long Meadow, toward rugged peaks, hints at wonders as yet unseen.

DAYS 3–4 (Sunrise High Sierra Camp to Cathedral Lakes Trailhead, 8.4 miles): Retrace your steps.

53 Lyell Canyon-PCT/JMT Trailhead

Trip Data: 11S 294306 4194865; 34 miles (shuttle) or 36.2 miles (loop); 5/1 days

Topos: *Merced Peak, Tenaya Lake, Merced Peak, Vogelsang Peak*

Highlights: This looping trip samples everything the Cathedral Range has to offer, from sweeping vistas from 10,000-foot passes to the deeply glaciated Merced River Canyon to forested side streams with secluded campsites. There's plenty of good fishing, too.

HEADS UP! *The last day is a very long one (10.8 miles). Hikers wishing an easier end to this trip could add a day and then adjust Day 4 to stop at Babcock Lake, Day 5 at Boothe Lake, and exit on a shorter final day, in this case the added Day 6.*

You can make a loop of this trip, mostly on trail, as described at the end of the last day. Note that doing so adds about 2.2 miles to your already long last day if you do this trip in 5 days. If you do the loop, you can reduce the last day's mileage by adding a day and adjusting the trip as described above.

Shuttle Directions: If you do this trip as a shuttle, the take-out is at the large backpackers' parking lot on the north side of the spur road that ends at Tuolumne Meadows Lodge (where you must be a paying guest to park overnight). This lot serves as a trailhead for the southbound PCT, soon to join the JMT. About 6.6 miles west of Tioga Pass on Hwy. 120 and just east of Lembert Dome, take the signed turnoff south toward Tuolumne Meadows Lodge. Almost immediately, another spur road darts right (southwest) to a wilderness-permit station and its parking lot. Avoiding that spur road, you continue toward the lodge as the road angles east, paralleling Hwy. 120. In a little more than 0.4 mile, look for the back-packers' parking lot on the north side of the road (on your left). Pull in here to leave your shuttle car (or to pick up your party).

DAY 1 (Cathedral Lakes Trailhead to Upper Cathedral Lake, 3.7 miles): *(Recap: Trip 51, Day 1.)* From the ex-parking lot, head generally southwest; in a few steps, the JMT joins your route at a step-across junction: Continue ahead (southwest) to begin to climb more steeply. After 0.75 mile of ascent, the trail levels off and descends to a small meadow where you can see the dramatically shaped tops of Unicorn Peak and the Cockscomb.

The trail undulates through meadow and hemlock forest and then dips near a stream. You presently meet a robust spring on a shady set of switchbacks. Beyond this climb, the tread levels off on Cathedral Peak's west slope and descends to a junction with the spur trail to Lower Cathedral Lake: ahead (southeast) to Upper Cathedral Lake; right (south) to Lower Cathedral Lake. (If camping is closed at Upper Cathedral Lake, head to Lower Cathedral Lake instead by going right here and descend to that lake: 9292'; 11S 286891 4191277.)

Continue ahead toward Upper Cathedral Lake and in a little over a half mile dip slight-ly into the bowl that holds the lake (9602'; 11S 287650 4190823). Tressider Peak lies south-west of the lake; Cathedral Peak is northeast. Camp well away from water.

DAY 2 (Upper Cathedral Lake to Echo Creek Crossing, 9 miles): *(Partial Recap: Trip 52, Day 2, from Upper Cathedral Lake to the junction with the trail to Echo Creek.)* Regain the JMT/Sunrise Trail and follow it up and south to Cathedral Pass and its excellent views. The JMT/Sunrise Trail continues climbing gradually along Tressider Peak's east flank to the actual high point of this trail, a marvelous viewpoint overlooking most of southern Yosemite National Park. Then the trail switchbacks quickly down to the north end of Long Meadow (may be dry by late season) and travels south down this long, gradually sloping valley to the junction with the trail to Echo Creek.

Now leave the Day 2 route for Trip 52 and turn left (east) to ford Long Meadow's stream. The trail quickly switchbacks up to top the ridge that separates this stream from Echo Creek and then descends through dense hemlock-and-lodgepole forest toward Cathedral Fork Echo Creek. Where the route approaches this stream, you have fine views of the creek's water gliding down a series of granite slabs. Then the trail veers away from the creek and descends gently above it for more than a mile. Even in late season, this shady hillside is well watered and abloom. On this downgrade, your route meets and again fords the Long Meadow stream, which has flowed out of that meadow through a gap between two large domes high above the trail.

At this point, the route levels out in a mile-long flat section of this valley where the wet ground yields an abundance of wildflowers and, sadly, of mosquitoes, too. Beyond this flat "park," the trail descends a more open hillside and passes above the confluence of Echo Creek's west and east forks. You can see across the valley the steep course of the east fork plunging down to join the west fork. Finally, the trail levels off and reaches the good camp-sites just before a metal bridge over Echo Creek (8153'; 11S 286787 4182449). Fishing in the creek is good for rainbow and golden trout.

DAY 3 (Echo Creek Crossing to Merced Lake, 4.9 miles): After crossing the bridge over Echo Creek, the trail leads down the forested valley and easily fords a tributary stream, staying well above the main creek. This pleasant, shaded descent encounters shaggy juniper trees and then tall, brittle red firs as it drops to another metal bridge 1 mile from the last one.

Beyond this sturdy span, the trail curves west-southwest as it rises slightly, and the creek drops precipitously, so that you are soon far above it. Then the sandy tread swings west away from Echo Creek and traverses down a hillside where views are excellent of Echo Valley, a wide place in the great Merced River canyon below. At the next junction, with the trail to Echo Valley, your route turns left (south).

Descend to a forested bench with a year-round stream before switchbacking down to Echo Valley and to another trail junction.

Here you meet and turn left (east) on the Merced River Trail. After crossing several forks of Echo Creek on wooden bridges, you pass a burn area where a 1966 fire killed most of the mature trees. But new, small lodgepoles grow by the hundreds, and the grassy valley floor is carpeted by the blue flowers of lupine and the white blossoms of yarrow and yampah. Leaving Echo Valley, the trail leads up immense granite slabs. This ascent offers travelers the sights and sounds of this dramatic part of the river: a long series of chutes, cascades, falls, cataracts, and pools that were all formed by the glacier that roughened the formerly smooth bed of the Merced River.

Above this turbulent stretch, the trail levels off beside the now quiet river and arrives at the outlet of Merced Lake. Follow the trail around the lake's north side to Merced Lake High Sierra Camp (7234'; 11S 287918 4179565) at its east end; a backpackers' campground in conjunction with the camp provides the only legal campsites in this area. You can buy a few provisions at the small store, or even rent a rowboat to try your luck for rainbow and brown trout. Be sure to bearproof your food.

DAY 4 (Merced Lake to Emeric Lake, 5.6 miles): Return to the trail and go eastward, away from the lake. The first short mile of this day's hike follows an almost level, wide, sandy path under a canopy of fir, pine, juniper, and aspen. You cross the roaring Lewis Creek on a bridge and arrive at the Merced Lake Ranger Station (emergency services available in summer) and a junction with the Lewis Creek Trail. Turn left (north) on the Lewis Creek Trail. This cobblestoned trail quickly becomes steep, and it remains so for a panting half mile plus. Fortunately, Sierra junipers and Jeffrey pines cast plenty of morning shade.

The trail levels momentarily as you pass a fine viewpoint for taking pictures of Merced Lake, far below, and Half Dome, due west. One more steep, cobblestoned climb leads to a junction with the Fletcher Creek Trail, and you turn left (northeast) onto this path.

Several switchbacks then descend to a wooden bridge over Lewis Creek. There is ample, hardened camping near the bridge. From here, the trail begins a 400-foot, moderate-to-steep ascent over unevenly cobblestoned, exposed trail—a grunt on a hot day. The path is bordered by mountain whitethorn and huckleberry oak shrubs. Just past a tributary a half mile from Lewis Creek, you have fine views of cataracts and waterfalls on Fletcher Creek where it rushes down open granite slopes dotted with lodgepole pines. The trail then passes very close to the creek before veering south and climbing, steeply at times, on the now-familiar cobblestones. Here there are more good views of Fletcher Creek, chuting and cascading down from a notch at the base of a granite dome before it leaps off a ledge in a free fall. The few solitary pine trees on this otherwise bald dome testify to nature's extraordinary tenacity.

The trail climbs up to the notch and then levels off near some nice but illegal campsites. Soon your path passes a side trail left (west and south) to small Babcock Lake (campsites). From this junction, you go ahead (north) on sandy trail that ascends steadily through moderate forest just east of Fletcher Creek. After a mile, the trail rises steeply via rocky switchbacks from which you can see, nearby in the north, the outlet stream of Emeric Lake—though not the lake itself, which is behind a dome just to the right of the outlet's notch.

On the less adventurous route to Emeric Lake, the switchbacks top out with the dome to the north, and the trail then follows Fletcher Creek northeast to a ford. Almost immediately beyond the ford, the track meets a junction with the spur trail to Emeric Lake. Go left

SHORTCUT TO EMERIC LAKE

For an adventurous shortcut to Emeric Lake, follow this outlet up to the lake. First, leave the trail and wade across granite-bottomed Fletcher Creek as best you can—there is no natural place to do so, and in a wet year you may get very wet yourself. Then follow up this outlet and stroll along the northwest shore of Emeric Lake to campsites.

(west) to Emeric Lake (9396'; 11S 290240 4183858) and follow anglers' trails to the excellent campsites midway along its northwest shore. The meadow north and northeast of the lake is carpeted with delicate wildflowers. Fishing is often good for rainbow.

DAY 5 (Emeric Lake to Lyell Canyon-PCT/JMT Trailhead, 10.8 miles for shuttle or 13 miles for loop): This is the longest hiking day on this trip, but the ascent to Tuolumne Pass is moderate and comes at the beginning. From Tuolumne Pass on the crest of the Cathedral Range, the rest is downhill.

Circle the head of Emeric Lake, crossing its inlet stream, and find the spur trail at the lake's northeast corner at the base of a granite knoll. Take the spur east-northeast for 0.6 mile to a junction in the valley of Fletcher Creek (if you took the less adventurous route to Emeric Lake, this is the junction from which you took the spur to the lake). Go left (northeast) on the main trail up the valley and follow a rocky-dusty trail to another junction where you go left (north-northeast) toward Boothe Lake.

Climb away from Fletcher Creek, passing northwest of a bald prominence that sits in the center of the upper valley of Fletcher and Emeric creeks, separating the two. Topping a minor summit, the trail descends slightly and then winds levelly past a long series of lovely ponds that are interconnected in early season. The Park Service is attempting to restore the meadows surrounding the ponds; numerous signs ask you to stay on the main trail. You soon pass a use trail to the south end of Boothe Lake (9845'), where there are some campsites.

At the top of a little swale, the trail reaches an overlook above Boothe Lake and then contours along a meadowy hillside, passing a junction with another use trail down to the lake. About a quarter mile farther, you reach Tuolumne Pass (9992') and a junction with a trail that goes sharply right (south) to Vogelsang High Sierra Camp. Enjoy the wonderful view ahead before continuing north and down.

Now on the Rafferty Creek Trail, you begin a gradual descent north along Rafferty Creek's headwaters, which rise in this high, boulder-strewn meadow. The year-round creek is always east of the trail, sometimes near and sometimes far, on this long, beautiful descent through sparse-to-moderate lodgepole forest; you don't ford Rafferty Creek (the topo is wrong). As the trail and the creek make their final drop into Lyell Canyon, you negotiate steep switchbacks as the trail loses about 400 feet.

On Lyell Canyon's forested floor, you meet the combined PCT/JMT just west of a substantial footbridge over Rafferty Creek. Camping is prohibited this close to Hwy. 120. Turn left (west) on the PCT/JMT and follow it about 0.6 mile to another junction. If you're taking this as a shuttle trip, the trip's end is about 1 mile ahead; those taking this as a loop should see the description below. For the shuttle trip, turn right (north) here, leaving the JMT but staying on the PCT, and soon cross Lyell Fork Tuolumne River on a double footbridge that offers excellent views up-canyon (a photo is almost mandatory).

Now on the river's north bank, curve slightly left past a large pine as you ascend a slight rise. Descend from the rise into forest and follow the PCT to the next junction. Go left (west) on the PCT to cross Dana Fork Tuolumne River on a stout footbridge; on the other side, the PCT turns northwest. Avoid a spur trail right (northeast) to Tuolumne Meadows Lodge. The PCT roughly parallels Dana Fork for a while before the curving west to meet a short, wide path on your right, uphill and northwest, to the spur road that ends at Tuolumne Meadows Lodge. Turn right on this path, ascend to the road, and cross the road to a large backpackers' parking lot with bear-resistant food-storage lockers (8701'; 11S 294306 4194865). Your car or shuttle ride should be waiting here.

> **LOOP OPTION**
>
> At the PCT/JMT junction just south of the double footbridge over Lyell Fork Tuolumne River, the shuttle trip's end is about 0.9 mile away on the PCT, while the loop trip's end is about 3.1 miles away on the JMT. Don't turn right (north) to the bridge. Instead, continue ahead (west-northwest) on the shady JMT, which presently angles west away from the river to meet a spur trail right (northwest) down into the far southeast corner of huge Tuolumne Meadows Campground, which has a walk-in section where you could camp (fee). To stay on the JMT, go ahead (west) here and follow the undulating path through pleasant though unremarkable forest. You soon meet a trail crossing yours almost at right angles (roughly north-south) from the campground and headed to Elizabeth Lake. Step across this trail and continue ahead (west) on the JMT to cross Unicorn Creek. At the next junction, with a spur right (north) to Hwy. 120 and the Tuolumne Meadow Visitors Center, again continue ahead (west) and eventually cross Budd Creek. Just beyond the creek, you meet the trail to Cathedral Lakes. Here, the JMT turns left (southwest), but you turn right (northeast) and shortly cross the bare area to Hwy. 120 (8576'; 11S 290424 4194431) and the shoulders along which you parked your car.

54 Tenaya Lake

Trip Data: 11S 282465 4189314; 25.4 miles; 4/1 days

Topos: *Merced Peak*, Merced Peak, Tenaya Lake

see map on p.184

Highlights: Although the first and last parts of this trip are along favorite, well-used trails, in between, you follow a little-used stretch of trail in the heart of Yosemite's spectacular glaciated highlands. Views of the immense domes and deep-cut canyons will leave lifetime memories.

Shuttle Directions: To reach the take-out trailhead, drive just 15.8 miles west of Hwy. 120's Tioga Pass and just past the west end of Tenaya Lake. There is a signed trailhead on the south side of the road at a turnout with a small parking lot and a toilet. The trailhead is at a closed, gated road.

DAY 1 (Cathedral Lakes Trailhead to Upper Cathedral Lake, 3.7 miles): *(Recap: Trip 51, Day 1.)* From the ex-parking lot, head generally southwest; in a few steps, the JMT joins your route at a step-across junction: Continue ahead (southwest) to begin to climb more steeply. After 0.75 mile of ascent, the trail levels off and descends to a small meadow where you can see the dramatically shaped tops of Unicorn Peak and the Cockscomb.

The trail undulates through meadow and hemlock forest and then dips near a stream. You presently meet a robust spring on a shady set of switchbacks. Beyond this climb, the tread levels off on Cathedral Peak's west slope and descends to a junction with the spur trail to Lower Cathedral Lake: ahead (southeast) to Upper Cathedral Lake; right (south) to Lower Cathedral Lake. (If camping is closed at Upper Cathedral Lake, head to Lower Cathedral Lake instead by going right here and descend to that lake: 9292'; 11S 286891 4191277.)

Continue ahead toward Upper Cathedral Lake and in a little over a half mile dip slightly into the bowl that holds the lake (9602'; 11S 287650 4190823). Tressider Peak lies southwest of the lake; Cathedral Peak is northeast. Camp well away from water.

DAY 2 (Upper Cathedral Lake to Echo Creek Crossing, 9 miles): *(Partial Recap: Trip 52, Day 2, from Upper Cathedral Lake to the junction with the trail to Echo Creek.)* Regain the JMT/Sunrise Trail and follow it up and south to Cathedral Pass and its excellent views. The JMT/Sunrise Trail continues climbing gradually along Tressider Peak's east flank to the actual high point of this trail. Then the trail switchbacks quickly down to the north end of Long Meadow (may be dry by late season) and travels south to the junction with the trail to Echo Creek.

(Partial Recap: Trip 53, Day 2, from the junction with the trail to Echo Creek to Echo Creek Crossing.) At the junction, you leave the Day 2 route of Trip 52 and turn left (east) and ford Long Meadow's stream. The trail quickly switchbacks up to top the ridge that separates this stream from Echo Creek and then descends through dense forest toward Cathedral Fork Echo Creek. Where the route approaches this stream, you have fine views of the creek's water gliding down a series of granite slabs. Then the trail veers away from the creek and descends gently above it for more than a mile. On this downgrade, your route meets and again fords the Long Meadow stream.

At this point, the route levels out in a mile-long flat section of this valley. Beyond this flat "park," the trail descends a more open hillside. Finally, the trail levels off and reaches the good campsites just before a metal bridge over Echo Creek (8153'; 11S 286787 4182449). Fishing in the creek is good for rainbow and golden trout.

DAY 3 (Echo Creek Crossing to Sunrise Creek, 5.1 miles): *(Partial Recap: Trip 53, Day 3, from Echo Creek Crossing to the junction with the trail to Echo Valley.)* After crossing the bridge, the trail leads down the forested valley and fords a tributary while staying above the main creek. In a mile, you cross another metal bridge and beyond it curve west-southwest as the trail rises and the creek drops so that you are soon far above the creek. Then the tread swings west away from Echo Creek and traverses down a hillside to the junction.

At this junction, you leave the Day 3 route of Trip 53 and turn right (west) to climb several hundred rocky feet before leveling off above the immense Merced River's canyon.

WAY BACK WHEN...

This trail segment was part of the route from Yosemite Valley to Merced Lake until a path up the canyon was constructed in 1931. Before that, the steep canyon walls coming right down to the river near Bunnell Point, the great dome to the southwest, had made passage impossible. Finally, a trail was built that bypasses the narrowest part of the canyon by climbing high on the south wall, and the trail you are now on fell into relative disuse.

With fine views of obelisk-like Mt. Clark in the south, you descend gradually for a half mile over open granite in a setting that is sure to give you a feeling of being above almost everything. Then the trail passes a stagnant lakelet and ascends to even better viewpoints of the immense, glaciated, granitic wonder that nature has spread out before you: Mt. Clark, Clouds Rest, Half Dome, Mt. Starr King, Bunnell Point, and the great unnamed dome across the canyon west of it.

The continuing ascent then rounds a ridge and veers north into a forest of handsome Jeffrey pines. Here, the trail levels off, and it remains level for a mile of exhilarating walking through Jeffreys, lodgepoles, and red firs that shade patch after patch of vivid green ferns and bright wildflowers. Still in forest, you descend slightly to meet the JMT/Sunrise Trail. To end this day, you go right on it for 150 yards to yet another junction, where you turn left (north) 200 yards up yet another trail (the Forsyth Trail) to Sunrise Creek to a ford—don't ford. You'll find fair campsites upstream some 200 yards on the south side of Sunrise Creek (8032'; 11S 281761 4182005). Fishing for small rainbow and brook is poor to fair.

DAY 4 (Sunrise Creek to Tenaya Lake, 7.6 miles): Return to the ford of Sunrise Creek and, back on yesterday's Forsyth Trail, go north to ford Sunrise Creek. The trail soon curves east and then northeast to climb steeply and ford a tributary of Sunrise Creek. Beyond this ford, the trail continues its steep climb to gentler terrain at about 8880 feet, where the now sandy trail rises more gently and soon begins a northward and then westward curve to a junction with a trail to Clouds Rest.

Go right (northeast) here, away from Clouds Rest, and stay on the Forsyth Trail as it descends a wet hillside, crosses three unnamed streams on the way, passes a lakelet, rises over a ridge, and descends a little before beginning a switchbacking, 320-foot climb northward to a saddle and junction with the trail that goes east to Sunrise Lakes and Sunrise High Sierra Camp.

At this junction, you continue ahead (north), staying on the Forsyth Trail. *(Recap in Reverse: Trip 49, Day 1, from the signed junction on the saddle on Sunrise Mountain with the trail to Sunrise High Sierra Camp, to Tenaya Lake.)*Beyond the junction on the saddle, your route begins a long, steep, switchbacking descent north-northwest. At the bottom of this descent, bear north to cross a couple of streams (may be dry by late season) and then follow the undulating trail northwest over the multi-stranded outlet of Mildred Lake, into a bouldery wash, and up to a little viewpoint.

Dropping north-northwest from the viewpoint, you briefly parallel Tenaya Lake's outlet upstream toward the lake and its campground site (closed for years) before reaching a junction where you go left (north-northeast) a short way. Curve left at a sign and meet a junction just before the trailhead with a closed dirt road and another trail. Go right (west) on the dirt road for about 150 feet to the trailhead and your shuttle ride or car (8150'; 11S 282465 4189314).

55 Yosemite Valley–Happy Isles Trailhead

Trip Data: 11S 274550 4179235;
22.4 miles; 3/0 days

Topos: *Merced Peak, Yosemite, Tenaya Lake, Merced Peak, Half Dome*

Highlights: This part of the JMT is also called the Sunrise Trail and takes you from Tuolumne Meadows to Yosemite Valley. It's one of the Park's most famous and most used backpack routes because its miles contain a magnificent range of flora and fauna, and the trail surveys some of the Park's best-known landmarks. This is a fine trip for backpackers who have a couple of shorter trips under their belts and want more.

Shuttle Directions: You cannot drive to the take-out Happy Isles Trailhead, but you can leave a car in Curry Village and take a shuttle to and from there. Whether you drive from the west or the east, get to the junction of highways 140 and 120 in Yosemite Valley. On what is now the Yosemite Valley Road, drive east and deeper into the valley—a somewhat confusing effort, as parts of this road are one way, and you must follow signs toward your prearranged pick-up point or, if you are leaving a car, toward overnight parking near Curry Village. Note that private cars cannot drive the Yosemite Valley Road east beyond the big parking lot at Curry Village. Weary hikers will probably want to ride the free shuttlebus from the Happy Isles bus stop to their pick-up point or to Curry Village parking. Or they can walk 1 mile more generally west on paved trail to Curry Village parking.

DAY 1 (Cathedral Lakes Trailhead to Sunrise High Sierra Camp, 8.7 miles): *(Partial Recap: Trip 51, Day 1, from Cathedral Lakes Trailhead to Upper Cathedral Lake.)* From the ex-parking lot, head generally southwest; in a few steps, the JMT joins your route at a step-across junction: Continue ahead (southwest) to begin to climb more steeply. After 0.75 mile of ascent, the trail levels off and descends to a small meadow where you can see the dramatically shaped tops of Unicorn Peak and the Cockscomb.

The trail undulates through meadow and hemlock forest and then dips near a stream. You presently meet a robust spring on a shady set of switchbacks. Beyond this climb, the tread levels off on Cathedral Peak's west slope and descends to a junction with the spur trail to Lower Cathedral Lake: ahead (southeast) to Upper Cathedral Lake; right (south) to Lower Cathedral Lake. (If camping is closed at Upper Cathedral Lake, head to Lower Cathedral Lake instead by going right here and descend to that lake: 9292'; 11S 286891 4191277.)

Continue ahead toward Upper Cathedral Lake and in a little over a half mile dip slightly into the bowl that holds the lake (9602'; 11S 287650 4190823). Stay on the JMT/Sunrise Trail.

(Recap: Trip 52, Day 2.) Now leave the Day 1 route of Trip 51 and follow the JMT/Sunrise Trail up and south to Cathedral Pass and its excellent views. The JMT/Sunrise Trail continues climbing gradually along Tressider Peak's east flank. Then the trail switchbacks quickly down to the north end of Long Meadow (may be dry by late season) and travels south down this long, gradually sloping valley.

At the junction with the trail to Echo Creek, your route continues ahead (south) and gradually down to fair campsites along the stream near Sunrise High Sierra Camp (9333'; 11S 285820 4185899). The views here are excellent.

DAY 2 (Sunrise High Sierra Camp to Sunrise Creek, 5.1 miles): Return to the JMT/Sunrise Trail and continue south through Long Meadow, almost immediately reaching a junction with the trail right (northwest) to Sunrise Lakes and Tenaya Lake. Go left (south) to continue on the JMT/Sunrise Trail on a long, traversing climb of Sunrise Mountain's east slope. More than a mile from Long Meadow, you reach a saddle from which the JMT descends steeply by switchbacks down a rocky moraine as the track roughly parallels Sunrise Creek's headwaters.

ABOUT THIS MORAINE

This moraine is the largest of a series of ridge-like glacial deposits in this area, and the gigantic granite boulders along their sides testify to the power of the mer de glace that once filled Little Yosemite Valley and its tributaries. One such "erratic," (a boulder that has been transported by a glacier from one place and deposited at another) about the size of a compact car, was found poised on the side of Moraine Dome to the southwest, and geologists have determined that it came from the slopes of the peaks at the northwest end of the Cathedral Range.

At the foot of the descent, the trail crosses Sunrise Creek and then descends westward to meet the Forsyth Trail from Tenaya Lake. Turn right (north, uphill) a short way on the Forsyth Trail toward a ford of Sunrise Creek (8032'; 11S 281761 4182005). Don't ford; look for fair campsites about 200 yards upstream along Sunrise Creek's south side. Fishing on Sunrise Creek is poor to fair for small rainbow and brook.

DAY 3 (Sunrise Creek to Yosemite Valley-Happy Isles Trailhead, 8.6 miles): *(Recap: Trip 50, Day 2.)* Return to the Forsyth Trail and turn left (west-southwest) on it to continue your trip. In less than 0.2 mile, after the trail swings southward, you reach a junction with the JMT/Sunrise Trail and go ahead (south) on it. After less than 0.2 mile, the JMT/Sunrise Trail meets the trail left (east) to Merced Lake; you go right (west), staying on the JMT.

A mile from the last junction, ford Sunrise Creek in a red fir forest. In another mile, you ford Sunrise Creek again (campsites), ford a tributary (more campsites) soon after that, and then meet the trail coming down from Clouds Rest at a T-junction. At this junction, go left (southwest) on the JMT/Sunrise Trail.

In less than a half mile from there, you meet the signed lateral right (northwest) to Half Dome (about 4 miles round trip). At this junction, turn left (briefly southeast) on the shady JMT/Sunrise Trail, beginning switchbacks down through a changing forest cover. After the trail levels out, it forks; you go right (southwest) on the JMT, leaving the old Sunrise Trail behind, on a shortcut into the west end of Little Yosemite Valley. A summer ranger may be on duty nearby.

The JMT soon meets the main route through Little Yosemite Valley to Merced Lake. At this junction, turn right (west), ascend out of Little Yosemite Valley, and then descend near the Merced River for about a half mile toward Nevada Fall. A few hundred yards before the roaring fall, the JMT meets the famous Mist Trail. Both descend toward Yosemite Valley, but this trip stays on the JMT by going left (south along the river) from this junction. Stay out of the rushing water or you'll be swept over 594-foot Nevada Fall to your death. Lookout points on the river's north side offer close-ups of the fall.

The JMT crosses above Nevada Fall on a footbridge to the river's south side and presently meets a couple of junctions with the Panorama Trail. At both junctions, go ahead (west) on the JMT to begin long, steep, mostly paved switchbacks, enjoying views across the river of Liberty Cap, Mt. Broderick, and the back of Half Dome. At Clark Point and a junction with the Clark Trail (on the right), continue down the JMT by going ahead (generally west).

After a long descent on switchbacks, the JMT levels out and meets a signed HORSE TRAIL coming in from the left. Avoid that and go ahead (west) on the JMT; the Mist Trail shortly joins the JMT from the right. The JMT then curves north to the Merced's south bank and crosses the river on a footbridge that offers a superb view of 317-foot Vernal Fall.

Cross the bridge to the river's north side, where the trail climbs a little before descending steeply again. The JMT presently passes above the Happy Isles and then a gauging station and the remains of a bridge to the Happy Isles. At last the trail levels out near its end, where it meets the road that curves through Yosemite Valley's floor (4023'; 11S 274550 4179235).

There's a bridge across the Merced to your left; cross it to the Happy Isles bus stop, where you can pick up a free Valley shuttle-bus to numerous Valley destinations, including Curry Village and its overnight parking lot where your car or a ride should be waiting. Or you can follow the paved path northwest beyond the bus stop for a mile to Curry Village—distance not included in this trip.

Liberty Cap

HWY 120

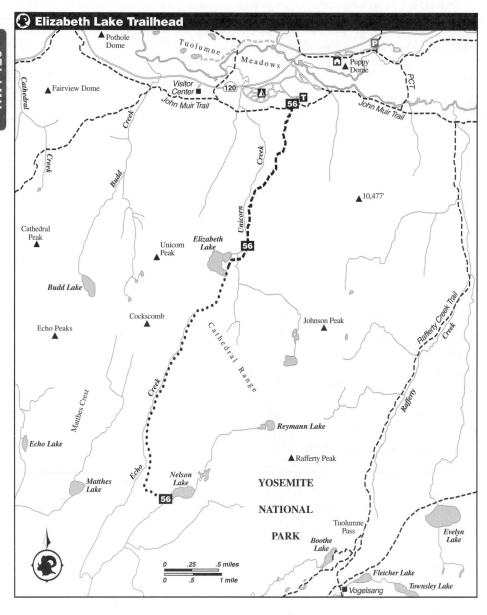

Elizabeth Lake Trailhead

Pothole Dome

Tuolumne Meadows

Cathedral Creek

Fairview Dome

Visitor Center

John Muir Trail

120

56

T

56

John Muir Trail

PCT

Puppy Dome

P

10,477'

Unicorn Creek

Budd Creek

Cathedral Peak

Unicorn Peak

Elizabeth Lake

Budd Lake

Cockscomb

Echo Peaks

Cathedral Range

Johnson Peak

Rafferty Creek Trail

Rafferty Creek

Matthes Crest

Echo Creek

Echo Lake

Reymann Lake

Rafferty Creek

Matthes Lake

Echo Creek

Nelson Lake

56

Rafferty Peak

YOSEMITE

NATIONAL

PARK

Tuolumne Pass

Boothe Lake

Evelyn Lake

Fletcher Lake

Townsley Lake

Vogelsang

0   .25   .5 miles

0   .5   1 mile

Elizabeth Lake Trailhead

8680'; 11S 292849 4194039

DESTINATION/ UTM COORDINATES	TRIP TYPE	BEST SEASON	PACE (HIKING/ LAYOVER DAYS)	TOTAL MILEAGE
56 Nelson Lake 11 S 290553 4187268	Out & back	Mid or late	2/1 Moderate, part cross-country	11.8

Information and Permits: These trips enter Yosemite National Park: Yosemite Permits, PO Box 545, Yosemite National Park, CA 95389; 209-372-0740; www.nps.gov/yose/wilderness/permits.htm. Bear canisters are required; pets and firearms are prohibited.

Driving Directions: Just 7.2 miles west of Tioga Pass on Hwy. 120 is the entrance to Tuolumne Meadows Campground. Turn south into the campground, stop at the entrance station to get permission to go to the Elizabeth Lake Trailhead, and then follow road signs to the group-campground loop. The trailhead is off the spur road to the group-campground loop, the second paved turnoff left from the main campground road. Follow the spur to a gate just before the signed HORSE CAMP; the trailhead is here, another 0.4 mile from the highway. Park in the adjacent lot. There are toilets and water in the campground when it's open. If the campground is closed, park outside it near the entrance and walk through the campground.

56 Nelson Lake

Trip Data: 11 S 290553 4187268; 11.8 miles; 2/1 days

Topos: *Vogelsang Peak, Tenaya Lake*

Highlights: This interesting and varied route visits the scenic Elizabeth Lake basin and then goes cross-country over the serrated Cathedral Range to Nelson Lake, where the fishing and camping are good and the scenery excellent.

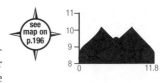

HEADS UP! *Between the Elizabeth Lake basin and Nelson Lake, there's a beaten path that fades out at times, leaving you to work cross-country. You need good navigation skills to find your way. Camping is prohibited within 4 miles of Hwy. 120 and throughout the Elizabeth Lake basin. You must go 1.5 miles beyond Elizabeth Lake before camping.*

DAY 1 (Elizabeth Lake Trailhead to Nelson Lake, 5.9 miles, part cross-country): The signed trail begins across from a masonry building near the campground's Horse Camp section. You head south and uphill from the trailhead and in a few hundred feet step across the JMT, which goes generally left (east) and right (west) to Lyell Canyon and Yosemite Valley. Avoiding the JMT, you continue ahead (south-southwest) on a steady ascent. The shade-giving forest cover is almost entirely lodgepole pine and mountain hemlock as the trail crosses several runoff streams that dry up by late summer.

More than a mile from the start, the route veers close to dashing Unicorn Creek, which flows out of the Elizabeth Lake basin. When the ascent finally ends, you emerge at the foot of a long meadow containing Elizabeth Lake, west of the trail but hidden by forest and at the foot of striking Unicorn Peak. This meadow is rapidly becoming a lodgepole pine forest.

The main trail branches right (west) across the creek to Elizabeth Lake (9487'; no camping permitted). Your route continues straight ahead and generally south on a well-beaten use trail along the stream running through this lovely meadow, soon meeting a second trail branching right (west) to the lake. Continue ahead (south) along the meadow's stream, which, late in the season, may be your last chance for water before upper Echo Creek.

The meadow gives way to a moderately dense forest cover of lodgepole interspersed with mountain hemlock, and the trail climbs very steeply, then moderately, and steeply again, getting fainter as it goes. A few hundred feet before you reach the ridgecrest, you come to a late-lingering snow bank (cross with care), beyond which the trail may appear to fork but doesn't really. If you notice the "fork," be sure to take the right fork south-southwest. (The left fork soon peters out; it used to lead to a much steeper, rockier route down to Echo Creek.)

Regardless of whether you notice the fork, follow the faint track as it veers right up a granite-sand slope sparsely dotted with stunted whitebarks. A few more steps bring you to a viewless, unnamed col (10,160'; 11S 291172 4190575), from which the very faint path begins a descent south-southwest, soon becoming a beaten track again.

The route now winds steeply down, first on sand and then through lovely pocket meadows on the headwaters of Echo Creek, along which it descends for about 2 miles. Near the floor of Echo Creek's valley, where you have a fine over-the-shoulder view of the Cockscomb atop the west valley wall, you pass through a maze of avalanche-downed tree trunks. Fortunately, seasons of hikers before you have beaten a circuitous but passable route through the trunks.

THE COCKSCOMB

Aptly named by François Matthes, this slender crest bears clear marks of the highest level reached by the ice of the last glacial episode. Its lower shoulders reveal the rounded, well-polished surfaces that betray glacial action, while its jagged, sharply etched crest shows no such markings. Further evidence of glacial action may be clearly seen on the steep descent into the head of long, typically U-shaped Echo Creek valley. The shearing and polishing action of the ice mass that shaped this rounded valley is evident on the cliffs on the west side.

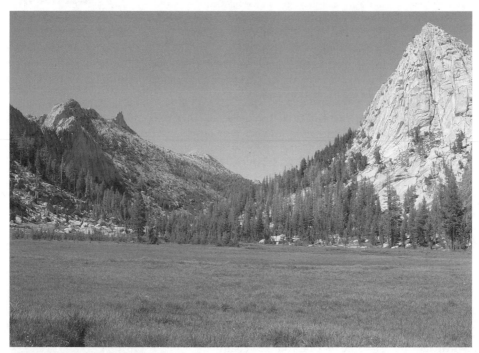

The Cockscomb (left) from Echo Creek

At last the trail reaches the valley floor, where the meadow is lush with seasonal wild-flowers: Davidson's penstemon, Douglas phlox, groundsel, red heather, lupine, and ranger's button. Going down the valley, the trail stays on the creek's east side.

As you approach the end of the second large meadow in this valley, the trail abruptly curves left (east) and leaves Echo Creek to veer up a low, rocky ridge—but don't top the ridge immediately. Instead, follow the undulating track a little below the ridgetop, through sparse forest, and finally up a trackless granite slot. At the slot's upper end, you are on the ridgetop (9532′; 11S 290080 4187464—field), without a trail and in a sort of Duck Hell: gran-ite slabs with way too many ducks, many of them misleading. Bear right (southeast), gen-erally toward prominent Peak 11357T, to cross the ridge and descend into an unnamed gully where you pick up a distinct track again.

The path shortly crosses the gully's intermittent stream and soon begins climbing the next ridge east on moderately steep switchbacks. At the sandy ridgetop, the track crosses over (eastward) and then, angling left (northeast), makes a very brief descent into the meadow along Nelson Lake's outlet. Bear left on the track through the meadow; the track vanishes as you near Nelson's shore near an overused campsite (9605′, 11S 290553 4187268—field).

Nelson Lake sits under imposing Rafferty Peak to the east-northeast, Peak 11105T of the Cathedral Range to the north-northeast, and an unnamed, south-trending spur of the Cathedral Range to the west (you just crossed one of the spur's low points). Good camp-sites may be found on the southeast and southwest sides. Anglers will find the lake's waters good fishing for brook trout.

DAY 2 (Nelson Lake to Elizabeth Lake Trailhead, 5.9 miles, part cross-country): Retrace your steps.

HWY 120

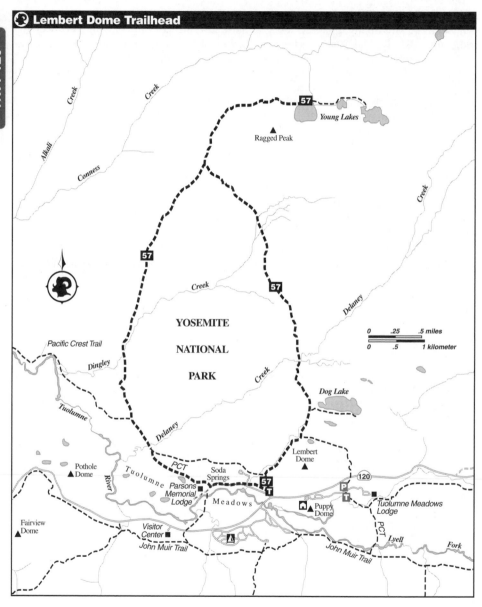

Lembert Dome Trailhead

Lembert Dome Trailhead

8584'; 11S 292591 4194973

DESTINATION/ UTM COORDINATES	TRIP TYPE	BEST SEASON	PACE (HIKING/ LAYOVER DAYS)	TOTAL MILEAGE
57 Young Lakes 11S 293594 4201417	Semiloop	Mid or late	2/1 Moderate	15.1

Information and Permits: These trips enter Yosemite National Park: Yosemite Permits, PO Box 545, Yosemite National Park, CA 95389; 209-372-0740; www.nps.gov/yose/wilderness/permits.htm. Bear canisters are required; pets and firearms are prohibited.

Driving Directions: From Hwy. 120 in Yosemite's Tuolumne Meadows, just 7 miles southwest of Tioga Pass and just east of the bridge over the Tuolumne River, turn west on a dirt road along Lembert Dome's western face. The road leads to a locked gate, which we consider the trailhead, and from here the road turns right toward the stables. Find a parking spot where permitted along the road between the highway and the gate. You may not park overnight in the lot at the base of Lembert Dome.

57 Young Lakes

Trip Data: 11S 293594 4201417; 15.1 miles; 2/1 days

Topos: *Tioga Pass, Falls Ridge*

Highlights: The three Young Lakes, cupped under soaring Ragged Peak, offer a large selection of campsites, some in heavy woods and some at timberline.

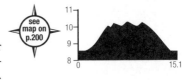

These camps provide a base for exciting excursions into the headwaters of Conness Creek and for climbing Mt. Conness itself.

DAY 1 (Lembert Dome Trailhead to Lowest Young Lake, 8.2 miles): Go around the locked gate and continue west along the lodgepole-dotted flank of Tuolumne Meadows, with fine views south across the meadows of Unicorn Peak, Cathedral Peak, and some of the Echo Peaks. Approaching a boulder-rimmed old parking loop, you veer right past a shelter around a rust-colored soda spring and climb slightly to what was once Soda Springs Campground.

> **SODA SPRINGS CAMPGROUND**
> This former campground was once the private holding of John Lembert, namesake of Lembert Dome. His brothers, who survived him, sold it to the Sierra Club in 1912, and for 60 years Club members enjoyed a private campground in this marvelous subalpine meadow. But in 1972 the Club deeded the property to the National Park Service so that everyone could use it.

Here the road forks, and you go right (northwest), now on the PCT. (To take a peek at the nearby buildings—McCauley Cabin, Parsons Memorial Lodge, and a restroom—briefly go left, and then return after having satisfied your curiosity.) The sandy PCT undulates northwest through a forest of sparse, small lodgepole pines and passes a trail to the right that leads southeast and back to the stables. You continue north-northwest and descend to a ford of Delaney Creek (the only year-round, reliable water in either Delaney or upcoming Dingley creeks). Immediately beyond the ford, you hop a branch of Delaney Creek and then hop another in 300 yards; by late season, these branches are dry.

Soon the trail almost touches the southwest arm of Tuolumne Meadows and then ascends to a signed trail junction where you go right (north) toward Young Lakes. From the junction, you ascend slightly and cross a broad expanse of boulder-strewn sheets of granite. An open spot affords a look south across broad Tuolumne Meadows to the line of peaks from Fairview Dome to the steeple-like spires of the Cathedral Range.

After crossing the open granite, the trail climbs a tree-clothed slope to a ridge, turns up the ridge for several hundred yards, and then veers down to cross Dingley Creek (may be dry by late season). Past floods have strewn this area with logs, and it is easy to lose the trail here. Head across directly perpendicular to the creek; you will find the clearly worn trail on the far side of the extensive flood debris. In the first mile beyond this small creek, you jump across its north fork (also likely to be dry late in the year) and then wind gently upward in shady pine forest carpeted with a fine flower display even into late season: groundsel, daisies, lupine, squawroot, gooseberries, and perhaps the delicate, creamy-white flowers of Mariposa lilies, with one rich brown spot in the throat of each petal. Near the ridgetop, breaks in the lodgepole forest allow you glimpses of the whole Cathedral Range.

On the other side of the ridge, a new panoply of peaks appears in the north: majestic Tower Peak, Doghead and Quarry peaks, the Finger Peaks, Matterhorn Peak, Sheep Peak, Mt. Conness, and the Shepherd Crest. From this viewpoint, a brief, moderate descent leads to a ford of a tributary of Conness Creek (may be dry by late season), where more varieties of flowers decorate the green banks of this icy, dashing stream.

At once, the descending trail reaches the signed Dog Lake Trail junction, temporarily ending the loop part of this trip. Turn left (generally north) and descend into thickening hemlock forest. On a level stretch of trail, you cross another branch of Conness Creek, and then switchback a half mile up to a plateau from where the view is fine of the steep north face of Ragged Peak.

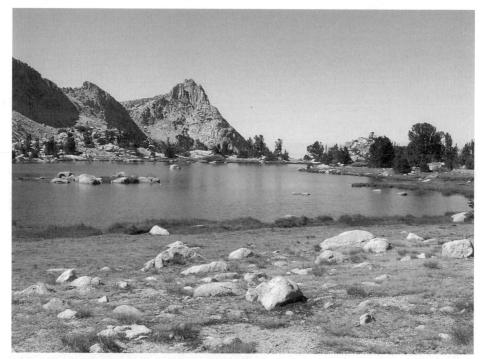

Highest Young Lake, with Ragged Peak just left of center

The trail curves east, and after passing a meadow that was the fourth Young Lake before it filled in with stream sediments, the path descends to the west shore of Lowest Young Lake (9894'; 11S 293594 4201417), the most popular destination of the three Young Lakes. (The mileage given for this trip is only to Lowest Young Lake.) There are both primitive and well-developed campsites along the north shore of this lake. More secluded campsites may be found on Middle Young Lake (9892') by following the trail east around the lower lake, fording the lower lake's outlet, and picking up a use trail east to the middle lake. From the middle lake, you can go up the inlet to the highest lake (10,218'), which is the most attractive and also the most exposed. Fishing on the Young Lakes is fair to good for brook trout.

DAY 2 (Lowest Young Lake to Lembert Dome Trailhead, 6.9 miles): From Lowest Young Lake, retrace your steps to the signed Dog Lake Trail junction. Turn left (southeast) toward Dog Lake, "reopening" the loop part of this trip, and climb the southwest spur of Ragged Peak on a sandy, boulder-scattered slope under a moderate lodgepole-and-hemlock forest cover. Views from this point are outstanding. From here, the trail descends through a very large, gently sloping meadow dotted with small lodgepoles. This broad expanse is a wildflower garden in season, laced with meandering brooks, but it may be almost dry late in a dry year. Paintbrush, lupine, and monkeyflower in the foreground set off the occasional views of the entire Cathedral Range, strung out on the southern horizon.

Near the lower edge of the meadow, you cross the headwaters of Dingley Creek (may be dry by late season) and then descend, steeply at times, some 300 feet through a moderately dense forest of lodgepoles and a few hemlocks. Then the trail levels off and veers east on a gently rolling course through more lodgepole forest where the sandy soil sprouts thousands of prostrate little lupine plants. Beyond is a very large, level meadow where the reddish peaks of Mt. Dana and Mt. Gibbs loom in the east, Delaney Creek meanders lazily through the grass, and Belding ground squirrels pipe away. The Delaney Creek ford is difficult in early season; you might look upstream. Beyond the creek, you will find the continuation of your trail.

After crossing a little ridge, the route drops once more toward Tuolumne Meadows. Lembert Dome can be glimpsed through the trees along this stretch of trail. The trail levels slightly before it fords Dog Lake's outlet and meets the signed 0.1-mile lateral left to Dog Lake; you continue ahead (south). Then it passes a junction with a trail that goes east; you go ahead (generally south) here. The 560-foot descent from here is terribly dusty, loose, rocky, and steep and is heavily used by dayhikers as it switchbacks down close under the steep west face of Lembert Dome. At the bottom of the deep dust, a lateral trail leads right (west) to the stables; you continue ahead (south-southeast) here. Soon, another lateral goes left, but you continue ahead (south-southeast) to cross slabs between parallel rows of rocks before passing through lodgepole forest and past restrooms to the Lembert Dome parking lot and the road you drove in on. Turn right on the road to find your car.

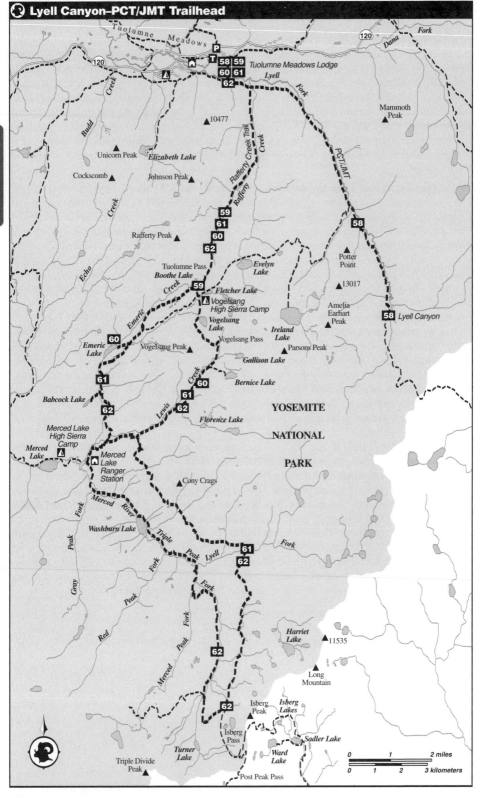

Tuolumne Meadows

120

10477

Budd Creek

Unicorn Peak

Elizabeth Lake

Cockscomb

Johnson Peak

Echo Creek

Rafferty Peak

59
61
62

Rafferty Creek Trail

Rafferty Creek

Tuolumne Pass
Boothe Lake

59

Evelyn Lake

Emeric Creek

Fletcher Lake

Vogelsang High Sierra Camp

Vogelsang Lake

Emeric Lake

60

Vogelsang Peak

Vogelsang Pass

Ireland Lake

Parsons Peak

61

Babcock Lake

Lewis Creek

60

Gallison Lake

61
62

Bernice Lake

62

Florence Lake

Merced Lake High Sierra Camp

Merced Lake

Merced Lake Ranger Station

Cony Crags

Merced River

Washburn Lake

Gray Peak Fork

Red Peak Fork

Triple Peak Fork

Lyell Fork

Fork

61
62

Merced Peak Fork

62

Harriet Lake

11535

Long Mountain

62

Isberg Peak

Isberg Lakes

Isberg Pass

Turner Lake

Ward Lake

Sadler Lake

Triple Divide Peak

Post Peak Pass

120

Dana Fork

58 **59**
60 **61**
62

Tuolumne Meadows Lodge

Lyell Fork

Mammoth Peak

PCT/JMT

58

Potter Point

13017

Amelia Earhart Peak

58 Lyell Canyon

YOSEMITE

NATIONAL

PARK

0   1   2 miles
0   1   2   3 kilometers

204

Lyell Canyon-PCT/JMT Trailhead   8701'; 11S 294306 4194865

DESTINATION/ UTM COORDINATES	TRIP TYPE	BEST SEASON	PACE (HIKING/ LAYOVER DAYS)	TOTAL MILEAGE
58 Lyell Canyon 11S 300785 4184806	Out & back	Early to late	2/1 Leisurely	18
59 Vogelsang High Sierra Camp 11S 293663 4185823	Out & back	Mid or late	2/1 Leisurely	15.4
60 Emeric Lake 11S 290240 4183858	Semiloop	Mid or late	4/1 Moderate	28.8
61 Lyell Fork Merced River 11S 294995 4175798	Semiloop	Mid or late	6/1 Leisurely	40.3
62 Triple Peak Fork Merced River 11S 293186 4170519	Semiloop	Mid or late	7/1 Moderate	51.3

Information and Permits: These trips enter Yosemite National Park: Yosemite Permits, PO Box 545, Yosemite National Park, CA 95389; 209-372-0740; www.nps.gov/yose/wilderness/permits.htm. Bear canisters are required; pets and firearms are prohibited.

Driving Directions: This is a trailhead for the southbound PCT, soon to join the JMT. About 6.6 miles west of Tioga Pass on Hwy. 120 and just east of Lembert Dome, take the signed turnoff south toward Tuolumne Meadows Lodge. Almost immediately, another spur road darts right (southwest) to a wilderness permit station and its parking lot. Avoiding that spur road, you continue toward the lodge as the road angles east, paralleling Hwy. 120. In a little more than 0.4 more mile, look for the backpackers' parking lot on the north side of the road (on your left).

58 Lyell Canyon

Trip Data: 11S 300785 4184806; 18 miles; 2/1 days

Topos: *Vogelsang Peak, Tioga Pass*

Highlights: The subalpine meadows of Lyell Canyon are the stuff of which favorite backpacking memories are made. Idyllic from beginning to end, this long, gentle grassland with its meandering river is a delight to travel.

see map on p.204

HEADS UP! *Park regulations prohibit camping within 4 miles of Hwy. 120. Bears are especially active in Lyell Canyon.*

DAY 1 (Lyell Canyon-PCT/JMT Trailhead to Lyell Base Camp, 9 miles): The trailhead is immediately across the spur road from the parking lot, a broad track signed for the JMT, though in fact the JMT is some distance ahead. Follow this path a short distance downhill to meet a trail that runs east-west, roughly paralleling the spur road. This trail is in fact the PCT, and you turn left (east) onto it, soon meeting Dana Fork Tuolumne River. Where the PCT curves right (south), a use trail darts left (north) off to Tuolumne Meadows Lodge; you continue on the PCT and cross Dana Fork on a footbridge. On the other side of the bridge, a trail goes left (east), but you go ahead (south) on the PCT, ascend a low rise, and, curving a little bit right past a large pine tree, descend slabs to Lyell Fork Tuolumne River.

The PCT crosses Lyell Fork on a substantial double bridge that offers splendid views upstream (eastward) to beautiful riverside meadows and beyond to Mt. Dana and Mt. Gibbs. There's good fishing here for brown trout. About 0.1 mile past the bridge and a little less than a mile from your trailhead, you meet the JMT. Turn left (east) onto it in dense

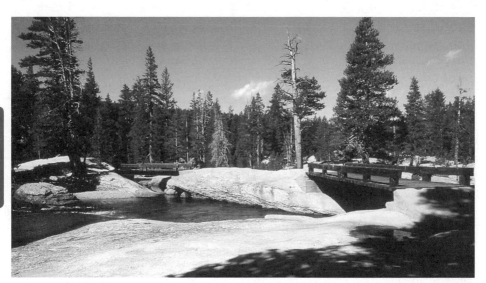

Lyell Fork's double bridge

forest and in a little under 0.75 mile, meet the Rafferty Creek Trail (right, south) at a junction just shy of a sturdy footbridge over Rafferty Creek (may be dry here by late season in a dry year).

> **REROUTING TRAILS**
>
> The preceding PCT/JMT leg once ran through the meadow along the river but has since been rerouted into the meadow's forested edge. The new trail was established because of extensive trail wear and subsequent erosion of the old route. Rerouting is one of several far-sighted policies the Park Service has adopted to allow areas in the wilderness a breather—a chance to recover from overuse.

At this junction, your route goes ahead (east) and crosses Rafferty Creek on the bridge. From this point on, the trail traverses alternating meadowed and forested sections as it veers southeastward, and lucky hikers may see grazing deer in the meadows and an occasional marmot that has ventured from the rocky hillside on the right. Fields of wildflowers color the grasslands from early to late season, but the best times of the year for seeing this color are generally early to mid season. From the more open parts of the trail, there are excellent views of the Kuna Crest as it slopes up to the southeast, and the river itself has delighted generations of mountain photographers.

The route then passes a trail branching right (south) to Ireland and Evelyn lakes, Vogelsang High Sierra Camp, and Tuolumne Pass; your route, the PCT/JMT, continues ahead (south-southeast) along the river. There are fair campsites around this junction. Beyond this junction, the trail fords Ireland Creek (difficult in early season), passes below Potter Point, and ascends moderately, gradually curving southward, for almost 3 miles to the fair campsites at Lyell Base Camp (not shown as such on the 7.5' topo; 9040'; 11S 300785 4184806). Fishing is fair for brook trout. This base camp, surrounded on three sides by steep canyon walls, marks the end of the meadowed sections of Lyell Canyon and is the traditional first-night stopping place for those who walk the JMT beginning at your trailhead.

DAY 2 (Lyell Canyon to Lyell Canyon-PCT/JMT Trailhead, 9 miles): Retrace your steps.

59 Vogelsang High Sierra Camp

Trip Data: 11S 293663 4185823; 15.4 miles; 2/1 days

Topos: *Vogelsang Peak*

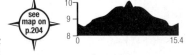

Highlights: Vogelsang Camp has the most dramatic
setting of all the famous High Sierra Camps. Located
right under the somber north face of Fletcher Peak, it offers eagle views of valleys, granite
domes, and lakes below. Many nearby lakes offer exciting side trips for anglers, swimmers,
and picnickers, and Fletcher Peak, a Class 2 scramble, invites climbers.

DAY 1 (Lyell Canyon-PCT/JMT Trailhead to Vogelsang High Sierra Camp, 7.7 miles): *(Partial Recap: Trip 58, Day 1, from Lyell Canyon-PCT/JMT Trailhead to the junction just shy of the bridge over Rafferty Creek.)* The trailhead is immediately across the spur road from the parking lot, a broad track signed for the JMT. Follow this path a short distance downhill to meet the PCT running west-east. Turn left (east) onto it, soon meeting Dana Fork Tuolumne River. Where the PCT curves right (south), a use trail darts left (north) off to Tuolumne Meadows Lodge; you continue on the PCT and cross Dana Fork on a footbridge. On the other side, a trail goes left (east), but you go ahead (south) on the PCT, ascend a low rise, and, curving right past a large pine tree, descend slabs to Lyell Fork Tuolumne River. Cross Lyell Fork on a double bridge and, about 0.1 mile past the bridge and a little less than a mile from your trailhead, you meet the JMT. Turn left (east) onto it in dense forest and in a little under 0.75 mile, meet the Rafferty Creek Trail (right, south) at a junction just shy of a sturdy footbridge over Rafferty Creek.

Leaving the Day 1 route of Trip 58, you turn right onto the Rafferty Creek Trail and begin climbing moderately to steeply about 400 feet on switchbacking trail under good forest shade. As the grade eases, you pass through high, boulder-strewn meadows. Soon the trail dips close to year-round Rafferty Creek. The path won't ford the creek but instead stays west of it—but rarely close to it—until just below Tuolumne Pass (contrary to what the 7.5' topo shows). The nearly level trail makes a very long, gentle ascent, skirting some large, rocky knolls as it traverses a sparse forest of lodgepole pines. The terrain is starkly beautiful, with huge, lichen-bearing boulders and meadows bounded by polished granite walls. On the way, you cross some tributaries of Rafferty Creek that may be dry by late season.

As you begin the final, gentle ascent to Tuolumne Pass, dense and varied wildflower displays nearby vie for your attention. Finally, the lodgepole pines give way to a few whitebark pines, and these trees diminish the force of the winds that often sweep through Tuolumne Pass (9992'), a major gap in the Tuolumne Range. In the pass, a signed trail junction indicates that the right fork goes to Boothe, Emeric, Babcock, and Merced lakes, while the left fork, your route, heads south to Vogelsang High Sierra Camp. Through breaks in this forest, you have intermittent views of cliff-bound, dark-banded Fletcher Peak and Vogelsang Peak in the south.

Taking the left fork, leave the forest as the trail leads out into an area of bouldery granite outcrop-

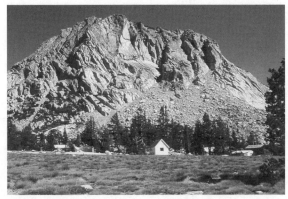

Day 1's destination, Vogelsang High Sierra Camp, beneath Fletcher Peak

pings dotted with a few trees. Now on the west side of saucer-shaped Tuolumne Pass, you follow a rocky-dusty path up a moderately steep hillside, below which are serene Boothe Lake and its surrounding meadows. Finally, the trail reaches the top of this climb, and suddenly you see the tents of Vogelsang High Sierra Camp (10,157') spread out before you. You can buy a few snacks and minor equipment items at the tiny store here and reserve a dinner or breakfast if the dining room has space for you.

There is a major junction here: right (southwest) down to Fletcher Creek, ahead (south) to Vogelsang Lake, and left (east) to Fletcher Lake, a short distance beyond the High Sierra Camp. Unless you have a reservation for the camp, turn left and follow a nearly level path past a use trail back to the High Sierra Camp and toward a raised pit toilet on the left, abreast of but well away from lovely Fletcher Lake, just below towering Fletcher Peak. There are backpacker campsites under the whitebark pines here (10159'; 11S 293663 4185823).

DAY 2 (Vogelsang High Sierra Camp to Lyell Canyon-PCT/JMT Trailhead, 7.7 miles): Retrace your steps.

60 Emeric Lake

Trip Data: 11S 290240 4183858; 28.8 miles; 4/1 days

Topos: *Merced Peak, Vogelsang Peak, Mt. Lyell, Merced Peak, Tenaya Lake*

Highlights: With Vogelsang High Sierra Camp as the beginning of the loop part of this semiloop, this trip "lassos" Vogelsang Peak by dashing down the valley of Lewis Creek and then cruising back up the valley of Fletcher Creek. The views are spectacular, and the fishing on creeks and lakes is good.

HEADS UP! The last day is a very long one (10.8 miles). Hikers wishing an easier end to this trip could add a day and then adjust Day 3 to stop at Babcock Lake, Day 4 at Boothe Lake, and exiting on a shorter final day, in this case the added Day 5.

DAY 1 (Lyell Canyon-PCT/JMT Trailhead to Vogelsang High Sierra Camp, 7.7 miles): *(Partial Recap: Trip 58, Day 1, from Lyell Canyon-PCT/JMT Trailhead to the junction just shy of the bridge over Rafferty Creek.)* The trailhead is immediately across the spur road from the parking lot, a broad track signed for the JMT. Follow this path a short distance downhill to meet the PCT running west-east here. Turn left (east) onto it, soon meeting Dana Fork Tuolumne River. Where the trail curves south, a use trail darts off to Tuolumne Meadows Lodge; you continue on the PCT and cross Dana Fork on a footbridge. On the other side, a trail goes left (east), but you go ahead (south) on the PCT, and, curving right past a large pine tree, descend slabs to Lyell Fork Tuolumne River. Cross Lyell Fork on a double bridge and, about 0.1 mile past the bridge and a little less than a mile from your trailhead, you meet the JMT. Turn left (east) onto it in dense forest and in a little less than 0.75 mile, meet the Rafferty Creek Trail (right, south) at a junction just shy of a sturdy footbridge over Rafferty Creek.

(Partial Recap: Trip 59, Day 1, from the junction just shy of the bridge over Rafferty Creek to Vogelsang High Sierra Camp.) Turn right onto the Rafferty Creek Trail and climb moderate-to-steep, shady switchbacks about 400 feet. As the grade eases to gradual, you pass through meadows and soon dip close to year-round Rafferty Creek. You won't ford this creek until just below Tuolumne Pass (contrary to what the 7.5' topo shows), but you will cross some of its tributaries, which may be dry by late season. At Tuolumne Pass (9992'), a major gap in the Tuolumne Range, there's a signed trail junction: The left fork, your route,

heads south to Vogelsang High Sierra Camp. Take that left fork to begin the loop part of this trip. Now on the west side of Tuolumne Pass, you follow a rocky-dusty path up a moderately steep hillside with Vogelsang High Sierra Camp (10,157') at the top. There is a major junction here: right (southwest) down to Fletcher Creek, ahead (south) to Vogelsang Lake, and left (east) to Fletcher Lake, a short distance beyond the High Sierra Camp (piped water available). Turn left and follow a nearly level path past a use trail back to the High Sierra Camp and toward a raised pit toilet on the left, abreast of but well away from Fletcher Lake (10159'; 11S 293663 4185823) and find campsites scattered under the whitebark pines here.

DAY 2 (Vogelsang High Sierra Camp to Florence Creek, 4.3 miles): Return to the trail junction next to the High Sierra Camp and take the trail left (south) to Vogelsang Lake and Pass. The track drops a little along Fletcher Creek, fords it, and begins a 550-foot moderate ascent with occasional steep sections toward the pass. Your climb is rewarded, as always in the Sierra, with increasingly good views. Fletcher Peak rises grandly on the left, and to the far north stands Mt. Conness. Clouds Rest and Half Dome come into view in the west-southwest.

Partway to the pass, the trail skirts the west shore of Vogelsang Lake (10,324), a timberline lake that offers windswept camping among the whitebarks bordering it. Nearer the pass, views to the north are occluded somewhat, but expansive new views appear in the south: From left to right are Parsons Peak, Simmons Peak, Mt. Maclure, the tip of Mt. Lyell behind Maclure, Mt. Florence and, in the south, the entire Clark Range from Triple Divide Peak on the left to Mt. Clark on the right.

From the windswept pass (10,650'), you look down to the east onto Gallison and Bernice lakes. The trail rises briefly northeast before it follows murderously steep switchbacks down into sparse lodgepole forest where many small streams provide moisture for thousands of giant lupine plants with their blossoms in shades of blue. The music of Gallison Lake's unnamed outlet stream becomes clear as the trail begins to level off, and then you reach a flat meadow through which the stream slowly meanders. There are some excellent campsites from here to Florence Creek.

Proceeding down a rutted, grassy trail for several hundred yards, you come to a brief, steep descent on a rocky path that swoops down to the meadowed valley of multi-braided Lewis Creek. In this little valley, in quick succession, you ford the Gallison Lake outlet and then Lewis Creek. In a few minutes, you pass the steep half-mile lateral east-southeast and uphill to Bernice Lake (incorrectly indicated as 1 mile on the sign); here, continue ahead (southwest). The shady trail winds gently down east of the creek under a moderate

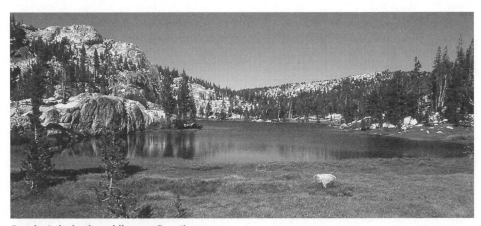

Boothe Lake beckons hikers on Day 4's route.

canopy of lodgepole pine mixed with some hemlock, crossing a little stream about a half mile from the last ford.

Then, after almost touching the creek opposite a steep, rusty west canyon wall, the trail veers away and fords another small tributary stream. Here the trail crosses the scars of invading avalanches as it winds through dense hemlock forest to the good campsites beside Florence Creek (9200'; 11S 292530 4181379), which flows into Lewis Creek nearby. This year-round creek cascades dramatically down to the camping area over steep granite sheets, and fishing in Florence and Lewis creeks is good for brook trout.

DAY 3 (Florence Creek to Emeric Lake, 6 miles): Leaving the hemlock forest, the trail descends a series of lodgepole-dotted granite slabs above Lewis Creek, which rumbles through chutes below on your right.

PEELING GRANITE?

Where the creek's channel narrows, you find on the left a lesson in exfoliation: granite layers peeling like an onion. This kind of peeling is typically seen on Yosemite's domes, but this fine example is located on a canyon slope.

As the bed of Lewis Creek steepens, so does the trail, and the descent reaches the zone of red firs and western white pines. After dipping beside the creek, the trail climbs away from it. At about 8700 feet, you meet a junction with the signed Isberg Trail. You continue ahead (generally west-southwest) and switchback down moderately to steeply under a sparse cover of red fir, juniper, lodgepole, and western white pine for 1 mile to a signed junction with the Fletcher Creek Trail. You turn right (northeast) onto this trail.

(Partial Recap: Trip 53, Day 4, from the junction with the Fletcher Creek Trail to Emeric Lake.) Now you descend to a wooden bridge over Lewis Creek (hardened camping near the bridge). From here, the trail climbs moderately to steeply for 400 feet on cobblestoned, exposed trail past a tributary a half mile from Lewis Creek, where there are views of cascades on Fletcher Creek. The trail then swings very close to the creek before climbing, steeply at times, on more cobblestones, until it finally levels off near some nice but illegal campsites. Soon your path meets a side trail left (west) to small Babcock Lake (campsites).

From this junction, you go ahead (north) on sandy trail that ascends steadily through moderate forest just east of Fletcher Creek. After a mile, the trail rises steeply via rocky switchbacks from which you can see, nearby in the north, the outlet stream of Emeric Lake—though not the lake itself, which is behind a dome just to the right of the outlet's notch.

The switchbacks top out with the dome to the north, and the trail then follows Fletcher Creek northeast to a ford. Almost immediately beyond the ford, the track meets a junction with the spur trail to Emeric Lake.

Go left (west) to Emeric Lake (9396'; 11S 290240 4183858) and follow angler's trails to the excellent campsites midway along its northwest shore. The meadow north and northeast of the lake is carpeted with delicate wildflowers. Fishing is often good for rainbow.

DAY 4 (Emeric Lake to Lyell Canyon-PCT/JMT Trailhead, 10.8 miles): *(Recap: Trip 53, Day 5.)* This is a very long day, so get an early start. Retrace your steps to the spur trail at the lake's northeast corner at the base of a granite knoll. Take the spur east-northeast for 0.6 mile to a junction in the valley of Fletcher Creek. Go left (northeast) on the main trail up the valley and follow a rocky-dusty trail to another junction where you go left (north-northeast) toward Boothe Lake (the right fork goes up Fletcher Creek's valley to Vogelsang). Climb away from Fletcher Creek and top a minor summit where the trail descends slightly and then winds levelly past a long series of lovely ponds; numerous signs ask you to stay on the main trail. You soon reach a junction with a use trail to the south end of Boothe Lake (9845'; campsites).

The trail shortly goes ahead, bypassing Boothe Lake and contouring above it, passing a junction with another use trail down to the lake. About a quarter mile farther, you reach Tuolumne Pass (9992') and close the loop at the junction with the trails to Vogelsang High Sierra Camp (sharp right) and down the Rafferty Creek Trail (ahead, north). Go ahead on the Rafferty Creek Trail and retrace your steps of Day 1 of this trip to the Lyell Canyon-PCT/JMT Trailhead (8701'; 11S 294306 4194865).

61 Lyell Fork Merced River

Trip Data: 11S 294995 4175798; 40.3 miles; 6/1 days

Topos: *Merced Peak, Vogelsang Peak, Mt. Lyell, Merced Peak, Tenaya Lake*

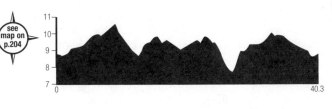

see map on p.204

Highlights: Beginning backpackers sooner or later want to try their newfound skills on a challenging trip of some length. This excursion is made to order for them: long mileage, but not too long; tough but manageable climbs; lonely stretches, but two popular camp-sites in between. And it encompasses some of the best scenery in Yosemite National Park.

DAY 1 (Lyell Canyon-PCT/JMT Trailhead to Vogelsang High Sierra Camp, 7.7 miles): *(Partial Recap: Trip 58, Day 1, from Lyell Canyon-PCT/JMT Trailhead to the junction just shy of the bridge over Rafferty Creek.)* The trailhead is immediately across the spur road from the parking lot, a broad track signed for the JMT. Follow this path a short distance downhill to meet the PCT running west-east here. Turn left (east) onto it, soon meeting Dana Fork Tuolumne River. Where the trail curves south, a use trail darts off to Tuolumne Meadows Lodge; you continue on the PCT and cross Dana Fork on a footbridge. On the other side, a trail goes left (east), but you go ahead (south) on the PCT, and, curving right past a large pine tree, descend slabs to Lyell Fork Tuolumne River. Cross Lyell Fork on a double bridge and, about 0.1 mile past the bridge and a little less than a mile from your trailhead, you meet the JMT. Turn left (east) onto it in dense forest and in a little less than 0.75 mile, meet the Rafferty Creek Trail (right, south) at a junction just shy of a sturdy footbridge over Rafferty Creek.

(Partial Recap: Trip 59, Day 1, from the junction just shy of the bridge over Rafferty Creek to Vogelsang High Sierra Camp.) Turn right onto the Rafferty Creek Trail and climb moder-ate-to-steep, shady switchbacks about 400 feet. As the grade eases to gradual, you pass through meadows and soon dip close to year-round Rafferty Creek. You won't ford this creek until just below Tuolumne Pass (contrary to what the 7.5' topo shows), but you will cross some of its tributaries, which may be dry by late season. At Tuolumne Pass (9992'), a major gap in the Tuolumne Range, there's a signed trail junction: The left fork, your route, heads south to Vogelsang High Sierra Camp. Take that left fork to begin the loop part of this trip. Now on the west side of Tuolumne Pass, you follow a rocky-dusty path up a mod-erately steep hillside with Vogelsang High Sierra Camp (10,157') at the top. There is a major junction here: right (southwest) down to Fletcher Creek, ahead (south) to Vogelsang Lake, and left (east) to Fletcher Lake, a short distance beyond the High Sierra Camp (piped water available). Turn left and follow a nearly level path past a use trail back to the High Sierra Camp and toward a raised pit toilet on the left, abreast of but well away from

Fletcher Lake (10159'; 11S 293663 4185823) and find campsites scattered under the white-bark pines here.

DAY 2 (Vogelsang High Sierra Camp to Florence Creek, 4.3 miles): *(Recap: Trip 60, Day 2.)* Return to the trail junction next to the High Sierra Camp and take the trail left (south) to Vogelsang Lake and Pass. The track drops a little along Fletcher Creek, fords it, and begins a 550-foot moderate ascent with occasional steep sections toward the pass. Partway to the pass, the trail skirts the west shore of Vogelsang Lake (10,324; windswept camping).

From windswept Vogelsang Pass, the trail rises briefly northeast before it follows murderously steep switchbacks down into sparse lodgepole forest. As the trail levels off, you reach a flat meadow through which Gallison Lake's outlet stream slowly meanders. There are some excellent campsites from here to Florence Creek.

You presently come to a brief, steep descent on a rocky path down the valley of Lewis Creek. In this little valley, in quick succession, you ford Gallison Lake's outlet and then Lewis Creek. In a few minutes, you pass the lateral east-southeast and uphill to Bernice Lake; here, continue ahead (southwest). The shady trail crosses a little stream about a half mile from the last ford.

Then ford another stream and wind through forest to the good campsites beside Florence Creek (9200'; 11S 292530 4181379), which flows into Lewis Creek nearby. Fishing in Florence and Lewis creeks is good for brook trout.

DAY 3 (Florence Creek to Lyell Fork Merced River, 7.4 miles): *(Partial Recap: Trip 60, Day 3, from Florence Creek to the junction with the Isberg Trail.)* Leaving the forest, the trail descends slabs above Lewis Creek. The trail becomes steeper, and the descent reaches the creek and then climbs away from it. At about 8700 feet, you meet a junction with the signed Isberg Trail.

Here, you leave the Day 3 route of Trip 60 and turn left (generally south), onto the switchbacking Isberg Pass Trail. The ascent from here is a tough, unrelieved 1000 vertical feet, but fortunately most of it is in shady forest of red fir and western white and lodgepole pine. Near the top, where the grade is a little less steep, the forest cover also includes altitude-loving whitebark pines.

At about 9000 feet, views to the west and north grow expansive, and you can make out Half Dome, Clouds Rest, the Cockscomb, and Unicorn Peak. After crossing a ridge, the sandy path descends into a meadow long since invaded by lodgepoles and reaches an all-year stream.

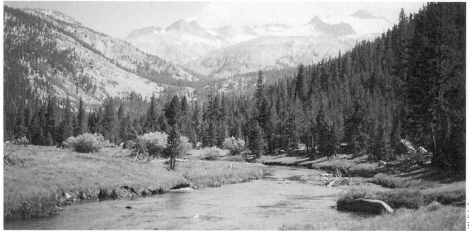

Lyell Fork Merced River, west side of Cathedral Range, with Rogers (left) and Electra (right) peaks in the background

Beyond this easy ford, your route, also known as the High Trail, traverses a broad bench at about 10,000 feet and fords a second, larger stream (may be difficult in early season). Then the trail climbs again, away from the lip of the main canyon, until it veers south back to the lip at a spectacular viewpoint for studying the headwaters of the Lyell Fork (in the east) and the Merced Peak Fork (in the south) of the Merced River. You could spend many days in these vast, trailless headwaters without seeing another human being.

From this overlook, the trail descends a bit steeply in places to ford a third all-year stream and then continues down to the cascading, chuting Lyell Fork Merced River (9125′; 11S 294995 4175798). The last segment of trail before the stream, over granite slabs, is a little hard to follow, but the route leads where you would expect it to. The campsites at the ford are poor, but good ones lie 150 yards downstream, where beautiful chutes and rapids flow over the sculpted granite bedrock. There are also good campsites a half mile upstream, a better base if you are going to explore the remote lake basins at the headwaters of the Lyell Fork. Fishing in the Lyell Fork is good for brook trout.

DAY 4 (Lyell Fork to Babcock Lake, 9.1 miles): First, retrace your steps to the Lewis Creek Trail. *(Partial Recap: Trip 50, Day 3, from the Isberg Trail junction to the side trail to Babcock Lake.)* Turn left (generally west-southwest) onto the Lewis Creek Trail. Switchback down moderately to steeply under a sparse forest for 1 mile to a signed junction with the Fletcher Creek Trail. Turn right (northeast) onto this trail.

(Partial Recap: Trip 53, Day 4, from the junction with the Fletcher Creek Trail to the Fletcher Creek Trail-Babcock Lake junction.) Now you descend to a wooden bridge over Lewis Creek (hardened camping near the bridge). From here, the trail climbs moderately to steeply for 400 feet on cobblestoned, exposed trail past a tributary a half mile from Lewis Creek, where there are views of cascades on Fletcher Creek. The trail then swings very close to the creek before climbing, steeply at times, on more cobblestones, until it finally levels off near some nice but illegal campsites. Soon your path meets a side trail left (west) to small Babcock Lake (campsites).

Leaving the Day 4 route of Trip 53, turn left and ford Fletcher Creek (difficult in early season). Then follow the winding trail 0.3 mile west to narrow, granite-bound Babcock Lake (8906′; 11S 289085 4181738). There are fine campsites all around this forested lake, and fishing is good for brook trout.

DAY 5 (Babcock Lake to Boothe Lake, 4.4 miles): Retrace your steps from Babcock Lake to the Fletcher Creek Trail-Babcock Lake junction. *(Partial Recap: Trip 53, Day 4, from the Fletcher Creek Trail-Babcock Lake junction to the Fletcher Creek Trail-Emeric Lake junction.)* From this junction, you go left (north) and ascend just east of Fletcher Creek. After a mile, the trail rises steeply via rocky switchbacks toward a dome near Emeric Lake. The switchbacks top out with the dome to the north, and the trail then follows Fletcher Creek northeast to a ford. Almost immediately beyond the ford, the track meets the spur trail to Emeric Lake (Fletcher Creek Trail-Emeric Lake junction).

(Partial Recap: Trip 53, Day 5, from the Fletcher Creek Trail-Emeric Lake junction to the junction with the use trail to the south end of Boothe Lake.) Go ahead (northeast) on the main trail a short distance to another junction, where you take the left fork northeast toward Boothe Lake (the right fork goes to Vogelsang). Climb away from Fletcher Creek, passing northwest of a bald prominence that sits in the center of the upper valley of Fletcher and Emeric creeks, separating the two. Topping a minor summit, the trail descends slightly and then winds levelly past a long series of lovely ponds; numerous signs ask you to stay on the main trail. At the junction with the use trail to the south end of Boothe Lake, leave the Day 5 route of Trip 53 again and bear left (north-northeast) to Boothe Lake's south end (9856′; 11S 293152 4186042), where there are some campsites.

DAY 6 (Boothe Lake to Lyell Canyon-PCT/JMT Trailhead, 7.4 miles): Retrace your steps to the main trail and turn left (northeast) on it. *(Partial Recap: Trip 53, Day 5, from the junction with* *the use trail to Boothe Lake's south end to the Lyell Canyon-PCT/JMT Trailhead.)* The trail shortly contours above Boothe Lake, passing a junction with another use trail down to the lake. About a quarter mile farther, you reach Tuolumne Pass (9992') and close the loop at the junction with the trails to Vogelsang High Sierra Camp (sharp right) and down the Rafferty Creek Trail (ahead, north). Go ahead on the Rafferty Creek Trail and retrace your steps for Day 1 of this trip to the Lyell Canyon-PCT/JMT Trailhead (8701'; 11S 294306 4194865).

62 Triple Peak Fork Merced River

Trip Data:
11S 293186
4170519;
51.3 miles;
7/1 days

see map on p.204

Topos: *Merced Peak,*
Vogelsang Peak,
Mt. Lyell, Merced Peak, Tenaya Lake

Highlights: The headwaters of the Triple Peak Fork Merced River are about as far as you can get from civilization, so this is a trip for those who feel they encounter too many people on most of their hikes. Their opportunity to view most of the High Sierra from the southern border of Yosemite is won by a long walk through grand high country.

HEADS UP! The last day is a very long one (10.8 miles). Hikers wishing an easier end to this trip could add a day and then adjust Day 6 to stop at Babcock Lake, Day 7 at Boothe Lake, and exiting on a shorter final day, in this case the added Day 8.

DAY 1 (Lyell Canyon-PCT/JMT Trailhead to Vogelsang High Sierra Camp, 7.7 miles): *(Partial Recap: Trip 58, Day 1, from Lyell Canyon-PCT/JMT Trailhead to the junction just shy of the bridge over Rafferty Creek.)* The trailhead is immediately across the spur road from the parking lot, a broad track signed for the JMT. Follow this path a short distance downhill to meet the PCT running west-east here. Turn left (east) onto it, soon meeting Dana Fork Tuolumne River. Where the trail curves south, a use trail darts off to Tuolumne Meadows Lodge; you continue on the PCT and cross Dana Fork on a footbridge. On the other side, a trail goes left (east), but you go ahead (south) on the PCT, and, curving right past a large pine tree, descend slabs to Lyell Fork Tuolumne River. Cross Lyell Fork on a double bridge and, about 0.1 mile past the bridge and a little less than a mile from your trailhead, you meet the JMT. Turn left (east) onto it in dense forest and in a little less than 0.75 mile, meet the Rafferty Creek Trail (right, south) at a junction just shy of a sturdy footbridge over Rafferty Creek.

(Partial Recap: Trip 59, Day 1, from the junction just shy of the bridge over Rafferty Creek to Vogelsang High Sierra Camp.) Turn right onto the Rafferty Creek Trail and climb moderate-to-steep, shady switchbacks about 400 feet. As the grade eases to gradual, you pass through meadows and soon dip close to year-round Rafferty Creek. You won't ford this creek until just below Tuolumne Pass (contrary to what the 7.5' topo shows), but you will cross some of its tributaries, which may be dry by late season. At Tuolumne Pass (9992'), a major gap in the Tuolumne Range, there's a signed trail junction: The left fork, your route, heads south to Vogelsang High Sierra Camp. Take that left fork to begin the loop part of this trip. Now on the west side of Tuolumne Pass, you follow a rocky-dusty path up a moderately steep hillside with Vogelsang High Sierra Camp (10,157') at the top. There is a major junction here: right (southwest) down to Fletcher Creek, ahead (south) to Vogelsang

Lake, and left (east) to Fletcher Lake, a short distance beyond the High Sierra Camp (piped water available). Turn left and follow a nearly level path past a use trail back to the High Sierra Camp and toward a raised pit toilet on the left, abreast of but well away from Fletcher Lake (10159'; 11S 293663 4185823) and find campsites scattered under the white-bark pines here.

DAY 2 (Vogelsang High Sierra Camp to Florence Creek, 4.3 miles): *(Recap: Trip 60, Day 2.)* Return to the trail junction next to the High Sierra Camp and take the trail left (south) to Vogelsang Lake and Pass. The track drops a little along Fletcher Creek, fords it, and begins a 550-foot moderate ascent with occasional steep sections toward the pass. Partway to the pass, the trail skirts the west shore of Vogelsang Lake (10,324; windswept camping).

From windswept Vogelsang Pass, the trail rises briefly northeast before it follows murderously steep switchbacks down into sparse lodgepole forest. As the trail levels off, you reach a flat meadow through which Gallison Lake's outlet stream slowly meanders. There are some excellent campsites from here to Florence Creek.

You presently come to a brief, steep descent on a rocky path down the valley of Lewis Creek. In this little valley, in quick succession, you ford Gallison Lake's outlet and then Lewis Creek. In a few minutes, you pass the lateral east-southeast and uphill to Bernice Lake; here, continue ahead (southwest). The shady trail crosses a little stream about a half mile from the last ford.

Then ford another stream and wind through forest to the good campsites beside Florence Creek (9200'; 11S 292530 4181379), which flows into Lewis Creek nearby. Fishing in Florence and Lewis creeks is good for brook trout.

DAY 3 (Florence Creek to Lyell Fork Merced River, 7.4 miles): *(Partial Recap: Trip 60, Day 3, from Florence Creek to the junction with the Isberg Trail.)* Leaving the forest, the trail descends slabs above Lewis Creek. The trail becomes steeper, and the descent reaches the creek and then climbs away from it. At about 8700 feet, you meet a junction with the signed Isberg Trail.

Here, you leave the Day 3 route of Trip 60 and turn left (generally south), onto the switchbacking Isberg Pass Trail. The ascent from here is a tough, unrelieved 1000 vertical feet, but fortunately most of it is in shady forest of red fir and western white and lodgepole pine. Near the top, where the grade is a little less steep, the forest cover also includes altitude-loving whitebark pines.

At about 9000 feet, views to the west and north grow expansive, and you can make out Half Dome, Clouds Rest, the Cockscomb, and Unicorn Peak. After crossing a ridge, the sandy path descends into a meadow long since invaded by lodgepoles and reaches an all-year stream.

Beyond this easy ford, your route, also known as the High Trail, traverses a broad bench at about 10,000 feet and fords a second, larger stream (may be difficult in early season). Then the trail climbs again, away from the lip of the main canyon, until it veers south back to the lip at a spectacular viewpoint for studying the headwaters of the Lyell Fork (in the east) and the Merced Peak Fork (in the south) of the Merced River. You could spend many days in these vast, trailless headwaters without seeing another human being.

From this overlook, the trail descends a bit steeply in places to ford a third all-year stream and then continues down to the cascading, chuting Lyell Fork Merced River (9125'; 11S 294995 4175798). The last segment of trail before the stream, over granite slabs, is a little hard to follow, but the route leads where you would expect it to. The campsites at the ford are poor, but good ones lie 150 yards downstream, where beautiful chutes and rapids flow over the sculpted granite bedrock. There are also good campsites a half mile upstream, a better base if you are going to explore the remote lake basins at the headwaters of the Lyell Fork. Fishing in the Lyell Fork is good for brook trout.

DAY 4 (Lyell Fork Merced River to Triple Peak Fork Meadow, 6.9 miles): This day's hike starts off strenuously up switchbacks on the south wall of Lyell Fork Merced River's canyon. Increasingly good views reward your struggle upward. In the northeast, on the Sierra Crest, are Mt. Maclure and Mt. Lyell, the highest point in Yosemite. After Lyell passes from view, Rodgers Peak, the second highest in the park, appears as the dark triangle beyond the right flank of Peak 12113. Other towering peaks in view this side of the crest don't even have names. Where the trail extends close to the lip of the Merced River's canyon, you can step off the path to an overlook for viewing most of the Clark Range in the southwest and Clouds Rest in the northwest.

Beyond the top of the ascent, the route winds among large boulders on *grus*—granite sand—that is the result of the breakup of just such boulders by the fierce erosion forces at work in these alpine climates. After crossing a seasonal stream, the trail ascends to a second broad ridge from which views through the whitebark pines continue to be excellent. About a half mile beyond this ridge, a trail to Foerster Lake (unnamed on the topo; trail not shown, either) veers off to the left. This unsigned trail is indicated by parallel rock borders and occasional flame-shaped blazes on trees. Secluded Foerster Lake has no fish, but swimming and camping there are excellent.

From this spur trail, the route makes a long descent, paralleling Foerster Lake's outlet part of the way, to a ford of Foerster Creek. The well-shaded trail then undulates past a number of pocket meadows, fording a couple of unmapped streams. A gentle traverse downward extends almost a mile to a small creek that winds through a flat area densely forested with hemlock and lodgepole pine. From this flat, the trail begins a climb that does not end until it reaches the Yosemite border at Isberg Pass. Very soon, the trail fords the outlet of the unnamed lake north of Isberg Peak, and in another 200 yards it reaches a large cairn that marks the junction with a trail down to the Triple Peak Fork. All hikers who arrive here with any surplus energy will greatly enjoy a 4-mile round trip to Isberg Pass before heading down to camp on the Triple Peak Fork (see sidebar).

SIDE TRIP TO ISBERG PASS

The mileage for this isn't included in the day's mileage above. The trail to Isberg Pass first climbs moderately for a quarter mile up a beautiful hillside covered with whitish broken granite in whose cracks a dozen species of alpine wildflowers grow. Looking west and north from this slope, you can see all the peaks of the Clark Range and most of the peaks of the Cathedral Range. You can probably make out Tenaya Peak, Tressider Peak, Cathedral Peak, Echo Peaks, Matthes Crest, and the Cockscomb. At the top of this little climb, a truly marvelous sight comes into view, for here you enter a large, high bowl nearly encircled by great peaks. The bowl contains an enormous meadow and two sparkling lakes. Here and there, clumps of whitebark and lodgepole pines help give scale to the vast amphitheater, and the delicacy of the meadow flowers is a perfect counterpoint to the massiveness of the encircling summits. The setting is magnificent—euphoria-inducing.

On the far side of the bowl, the trail begins to rise toward the crest and soon comes to a junction where the right fork leads to Post Peak Pass and the left to Isberg Pass, 0.75 mile away. The left fork ascends moderately a short way to reach the height of the pass, and then contours over to it. The best views—other than those you have already been enjoying for the last several miles—are to be had from a point on the ridgeline a few hundred yards beyond the sign-marked pass. You can see much of the northern High Sierra, from the Ritter Range close in the east, to peaks around Mt. Goddard southwest of Bishop.

Retrace your steps to the cairned junction, perhaps finding an exposed campsite in the high bowl to end this day.

Back at the cairned junction, your route turns west (left if you're returning from Isberg Pass; right if you didn't go to Isberg Pass) and starts straight downhill. It then veers southwest and switchbacks down into deep hemlock forest, turning north for the last 0.75 mile down to the river. There are good campsites around the junction of your trail and the trail to Red Peak Pass, which begins just across the placid Triple Peak Fork (9094'; 11S 293186 4170519) at the south end of long Triple Peak Fork Meadow. Fishing is good for brook and rainbow trout.

DAY 5 (Triple Peak Fork Meadow to Washburn Lake, 6.9 miles): Stroll north-northeast and then north for 1 mile through the meadow and then for another mile along the meandering Triple Peak Fork Merced River. Then make a short but steep descent to a verdant, forested flat through which the river winds slowly. The polished granite all around is a reminder that the mighty Merced glacier began in these upper reaches of the river.

At a switchback turn's overlook beneath a cascade and waterfall on the river, you begin zigzagging down out of the hanging valley through which you've been traveling, bearing generally northwest and then west down the north side of another of Triple Peak Fork's hanging valleys. Down in the valley, the trail momentarily levels as it meets Merced Peak Fork Merced River and, between roaring cascades above and below, crosses a quiet stretch of the river on a footbridge.

Descending northward on the river's west side through red fir and juniper, the trail soon passes the confluence of Merced Peak Fork and Triple Peak Fork Merced River. Continuing down, you shortly pass the confluence of the fork you've been walking along with Lyell Fork Merced River. Curving right, cross below the confluence on yet another footbridge (campsites in the vicinity).

Now the trail arcs northwest and west along the east and then north sides of the joined forks, descending gradually through an idyllic setting: bracken ferns under a forest of huge white firs and Jeffrey pines, with smaller lodgepoles and aspens, and occasional brushes with the emerald-green, placid river. By a lovely waterfall, the trail begins to descend a dry slope and soon reaches shaded campsites near a sandy beach at the head of Washburn Lake (7624'; 11S 291161 4176551).

DAY 6 (Washburn Lake to Emeric Lake, 7.3 miles): The sandy trail along the east side of Washburn Lake leads over slopes dotted with white fir, aspen, juniper, lodgepole pine, and Jeffrey pine, and from these slopes on a typical morning, the still water mirrors the soaring granite cliffs across the lake. Beyond this lake, the descending trail stays near the river in open forest, fording a small stream every quarter mile or so as it descends on a moderate grade. Then the canyon floor begins to widen, and the trail proceeds levelly under forest to a junction with the Lewis Creek Trail beside the Merced Lake Ranger Station (emergency services available in summer) and a junction with the Lewis Creek Trail.

Turn right (north) on the Lewis Creek Trail (left goes to Merced Lake). This cobblestoned trail quickly becomes steep, and it remains so for a half mile plus, but it is shaded. The trail levels momentarily as you pass a fine viewpoint of Merced Lake, far below, and Half Dome, due west. One more steep, cobblestoned climb leads to a junction with the Fletcher Creek Trail, and you turn left (northeast) onto this path.

(Partial Recap: Trip 53, Day 4, from the junction with the Fletcher Creek Trail to Emeric Lake.) Now you descend to a wooden bridge over Lewis Creek (hardened camping near the bridge). From here, the trail climbs moderately to steeply for 400 feet past a tributary a half mile from Lewis Creek. The trail then swings very close to the creek before climbing, steeply at times, until it finally levels off near some nice but illegal campsites. Soon your path passes a side trail left (west and south) to small Babcock Lake (campsites). From this junction, you go ahead (north) on sandy trail that ascends steadily through moderate forest just east of Fletcher Creek. After a mile, the trail rises steeply via rocky switchbacks

from which you can see, nearby in the north, the outlet stream of Emeric Lake—though not the lake itself, which is behind a dome just to the right of the outlet's notch.

The switchbacks top out with the dome to the north, and the trail then follows Fletcher Creek northeast to a ford. Almost immediately beyond the ford, the track meets a junction with the spur trail to Emeric Lake. Go left (west) to Emeric Lake (9396'; 11S 290240 4183858) and follow angler's trails to the excellent campsites midway along its northwest shore. The meadow north and northeast of the lake is carpeted with delicate wildflowers. Fishing is often good for rainbow.

DAY 7 (Emeric Lake to Lyell Canyon-PCT/JMT Trailhead, 10.8 miles): *(Recap: Trip 53, Day 5.)* This is a very long day, so get an early start. Retrace your steps to the spur trail at the lake's northeast corner at the base of a granite knoll. Take the spur east-northeast for 0.6 mile to a junction in the valley of Fletcher Creek. Go left (northeast) on the main trail up the valley and follow a rocky-dusty trail to another junction where you go left (north-northeast) toward Boothe Lake (the right fork goes up Fletcher Creek's valley to Vogelsang). Climb away from Fletcher Creek and top a minor summit where the trail descends slightly and then winds levelly past a long series of lovely ponds; numerous signs ask you to stay on the main trail. You soon pass a use trail to the south end of Boothe Lake (9845'; campsites).

The trail shortly contours above Boothe Lake, passing a junction with another use trail down to the lake. About a quarter mile farther, you reach Tuolumne Pass (9992') and close the loop at the junction with the trails to Vogelsang High Sierra Camp (sharp right) and down the Rafferty Creek Trail (ahead, north). Go ahead on the Rafferty Creek Trail and retrace your steps for Day 1 of this trip from here.

Mono Pass Trailhead

9692'; 11S 301048 4196126

DESTINATION/ UTM COORDINATES	TRIP TYPE	BEST SEASON	PACE (HIKING/ LAYOVER DAYS)	TOTAL MILEAGE
63 Alger Lakes 11S 308715 4185106	Shuttle	Mid or late	3/1 Moderate	20

Information and Permits: This trips enters Yosemite National Park: Yosemite Permits, PO Box 545, Yosemite National Park, CA 95389; 209-372-0740; www.nps.gov/yose/wilderness/permits.htm. Bear canisters are required; pets and firearms are prohibited.

Driving Directions: Just 1.5 miles west of Tioga Pass on Hwy. 120, there's a large turnout and parking area with a toilet on the south side of the road, signed as the Mono Pass Trailhead.

63 Alger Lakes

Trip Data: 11S 308715 4185106; 20 miles; 3/1 days

Topos: *Tioga Pass, Mount Dana, Koip Peak*

Highlights: This short trip offers a superb combination of views, alpine landscapes, and peaceful forests. Koip Peak Pass is the only major obstacle, and it's easier than you think.

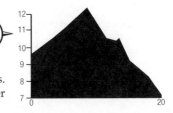

see map on p.220

HEADS UP! Yosemite National Park does not permit camping in the drainage of Dana Fork Tuolumne River, which includes all the lakes and streams on the Yosemite side of Parker and Mono passes. You must be on the Ansel Adams Wilderness side of Parker Pass before you camp.

Shuttle Directions: The take-out trailhead is off Hwy. 395 near the community of June Lake, which is south of the junction of highways 395 and 120. Two turnoffs, a north and a south, loop through June Lake. This trailhead is closer to the south turnoff, also known as the June Lakes Junction. At this intersection, turn southwest on Hwy. 158 toward the Sierra. Drive through June Lake Village, past June Lake Ski Area, and past Silver Lake and Silver Lake Resort. Just beyond the resort, between 5.2 and 5.3 miles from the turnoff, find the poorly signed RUSH CREEK TRAILHEAD on your left. Turn left here and go about 100 yards to a dirt parking lot near a cinderblock building housing toilets.

DAY 1 (Mono Pass Trailhead to Parker Creek, 5.5 miles): Pick up the trail from the parking lot and head south-southeast gradually downhill on an old road. Forest and meadow alternate, and a footpath presently branches left (east) from the old road. Take the footpath and cross two forks of a stream, climb a low ridge, veer east, and descend to skirt another meadow before ascending the next ridge. A little beyond 1 mile there's a beautiful view of Mammoth Peak over Parker Pass Creek.

You pass a ruined cabin to the left of the trail, make a long, gradual climb, and a little beyond 1.75 miles, ford a tributary just before reaching a junction. Go left (southeast) toward Mono Pass to find that the trail grows rockier as the climb becomes moderate to steep and the forest closes in. At 2.75 miles, you pass another ruined cabin.

At an obvious but unsigned junction a little shy of 3.25 miles, turn right (south) on the Parker Pass Trail. The first few feet of this trail may be picked out by stones lining it on both sides. Descending into a meadow, you enjoy beautiful views of the surrounding peaks: Mt. Gibbs and Mt. Lewis over your shoulder, unnamed peaks to the south, and the Kuna Crest ahead. You wind through low willows and hop over a couple of tiny streams that may be dry by late season.

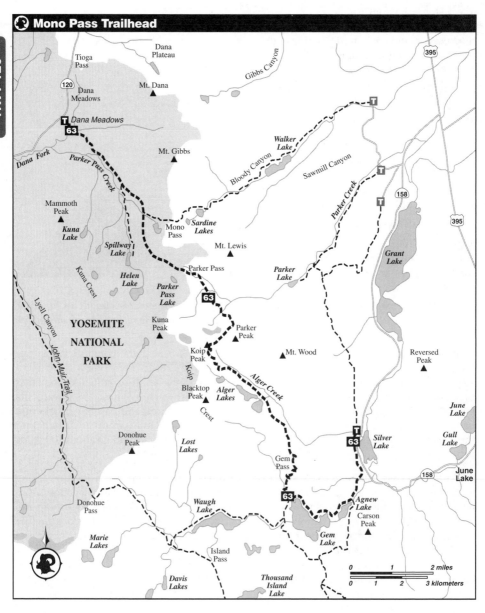

Mono Pass Trailhead

As the trail begins to rise again, it's blocked by fallen logs. Turn left (southeast) here—there may be a duck—onto a faint track and begin an easy traverse along a low ridge amid stunted whitebarks and lodgepoles. As you gain and follow the ridgeline, whitebarks come to dominate the increasingly dwarfed trees, and Spillway Lake comes into view in the distance on your right.

The trail gradually drifts rightward off the ridge and into a splendid alpine meadow. The easy, faint path presently reaches signed PARKER PASS (11,100'), and you step out of Yosemite National Park, across the Sierra Crest, and into Ansel Adams Wilderness.

Descending gradually, you soon spot ponds, streams, and dashing cascades fed by the year-round snowfields between Kuna, Koip (KO-ip), and Parker peaks. The ponds are tinted a magical, milky turquoise from the finely ground rock suspended in the snowmelt. There are some Spartan, scenic campsites between the trail and the ponds in this little valley (around 10,975'; 11S 306737 4189423).

DAY 2 (Parker Creek to Alger Lakes, 5.8 miles): Regain the trail and head generally southeast, gradually descending toward massive, brownish Parker Peak and hulking, gray Koip Peak; Koip Peak Pass lies between them. Watch your footing when fording: The rocks may be slippery with algae, the water icy and swift. The trail climbs over a low ridge, and from the summit you can see east over the headwaters of Parker Creek to the June Lake Loop.

Now the trail descends toward a lovely oval lake, passing a draw up which there's a sandy campsite. Angle slightly right across the lake's broad, stony outlet to find the trail on the other side as a faint dent in the alpine grasses. Ducks may help here.

Beyond the outlet, the trail begins its long climb to Koip Peak Pass. Expanding views eastward reveal Parker Lake as a sparkling blue teardrop far below, Parker Bench, long Grant Lake on the June Lake Loop, the otherworldly Mono Cones (lava domes just a few hundred years old), and the distant White Mountains. Mono Lake soon comes into view, too.

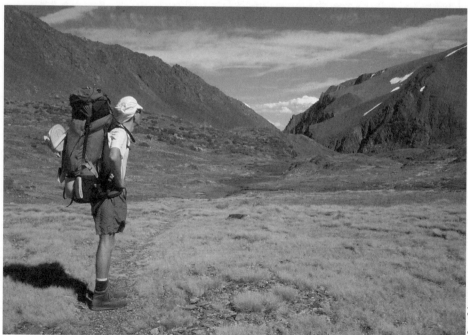

Hiker on Parker Pass Trail

Curving into the cirque between Koip and Parker peaks, you note the rushing, braided stream issuing from their snowfields. Soon you cross the stream's multiple channels, heading for the north-trending ridge of Parker Peak. This stream is your last reliable chance for water before Alger Lakes.

Although the trail is very exposed, narrow, and in scree, the footing is solid, and the grade is mostly gradual, occasionally moderate, and rarely steep. Best of all, the views just get better and better. Keep your eyes peeled for the switchback turns, as they can be hard to see amid all this scree. After the final switchback, the trail angles southwest on a long, gradual, ascending traverse to the Parker-Koip plateau.

Just before windy Koip Peak Pass (12,260'), you enjoy splendid views of Mono Lake, Koip and Parker peaks, nearby Mt. Lewis and Mt. Gibbs, the tips of Mt. Conness and its fellow peaks far to the north, and the dark rubble of Blacktop Peak ahead.

The Alger Lakes aren't visible from the pass, but shortly after you begin your descent, they appear—spectacular! Long, gradual switchbacks carry you down into this lovely basin with its several lakes, especially the two big ones on the southwest.

At the foot of the switchbacks, the track briefly parallels one small stream and soon crosses another as you glimpse the first stunted, shrub-like trees since your last crossing of Parker Creek. A sandy ridge separates your trail from the larger lakes. Where the trail abruptly ends, an obvious use trail climbs the ridge. Don't take it! Continue ahead to pick up the main trail again in 100 feet.

As the trees assume more normal proportions, you may want to make your way over the ridge to the north end of the largest Alger Lake to start looking for campsites. Staying on the trail, you begin to see huge ducks and many hoof prints as the trail fades out while crossing a low point in the ridge. Follow ducks toward the outlet of the southern large lake, near which a sign points out the trail to Gem Lake. Here, you meet the anglers' trail around the lakes—go hard right here (10,610'; 11S 308715 4185106) to follow it toward campsites on the isthmus and along the northern large lake.

Or cross the outlet (may be difficult in early season) and climb to seek a campsite high above the lake. Just across the outlet, an anglers' trail peels off left along the stream. In another 66 yards, an unsigned spur trail broader than your sandy main trail hooks sharply left to a large packer campsite. Clark's nutcrackers abound here, foraging noisily for whitebark cones in the trees around your campsite.

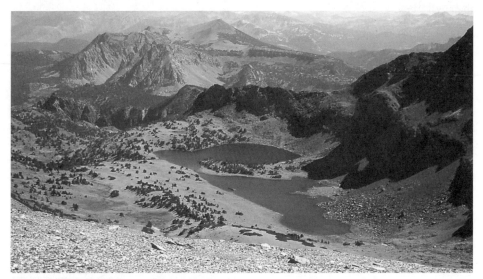

Alger Lakes from the descent of Koip Peak Pass

DAY 3 (Alger Lakes to Silver Lake, 8.7 miles): Climb southeast above the southern large lake, passing a trio of ponds, and begin descending toward views of distant June Mountain Ski Area, Carson Peak, San Joaquin Ridge, and a small oval lake that your trail will pass. The dusty trail drops to a lush meadow and then climbs to that lovely oval lake (10,400'), which lacks campsites.

You step across a tiny stream and climb to skirt a pretty pond on your right; there's a campsite on the left. Climb again to start a gradually ascending traverse high on the steep southwest wall of Alger Creek's canyon. At a Y-junction before Gem Pass, the trail splits. Both forks go to Gem Pass: One is lower than the other. Take whichever one appeals to you; snow cover may dictate your choice.

Cross unsigned Gem Pass in whitebark pines to find a rewarding view of Banner Peak. Now the sandy-dusty trail switchbacks down into moderate forest increasingly dominated by lodgepoles, crossing a couple of streamlets (may be dry by late season) and soon fording year-round Crest Creek.

The trail resumes its dusty descent amid willow, currant, senecio, ranger's button, and red heather. Crest Creek bubbles along in a deep ravine on the left, and you presently glimpse sun-dappled Gem Lake far below. Now curve away from the creek and into moderate forest, where you ford a seasonal stream and begin a long series of switchbacks.

Just a few steps after the trail meets Crest Creek again, you reach the junction with the Rush Creek Trail: right (southwest) to Waugh Lake and the JMT; left (north-northeast) across the creek to Agnew and Silver lakes. A use trail leads ahead to poor-to-fair campsites on Gem Lake (9058') at this junction (9080'). Carson Peak and interesting volcanic cliffs rise across this large, dammed lake.

Go left to ford Crest Creek, which provides the last readily accessible water and campsites until you are below Agnew Lake's dam. From here, you climb to a viewpoint above a little peninsula that's closed to camping. The trail makes an undulating traverse of the lake's north shore. A few spots seem like they offer good camping, but they're high above the lake, and the descent to water is long and steep.

As the main trail tops an outcrop, it curves left as indicated by a row of rocks; avoid an obvious use trail that goes right (ahead) and steeply down. Staying on the main trail, you descend into patchy lodgepole forest and then make a sunstruck curve around Gem's northeasternmost bay. At a Y-junction most of the way around the bay, take the left fork (southeast) to wind steeply up a knob that provides one last view of lovely Gem Lake and the High Sierra west of it.

Begin descending toward green Agnew Lake, whose steep, rugged slopes offer no campsites. Several switchbacks precede a long, moderate traverse high above the lake. Check out over-the-shoulder views of Rush Creek's showy cascade from Gem to Agnew.

The trail levels briefly as it passes Agnew's dam and reaches a junction signed CLARK LAKE. If you need water or are desperate to camp, descend to Rush Creek here. Otherwise, continue ahead (left, north) to begin a series of switchbacks. Twice, the trail crosses the tracks of a cable railway used to haul personnel and materiel to the dams on Rush Creek. Signs caution you to watch for moving cars and to stay off the tracks. The trail has been blasted out of the rock here; tall, poured concrete "steps" hold the tread in place. At a juniper-shaded overlook, you can see the creek's long, white ribbon dashing down to the Southern California Edison buildings below; the mountain ahead is Reversed Peak.

Now make a long, steady, shadeless descent north toward Silver Lake. Almost at its end, the trail plunges into aspens behind Silver Lake Resort, to which several use trails lead. Hook right (southeast) to step across a distributary of Alger Creek, and then cross its gravelly main channel on a bridge. From here, a dusty road leads leftward a short distance to the Rush Creek Trailhead (7241'; 11S 312546 4183792)—just head for the cinder-block restroom to end this trip.

HWY 120

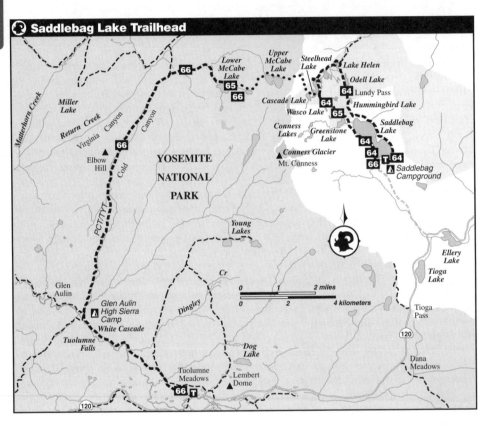

Saddlebag Lake Trailhead

Matterhorn Creek

Miller
Lake

Return Creek

Virginia Canyon

Cold Canyon

Elbow
Hill

YOSEMITE

NATIONAL

PARK

PCT/TYT

66

66

65

66

Lower
McCabe
Lake

Upper
McCabe
Lake

Steelhead
Lake

Lake Helen

Odell Lake

Lundy Pass

Hummingbird Lake

Cascade Lake

Wasco Lake

64

64

65

Conness
Lakes

Greenstone
Lake

Saddlebag
Lake

64

64

66

64

T

Conness Glacier

Mt. Conness

Saddlebag
Campground

Young
Lakes

Cr

Glen
Aulin

Glen Aulin
High Sierra
Camp

White Cascade

Tuolumne
Falls

Dingley

Dog
Lake

Tuolumne
Meadows

66

T

Lembert
Dome

120

Ellery
Lake

Tioga
Lake

Tioga
Pass

120

Dana
Meadows

0   1   2 miles

0   2   4 kilometers

Saddlebag Lake Trailhead

10,127'; 11S 300347 4204294

DESTINATION/ UTM COORDINATES	TRIP TYPE	BEST SEASON	PACE (HIKING/ LAYOVER DAYS)	TOTAL MILEAGE
64 20 Lakes Basin Loop 11S 297572 4207082	Loop	Mid or late	2/0 Leisurely	8.5
65 Lower McCabe Lake 11 293546 4207840	Out & back	Mid or late	2/0 Leisurely, part cross-country	11 or 13.8
66 Tuolumne Meadows 11 292557 4195059	Shuttle	Mid or late	3/1 Leisurely, part cross-country	20.2

Information and Permits: Saddlebag Lake and 20 Lakes Basin are part of Hoover Wilderness and are managed by Inyo National Forest. Wilderness permits are required, and trailhead quotas may be in effect. Contact Inyo National Forest, 351 Pacu Lane, Suite 200, Bishop, CA 93514; 760-873-2500; www.fs.fed.us.r5/inyo. Bear canisters are not required but are highly recommended. Two of the trips described here start in Hoover Wilderness and end in Yosemite National Park. All Yosemite rules and regulations (e.g., bear canisters required; pets and firearms prohibited) apply once you cross the park boundary.

Driving Directions: The turnoff to Saddlebag Lake on Hwy. 120 is 2 miles east of the Tioga Pass entrance to Yosemite National Park. From there, turn north-northwest and continue 2 miles on a dirt road to reach the trailhead parking lot, campground, and Saddlebag Lake Resort (café, store, water-taxi across Saddlebag Lake, and toilets).

64 20 Lakes Basin Loop

Trip Data: 11S 297572 4207082; 8.5 miles; 2/0 days

Topos: *Tioga Pass, Dunderberg Peak*

see map on p.224

Highlights: A short jaunt brings backpackers to a scenic granite sub-basin for an overnight in the shadow of beautiful peaks. Sturdy dayhikers will have no trouble taking this trip in a single day, with or without the ferry's help.

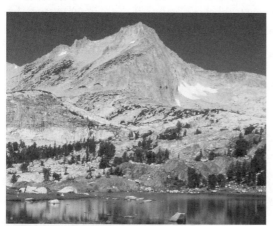

Day 1's route offers this view of North Peak over Greenstone Lake

HEADS UP! *Most of 20 Lakes Basin, which is "carpeted" by shards of the metamorphic rock out of which most of the basin is carved, offers no camping. This means that legally there's nothing but those shards (ouch!) on which to pitch a tent. The granitic sub-basin holding Cascade Lake is an exception.*

DAY 1 (Saddlebag Lake Trailhead to Cascade Lake, 3 miles): Those preferring to walk rather than take the water-taxi will find the trailhead a few steps past the summer ranger station south of Saddlebag's dam, where the trail begins as an old road that dips below the face of the dam.

(Crossing on the dam isn't recommended.) Climbing up on the other side, the road becomes a footpath north-northwest along Saddlebag Lake's west side, over shattered rocks and through a surprising array of flowers. The splendid peaks around the head of 20 Lakes Basin come into view, with North Peak and Mt. Scowden particularly striking. To the east are the gently rounded, metamorphic summits of the Tioga Crest.

The trail fades out as you approach the stream that's the outlet of Greenstone Lake (10,120') at 1.25 miles. Avoiding a spur trail around Greenstone's southwest side, you cross the stream to pick up the trail coming up from the water-taxi landing at Saddlebag's head, and then bear west above Greenstone Lake to enter Hoover Wilderness at just over 1.3 miles.

Here you begin a gradual-to-moderate climb on this wide, dusty trail that was once a road to a now-defunct mine deep in the basin. You traverse above skinny, rock-rimmed Wasco Lake, crossing a divide: Behind you, streams drain southeast through Saddlebag Lake and Lee Vining Creek; ahead, streams drain north into Mill Creek and through Lundy Canyon. The trail reaches lovely Steelhead Lake (10,270', 11S 297844 4207212) at a little over 2.3 miles. The stream from higher, unseen Cascade Lake spills noisily into Steelhead's southwest side, and a use trail branches left (west) across the inlet at Steelhead's south end.

Pick up that use trail to cross Steelhead's inlet and head west for about a half mile, wandering up ledges along the headwaters of Mill Creek, passing unnamed lakes west of Steelhead, into a handsome granite sub-basin around beautiful Cascade Lake (10,327'; 11S 297572 4207082) at about 3 miles. Exposed campsites are scattered here and there in this treeless basin beneath North Peak, and a layover day offers fine off-trail exploring and fishing for golden trout.

DAY 2 (Cascade Lake to Saddlebag Lake Trailhead, 5.5 miles): Return to the main trail near Steelhead Lake and turn left (north) along the lake's east shore. After crossing Steelhead's outlet, reach a signed trail junction: Go right (northeast) to Lake Helen and Lundy Canyon, climbing steeply but briefly on a trail that's well-beaten but not yet on the 7.5' topo. You reach islet-filled Shamrock Lake (10,250') at just over 4 miles. Climb up and over a talus slope on Shamrock's north side and then ascend a knob (don't stay on the talus slope) to an overlook of beautiful Lake Helen, Lundy Canyon, and some Great Basin peaks far to the east.

From this overlook, the trail curves right (northeast) to descend the knob's north face. You pass some lovely cascades and ponds on the way to Lake Helen and then curve around the lake's northwest bay to its outlet. Ford Helen's outlet to find a junction: Go left (northeast) to Lundy Canyon—take a five-minute detour here for views of Lundy Canyon and its waterfalls—and then return to your 20 Lakes Basin trail to continue the loop by turning left (south) at the junction (or continuing ahead, south) if you didn't detour to the overlook.

After climbing a rocky slot, the trail tops out briefly above Odell Lake (10,267') and then climbs gradually to a high point, unsigned Lundy Pass (10,320'). Now you begin a gradual descent to Saddlebag Lake, crossing the outlet of little Hummingbird Lake, and soon leaving Hoover Wilderness. Not long after, you reach a junction: Continue straight ahead (south) on a use trail if your destination is the ferry landing, or turn left (initially east) to begin traversing Saddlebag Lake's east side.

On an old road above the lakeshore, you stroll through an open lodgepole forest, climbing a little on a gradual grade. The forest vanishes as you cross above the peninsula that juts south into the lake, and then reappears as you near the south end of Saddlebag Lake. The old road curves around a meadow, rising slightly to a gate that separates the trail from the parking lot, where you close the loop.

65 Lower McCabe Lake

Trip Data: 11 293546 4207840; 11 or 13.8 miles; 2/0 days

Topos: *Tioga Pass, Dunderberg Peak*

Highlights: This adventurous cross-country trek climbs out of 20 Lakes Basin over a south-trending spur of Shepherd Crest and into Yosemite to the lightly visited McCabe Lakes. Breathtaking views and alpine scenery await you.

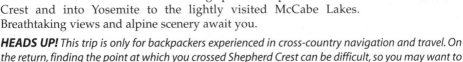

see map on p.224

HEADS UP! This trip is only for backpackers experienced in cross-country navigation and travel. On the return, finding the point at which you crossed Shepherd Crest can be difficult, so you may want to set up a few ducks or take a few GPS readings to help guide you back.

DAY 1 (Saddlebag Lake Trailhead to Lower McCabe Lake, 5.5 miles, part cross-country): (Partial Recap: Trip 64, Day 1, from Saddlebag Lake to Cascade Lake.) From Saddlebag Lake, traverse the west shore of Saddlebag, passing Greenstone Lake, entering Hoover Wilderness, passing Wasco Lake, and turning left (west) on the use trail across Steelhead Lake's inlet to go cross-country for about a half mile into the granite sub-basin to Cascade Lake (10,327'; 11S 297572 4207082), 3 miles from the trailhead.

At Cascade Lake, you leave the Day 1 route of Trip 64 and begin heading cross-country up the granite wall west of Cascade Lake (the wall is a south-trending extension of Shepherd Crest). Your first goal is to get to a small, unnamed lake high on the wall: Around the north side of Cascade Lake, find a tiny, unmapped, flower-lined inlet to the lake. Begin angling northwest along this streamlet, where there may be a use trail or ducks. As the streamlet curves northward, follow it upward as best you can to the small, unnamed lake the streamlet flows out of, locally called Secret Lake (10,889'; 11S 297133 4208107; located on the 7.5' *Tioga Pass* topo at just over 1.25 inches north-northwest of the north end of Cascade Lake).

Pause at Secret Lake to study your choices for the next section of the route and pick the one that best suits you; we offer three suggestions in the sidebar "Three Ways Up Shepherd Crest." Whichever route you take—and that depends on your skills—your next goal is to get to the top of Shepherd Crest, find the low point on this south-trending part of the crest, and from there make your way down to Upper McCabe Lake. The low point is north-

---

THREE WAYS UP SHEPHERD CREST

Here are three suggestions for getting to the low point atop Shepherd Crest:

1. Adept mountaineers can attack the wall directly, preferably keeping just to the right of the black, lichen-stained vertical streak on the wall. Once on top, walk to the low point on the crest, where you will find the route that descends the west side of the ridge to Upper McCabe Lake.

2. Hikers who want to put out some extra effort to achieve certainty and avoid steep exposure can arduously pick their way up the scree-laden part of the wall north of Secret Lake to the lip of what looks like but isn't a lake basin. From there, traverse slightly upward to the left (almost south), under the solid face of the east end of the main ridge of Shepherd Crest, to the low point on the crest, where you find the route described above, down to Upper McCabe Lake.

3. Most people choose the third way: From the south side of Secret Lake, walk directly up the increasingly steep wall until, about halfway up, you come to a long ledge that slopes slightly up to the south. Follow this ledge for about 200 yards south, and then leave it to climb almost directly up to the top of the ridge. Follow the top of the ridge north to the low point of the crest, where you find the route described above, down to Upper McCabe Lake.

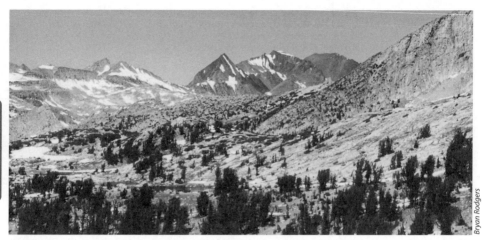

Bryan Rodgers

View from Shepard Crest; Upper McCabe Lake on the lower left

northwest of Secret Lake at just under 11,200 feet. There is a well-defined, though steep and eroded, route from that low point down to Upper McCabe Lake. Views from the top of the crest are outstanding.

Descend from the top of the crest at the crest's low point into Yosemite on a well-defined route that follows the gully northeast of Upper McCabe Lake. This section levels out near some small tarns, and the route continues to the north shore of Upper McCabe Lake. There are fair campsites at the lake's west end, and other, scattered, isolated ones. Follow Upper McCabe Lake's north shore westward, ford the outlet, and then strike out for the low, ducked saddle due west of the outlet and about 0.3 mile away.

Beyond this saddle, the best route heads generally west-southwest, remaining north of and well above Middle McCabe Lake. It drops past snowmelt tarns not shown on the topo map, and then winds down through a dense forest cover of lodgepole and whitebark pine and hemlock to the east shore of beautiful Lower McCabe Lake. The best campsites on the lake are near the outlet (9820'; 11S 293546 4207840). Fishing for eastern brook is excellent.

DAY 2 (Lower McCabe Lake to Saddlebag Lake Trailhead, 5.5 or 8.3 miles, part cross-country): Retrace your steps to Upper McCabe Lake and then over Shepherd Crest and down through the Cascade Lake sub-basin.

On reaching the main 20 Lakes Basin Trail at Steelhead Lake, you can either retrace your steps right (south) for 2.3 more miles past Wasco and Greenstone lakes and then along Saddlebag's west side (5.5 miles).

(Partial Recap: Trip 64, Day 2, from Steelhead Lake to Saddlebag Lake Trailhead.) Or, to make this trip a semiloop (and to add 2.8 miles to the trip's total), you can turn left (north) and take the 20 Lakes Basin Trail past Shamrock and Helen lakes on your return via Saddlebag's east side. At Helen's outlet, this trip's route goes ahead (south) and up to Odell; don't go left and down into Lundy Canyon. Pass high above Odell Lake, cross over unsigned Lundy Pass, pass Hummingbird Lake, and soon reach a junction on Saddlebag Lake's northeast shore. Go left (initially east) through lodgepole forest to walk around Saddlebag's east shore. Walking along the east shore on what is actually a closed old road, you leave the forest behind as you cross above a peninsula that juts south into the lake. The trail curves around a meadow and rises slightly to a gate that separates it from the parking lot, where you close the loop.

66 Tuolumne Meadows

Trip Data: 11 292557 4195059;
20.2 miles; 3/1 days

Topos: *Tioga Pass, Dunderberg Peak, Falls Ridge*

Highlights: This trip picks up the PCT and heads for Tuolumne Meadows via Glen Aulin High Sierra Camp.

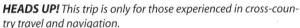

HEADS UP! *This trip is only for those experienced in cross-country travel and navigation.*

Shuttle Directions: From Hwy. 120 in Yosemite's Tuolumne Meadows, just 7 miles southwest of Tioga Pass and just east of the bridge over the Tuolumne River, turn west on a dirt road along Lembert Dome's western face. The road leads to a locked gate, where this trip ends, and from here the road turns right toward the stables. Find a parking spot where permitted along the road between the highway and the gate. You may not park overnight in the lot at the base of Lembert Dome.

DAY 1 (Saddlebag Lake Trailhead to Lower McCabe Lake, 5.5 miles, part cross-country): *(Partial Recap: Trip 64, Day 1, from Saddlebag Lake to Cascade Lake.)* From Saddlebag Lake, traverse the west shore of Saddlebag, passing Greenstone Lake, entering Hoover Wilderness, passing Wasco Lake, and turning left (west) on the use trail across Steelhead Lake's inlet to go cross-country for about a half mile into the granite sub-basin to Cascade Lake (10,327'; 11S 297572 4207082), 3 miles from the trailhead.

(Partial Recap: Trip 65, Day 1, from Cascade Lake to Lower McCabe Lake.) At Cascade Lake, you leave the Day 1 route of Trip 64 and begin heading cross-country up the granite wall west of Cascade Lake (the wall is a south-trending extension of Shepherd Crest). Your first goal is to get to a small, unnamed lake high on the wall: Around the north side of Cascade Lake, find a tiny, unmapped, flower-lined inlet to the lake. Begin angling northwest along this streamlet, where there may be a use trail or ducks. As the streamlet curves northward, follow it upward as best you can to the small, unnamed lake the streamlet flows out of, locally called Secret Lake (10,889'; 11S 297133 4208107; located on the 7.5' *Tioga Pass* topo at just over 1.25 inches north-northwest of the north end of Cascade Lake).

Pause at Secret Lake to study your choices for the next section of the route and pick the one that best suits you; we offer three suggestions in the sidebar "Three Ways Up Shepherd Crest" on page 227. Whichever route you take—and that depends on your skills—your next goal is to get to the top of Shepherd Crest, find the low point on this south-trending part of the crest, and from there make your way down to Upper McCabe Lake. The low

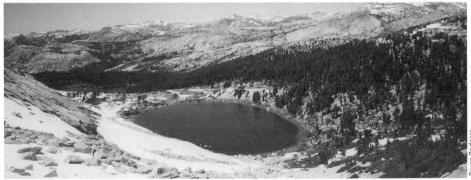

Middle McCabe Lake (center), Lower McCabe Lake (left of center)

point is north-northwest of Secret Lake at just under 11,200 feet. There is a well-defined, though steep and eroded, route from that low point down to Upper McCabe Lake.

Now take the steep, eroded trail from this low point. Descending from the top of the crest the trail follows the gully northeast of Upper McCabe Lake. This section levels out near some small tarns, and the route continues to the north shore of Upper McCabe Lake (campsites). Follow Upper McCabe Lake's north shore westward, ford the outlet, and then strike out for the low, ducked saddle due west of the outlet and about 0.3 mile away.

Beyond this saddle, the best route heads generally west-southwest, remaining north of and well above Middle McCabe Lake. It drops past snowmelt tarns not shown on the topo map, and then winds down through a forest cover to the east shore of Lower McCabe Lake (9820'; 11S 293546 4207840). Fishing for eastern brook is excellent.

DAY 2 (Lower McCabe Lake to Glen Aulin High Sierra Camp, 9 miles, part cross-country): From the campsites at the outlet of Lower McCabe Lake, the trail descends along the west side of the stream through a moderate-to-dense forest cover of hemlock, lodgepole, white-bark, western white pine, and occasional red fir. In late season or during a drier summer, be sure to get water at the lake or stream, as this may be your last chance before Glen Aulin. The upper portion of the trail from Lower McCabe Lake is usually very wet and swampy, drying out as it veers west. Flowers here include wallflower, Douglas phlox, lupine, buck-wheat, aster, and pussypaws.

The descent becomes gentle as the trail passes through a "ghost forest" caused by the needleminer moth. At the signed junction with the Virginia Canyon Trail (11S 291158 4208067); turn left (south-southwest) onto the PCT/TYT toward Glen Aulin.

(Partial Recap: Trip 40, Day 10, from the PCT/TYT junction with the trail up McCabe Creek to McCabe Lakes, to Glen Aulin.) Go right (southwest) into Cold Canyon for a long, gentle descent. When there's water in Cold Canyon, you may be able to camp in the occasional dry, forested patch. Continuing the Cold Canyon descent, the trail passes through long, broad meadows that are usually dry by late season. Then the trail climbs over a saddle and gently descends for about a half mile. Over the next mile, always near Cold Canyon's creek (mostly dry in late season), the path passes a few possible campsites.

From here, the trail leaves the creek and descends south-southwest to the Tuolumne River. On the final, rocky descent to the river, you glimpse and hear Tuolumne Falls and the White Cascade. Within sight of Glen Aulin High Sierra Camp, you reach a junction with the Tuolumne River Trail heading right (northwest; poor, unsafe camping), and in 15 more yards, you take a trail that goes left (east) to cross Conness Creek on a footbridge to Glen Aulin High Sierra Camp (7910'; 11S 287493 4198572) with its backpackers' camp-ground. Camping along the PCT/TYT is prohibited between Glen Aulin and the TYT's end at Tuolumne Meadows.

DAY 3 (Glen Aulin High Sierra Camp to Tuolumne Meadows, 5.7 miles): *(Recap: Trip 40, Day 11.)* Return to the PCT/TYT and go briefly ahead (southwest) to cross the Tuolumne River on a footbridge just below the White Cascade. Now turning southeast, the PCT/TYT climbs to a junction with a trail right (southwest) to McGee and May lakes; here, you go ahead (southeast) on the PCT/TYT and climb past Tuolumne Falls. Shortly, you cross the river on one last footbridge before beginning a ducked route over slabs along the river.

After the PCT/TYT's tread resumes, the trail gradually curves southeast away from the river and crosses the three branches of Dingley Creek. In a half mile, you meet the Young Lakes Trail going left (north), while you go ahead (south-southeast) on the PCT/TYT toward Tuolumne Meadows. Stay on the PCT/TYT at any more junctions as you touch the northwest edge of Tuolumne Meadows, cross three branches of Delaney Creek, ascend and cross a long, sandy ridge, and finally descend to pass Soda Springs. Remain on the PCT/TYT as it becomes an eastbound dirt road and reaches a locked gate (8590'; 11S 292581 4194990), beyond which, along a spur road from Hwy. 120 (Tioga Road), your pick-up ride or shuttle car should be waiting.

WESTERN YOSEMITE TRIPS

The three trailheads in this section are south of Hwy. 120 within the western part of Yosemite National Park: Yosemite Valley's Happy Isles Trailhead and, from the Glacier Point Road, the Bridalveil Creek Trailhead and the Glacier Point—Panorama Trailhead. There's another Yosemite waiting for you in the park's southern backcountry, and these trailheads are your gateways to it.

The Happy Isles Trailhead is probably the prettiest in Yosemite Valley, situated as it is near the cascading Merced River and near the Happy Isles—be sure to visit them if time permits.

Beyond the Bridalveil Creek Trailhead, you'll find not only the creekside meadows and abundant wildflowers for which the Bridalveil Creek area is rightly famous but also remote, peaceful lakes and high, rugged peaks.

Yosemite's Glacier Point is justly famed for its incomparable views of Yosemite Valley and of the great waterfalls on the Merced River. And it's a popular starting point for day-hikes down into the valley. But had you thought of it as a trailhead for backpacks? If not, prepare to be surprised at the wonderful overnighters possible from the Glacier Point—Panorama Trailhead. But whatever you do, don't leave this trailhead without enjoying the world-renowned views from Glacier Point proper.

W. YOSEMITE

TRAILHEADS: Happy Isles
Bridalveil Creek
Glacier Point—Panorama

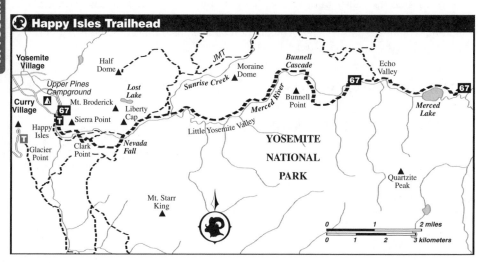

Happy Isles Trailhead   4023';11S 274550 4179235

T	DESTINATION/ UTM COORDINATES	TRIP TYPE	BEST SEASON	PACE (HIKING/ LAYOVER DAYS)	TOTAL MILEAGE
	67 Merced Lake 11S 287918 4179565	Out & back	Early	4/1 Leisurely	27.8

Information and Permits: These trips enter Yosemite National Park: Yosemite Permits, PO Box 545, Yosemite National Park, CA 95389; 209-372-0740; www.nps.gov/yose/wilderness/permits.htm. Bear canisters are required; pets and firearms are prohibited.

Driving Directions: You cannot drive to this trailhead, but you can leave a car in Curry Village's big overnight parking lot and take a shuttle to and from there. Whether you drive from the west or the east, get to the junction of highways 140 and 120 in Yosemite Valley. On what is now the Yosemite Valley Road, drive east and deeper into the valley—a somewhat confusing effort, as parts of this road are one way, and you must follow signs to Curry Village. Note that private cars cannot drive the Yosemite Valley Road east beyond the big parking lot at Curry Village. You can catch a shuttle from near here to the Happy Isles Trailhead. From the Happy Isles bus stop on the Merced River's west bank, cross the Merced River on a nearby bridge and find your trailhead on the Merced's east bank.

67 Merced Lake

Trip Data: 11S 287918 4179565; 27.8 miles; 4/1 days

see map on p.232

Topos: *Yosemite, Merced Peak, Half Dome, Merced Peak*

Highlights: An early-season trip (low altitude, early snowmelt), this route offers all the scenic grandeur of the Valley attractions, plus the intimate knowledge of the backcountry that only the backpacker can have. Fishing is good during early season on the Merced River and at Merced Lake. Swimming is poor in early season due to cold water, but the route is a joy for photographers and naturalists.

HEADS UP! *Though this trip is graded leisurely, the first hiking day is rigorous, with more than 2000 feet of hot, steady climbing. However, the route is so spectacular you'll forget those aches and pains.*

DAY 1 (Happy Isles Trailhead to Little Yosemite Valley, 4.7 miles): *(Recap in Reverse: Trip 50, Day 2.)* Follow the paved JMT as it passes above the Happy Isles and then a gauging station and the remains of a bridge. The trail climbs for some time before descending to cross the Merced on a bridge with great views of Vernal Fall upstream. Pass by a drinking fountain and restrooms on the river's west side as the JMT goes right (south) where the Mist Trail comes in on the left. Avoid a signed HORSE TRAIL as the JMT resumes climbing steeply up the Merced's gorge on eastbound switchbacks. At Clark Point, enjoy the view but avoid the Clark Trail (left and down to the Mist Trail) by going ahead (generally east), still climbing stiffly; views of Nevada Fall are superb.

Nearing the climb's top, the grade eases as the JMT passes two junctions with the Panorama Trail; at each, go ahead (northeast) to stay on the JMT. The trail soon emerges on the Merced's south bank on granite slabs, near a sturdy bridge, and just above Nevada Fall. Cross the bridge and pause to take in the view here before curving east on the sandy trail, soon passing the upper end of the Mist Trail on your left near restrooms. Go ahead to stay on the eastbound JMT as it rises a little before descending into Little Yosemite Valley and meeting a shortcut: left (northeast) on the JMT and out of the valley; right (east-northeast) into the valley with its improved but overused campsites near Sunrise Creek and the Merced. Go right to the camping area (where the trail crosses Sunrise Creek, 6095'; 11S 278493 4179091). There are toilets, a ranger station, and bear boxes. There are less-crowded sites about 2 level miles farther on at the east end of Little Yosemite Valley.

DAY 2 (Little Yosemite Valley to Merced Lake, 9.2 miles): Leave the camping area behind as you travel under shade and without a significant grade across the floor of Little Yosemite Valley toward its east end. The broad trail stays well away from the river here.

GEOLOGY LESSON

As an indication of how thick glaciers were here, look up at Moraine Dome to the east: Ice filled the valley almost to its summit 750,000 years ago. Since then, glaciers have repeatedly entered this valley, but none that thick.

At the valley's east end, the trail swings close to the river again as the canyon walls converge, and the grade steepens as you pass another camping area. You climb through a short, narrow gorge leading to Lost Valley, where glaciers did very little to modify the preexisting, V-shaped, stream-cut canyon, whose vertical walls reflect the vertical jointing in the bedrock. At Lost Valley's east end, the canyon narrows again, and you climb eastward under Bunnell Point (to the south) and past Bunnell Cascade to another, smaller valley. Before leaving this valley, the trail crosses one branch of the Merced via an island and a second branch on a wooden bridge whose lumber came from a 175-year-old sugar pine that once stood just below the trail.

Now the trail curves southward near the river before beginning the steep stretch up to Echo Valley, climbing 400 feet south and traversing over open slabs where glacial erratics mark your path. Curving north, the trail descends to cross the river on a bridge at the west end of Echo Valley. Following the river before angling away and northeast, the trail arrives at a junction and a multi-bridged crossing of Echo Creek. Cross the creek and bear southeast through a very dense young forest of lodgepole pines.

Soon the route winds up slabs, and, where the river is confined in yet another gorge, you walk right above the fast-moving water. The grade eases once again as the trail arrives at yet another wide, flat valley, this one containing Merced Lake. Following the lake's north shore, the trail passes a drift fence and arrives at lake's east end, where you find the camping area in conjunction with Merced Lake High Sierra Camp (7234'; 11S 287918 4179565), which offers tent-cabins, showers, and meals—if you have a reservation. Bears are plentiful; the lake contains brook and rainbow trout.

DAYS 3–4 (Merced Lake to Happy Isles Trailhead, 13.9 miles): Retrace your steps.

Bridalveil Creek Trailhead

6942'; 11S 268970 4171486

DESTINATION/ UTM COORDINATES	TRIP TYPE	BEST SEASON	PACE (HIKING/ LAYOVER DAYS)	TOTAL MILEAGE
68 Royal Arch Lake 11S 278975 4161785	Semiloop	Early or mid	5/1 Leisurely	27.9
69 Glacier Point— Panorama Trailhead 11S 273227 4178778	Shuttle	Early or mid	4/1 Moderate	29.1
70 Yosemite Valley- Happy Isles Trailhead 11S 274550 4179235	Shuttle	Early or mid	4/1 Leisurely	32.7

Information and Permits: These trips enter Yosemite National Park: Yosemite Permits, PO Box 545, Yosemite National Park, CA 95389; 209-372-0740; www.nps.gov/yose/wilderness/permits.htm. Bear canisters are required; pets and firearms are prohibited.

Driving Directions: Take Hwy. 41 to a junction near its summit, Chinquapin Junction, with the Glacier Point Road. Turn onto that road and follow it generally north and then east 7.6 miles to the Bridalveil Campground road. Turn right (south) onto that road and follow it past the camping loops to its end, where the trailhead is on your right at a tiny lot with room for perhaps three cars.

68 Royal Arch Lake

Trip Data: 11S 278975 4161785; 27.9 miles; 5/1 days

Topos: *Yosemite, Half Dome, Mariposa Grove*

see map on p.236

Highlights: In early season, this route is lush with wildflowers of every variety, and the fishing at Royal Arch Lake is excellent. The generally gentle grades make this a fine early-season choice for out-of-shape hikers.

DAY 1 (Bridalveil Creek Trailhead to Turner Meadow, 6.3 miles): From the trailhead, the trail scrambles over a low dome and begins winding southeastward along meandering Bridalveil Creek's south bank. The grade is gentle as the trail winds through the dense lodgepole forest. Periodically, the thick undergrowth gives way to intimate meadows filled with mountain bluebells. At a junction where a spur to Glacier Point Road hooks sharply left (north), you continue ahead (southeast). Beyond, the trail veers south beside one of the larger tributaries of Bridalveil Creek. It fords this tributary and meets a lateral left (northeast) to the Ostrander Lake Trail. Go right (south), and in a half mile ford the tributary again. Each ford is heralded by banks covered with lavender shooting stars.

The second ford marks the beginning of an easy, 400-foot climb over the ridge that separates the Bridalveil Creek and Alder Creek watersheds. In early and mid season, this ridge is colorfully decked out in lush pink and white fields of pussypaws, brodiaea, mat lupine, and Douglas phlox. From the top of this ridge, the trail drops south-southeast to meet the Deer Camp Trail (right, northwest) to Empire Meadows. Go ahead (southeast), climb over Turner Ridge, and descend to ford a tributary of Turner Meadow. Bill Turner, a European-descended pioneer, occupied these grasslands while running cattle around the turn of the 20th century. There is water here except in late season; there are no campsites.

In early season, you'll ford many little rills as you continue descending from that ford, and soon you'll trace the east side of long Turner Meadow. Just before the ford of a sizeable tributary to the meadows (7485'; 11S 270734 4164202), there's a large packer campsite

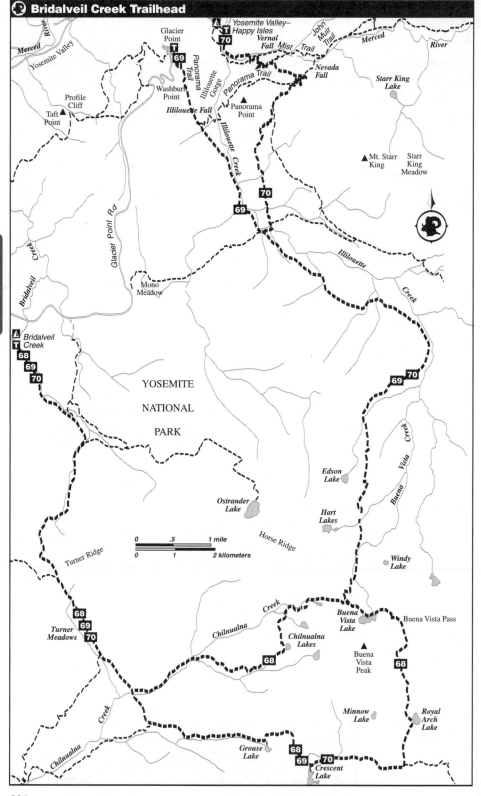

Merced River

Yosemite Valley

Glacier Point

T

69

Panorama Trail

Illilouette Gorge

Washburn Point

Profile Cliff

Taft Point

Illilouette Fall

A T

Yosemite Valley–
Happy Isles

70

Vernal Fall Mist Trail

John Muir Trail

Merced River

Panorama Trail

Nevada Fall

Starr King Lake

Panorama Point

Illilouette Creek

▲ Mt. Starr King

Starr King Meadow

70

69

Illilouette Creek

Glacier Point Rd

Bridalveil Creek

Mono Meadow

YOSEMITE

NATIONAL

PARK

A T
68
69
70
Bridalveil Creek

69 70

Edson Lake

Buena Vista Creek

Ostrander Lake

Hart Lakes

Horse Ridge

Turner Ridge

0 .5 1 mile
0 1 2 kilometers

Windy Lake

Creek

Chilnualna

Chilnualna Lakes

Buena Vista Lake

Buena Vista Pass

68
69
70
Turner Meadows

68

Buena Vista Peak

68

Chilnualna Creek

Minnow Lake

Royal Arch Lake

Grouse Lake

68
69
70
Crescent Lake

236

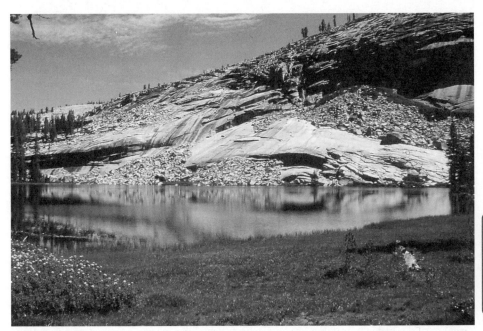

Royal Arch Lake

on your right (southwest) in the trees fringing the meadow. If that's full, then beyond the ford a short distance, there's a slender, open, sandy flat on the trail's right. Make some time to sit quietly by the meadow, especially in the early morning, to see wildlife. Wildflowers are abundant in early season—and so are mosquitoes.

DAY 2 (Turner Meadow to Royal Arch Lake, 6.7 miles): Resume your descent and soon meet the Wawona Trail coming up from Wawona on your right (south) at a fork. Go left (southeast) here, and in a little over 0.75 mile, meet the Chilnualna (chill-NWAHL-nah) Lakes Trail branching left (east) near a campsite. The loop part of this trip begins here. You take the right fork southward to ford swirling Chilnualna Creek (difficult in early season). From the ford, climb southeast on switchbacks over an eastward-rising ridge to a junction with a second lateral trail to Wawona, leading right (west). Take the left fork eastward here.

South of the ridgecrest, where views to the south open up, you turn east up the valley of Grouse Lake's little outlet stream and ascend gently for 2.25 miles to a junction with a hard-to-spot use trail leading right (south) to little Grouse Lake. Your trail jogs briefly left (north) to cross a small rise, turns east again, soon drops almost southward, and then descends to ford the inlet of shallow Crescent Lake, just out of sight to the south. Eastbound again, another mile of level walking into increasingly mosquito-infested forest brings you to the north edge of Johnson Lake (good fishing for brook and rainbow). Johnson Lake and its perimeter were one of the last acquisitions of private property within the park's boundaries, and two crumbling cabins remain to remind you of the homesteading era.

The next 0.75 mile, to a junction with the Royal Arch Lake Trail, is a 250-foot ascent up a lodgepole-covered slope. Here, you meet a junction with the Buck Camp Trail continuing ahead (east) to Buck Camp. You turn left (north) for a 0.75-mile climb through dense forest that gives way to open hillside as you approach dramatic, small, deep Royal Arch Lake. A seasonal tarn between the trail and the lake may be warm enough for good swimming by mid season. The best campsites are probably in the forest fringe on the lake's south shore (8729'; 11S 278975 4161785). Fishing is good for rainbow and brook.

ROYAL ARCH?

This lake probably got its name from the arching pattern of exfoliation on the granite dome on the lake's east side, which strongly resembles that of the famous Royal Arches—also exfoliation features—in Yosemite Valley.

DAY 3 (Royal Arch Lake to Lowest Chilnualna Lake, 4.6 miles): From Royal Arch Lake, resume your northward climb, traversing an idyllic meadow and fording its creek just below Buena Vista Pass on Buena Vista Peak's northeast ridge.

CLIMBING BUENA VISTA PEAK

From the pass (9300'), it is an easy 0.75-mile climb to the top of aptly named Buena Vista Peak (9709'). As the highest point for miles around, this peak offers some of the most expansive views in this part of the Sierra.

From the pass, the trail quickly descends to lightly forested Buena Vista Lake, dramatically situated beneath the peak and with several very scenic but mostly overused campsites. Nevertheless, the temptation to cut the day short and stay here is almost irresistible.

But resisting, you skirt the lake's north shore and descend to a junction where the right fork descends generally north into the drainage of Buena Vista Creek, on its way to Glacier Point. Take the left fork westward as it drops 480 forested feet on switchbacks to the northernmost of the little Chilnualna Lakes. Each of these little lakes is forested and meadow-edged, and each has the occasional good campsite. They are the headwaters of named Chilnualna Creek. Fishing is good for brook and rainbow except at the lowest lake. The trail skims the shores of this northernmost lake and, later on, the lowest lake. The other two Chilnualna Lakes are off trail and, especially the southernmost one, offer better and more secluded camping if you're up to the cross-country leg to get to them.

In dense forest now, trace the northernmost lake's outlet for a short distance before stepping over it and curving south, then west, and then south again on a pleasant ramble that's mostly a gentle descent. It's not long before you step over the off-trail middle lake's outlet (following it is a possible route to that lake). Going west and then south from here, you soon find the lowest lake with its good campsites on its north side (8381'; 11S 275674 4163773). This little lake is quite shallow and is one of this trip's warmest lakes for a dip.

DAY 4 (Lowest Chilnualna Lake to Turner Meadow, 4 miles): From the lowest lake, resume your gentle, forested descent out of sight of the creek that's the outlet of the southernmost Chilnualna Lake, though you won't meet it or the named Chilnualna Creek for a while. You soon curve west, and presently, as you near the outlet creek, you ford named Chilnualna Creek shortly before the confluence of the outlet creek and Chilnualna Creek. Fishing along the creek is fair for small brook and rainbow. The trail curves southwest, generally along the creek and then turns west just before reaching the junction where the loop part of this trip began on Day 3, 3.1 miles from the lowest Chilnualna Lake (yesterday's destination).

From here, turn right (northwest) and retrace your steps for about 0.9 mile to camping along Turner Meadow (7485'; 11S 270734 4164202 at the tributary crossing).

DAY 5 (Turner Meadow to Bridalveil Creek Trailhead, 6.3 miles): Retrace the steps of Day 1 of this trip.

69 Glacier Point—Panorama Trailhead

Trip Data: 11S 273227 4178778;
29.1 miles; 4/1 days

Topos: *Yosemite, Half Dome,
Mariposa Grove*

Highlights: On this trip, early- and mid-season travelers will find splendid forests, lush meadows, delightful wildflower displays, beautiful creeks, and excellent angling, all topped off with thrilling vistas of Yosemite's most famous scenery.

Shuttle Directions: Follow Hwy. 41 to a junction near its summit, Chinquapin Junction, with the Glacier Point Road. Turn east onto that road and follow it 15.5 miles generally north and then east to its end at Glacier Point. Turn right into the large, two-level parking lot. Here you'll find toilets, a snack bar, a gift shop, and knock-your-socks-off views at Glacier Point proper. Hikers will finish this trip at the Panorama Trailhead, which is well signed and almost opposite the toilets.

DAY 1 (Bridalveil Creek Trailhead to Turner Meadow, 6.3 miles): *(Recap: Trip 68, Day 1.)* From the trailhead, the trail scrambles over a low dome and then winds along Bridalveil Creek's south bank. At a junction where a spur to Glacier Point Road hooks sharply left (north), you continue ahead (southeast). Beyond, the trail veers south beside one of the larger tributaries of Bridalveil Creek, fords it, and meets a lateral left (northeast) to the Ostrander Lake Trail. Go right (south), and in a half mile ford the tributary again.

Now make an easy, 400-foot climb over a ridge. From its top, the trail drops south-southeast to meet the Deer Camp Trail (right, northwest). Go ahead (southeast), climb over Turner Ridge, and descend to ford a tributary of Turner Meadow.

Continue descending until you are tracing the east side of long Turner Meadow. Just before the ford of a sizeable tributary to the meadows (7485'; 11S 270734 4164202), there's a large packer campsite on your right (southwest), and beyond the ford a short distance, there's a slender, open, sandy flat on the trail's right.

DAY 2 (Turner Meadow to Royal Arch Lake, 6.7 miles): *(Recap: Trip 68, Day 2.)* Resume your descent and soon meet the Wawona Trail (right, south). Go left (southeast) here, and in a little over 0.75 mile, meet the Chilnualna (chill-NWAHL-nah) Lakes Trail branching left (east) near a campsite. Take the right fork southward to ford swirling Chilnualna Creek (difficult in early season). From the ford, climb southeast over an eastward-rising ridge to a junction with a second lateral trail to Wawona, leading right (west). Take the left fork eastward here.

South of the ridgecrest, turn east up the valley of Grouse Lake's outlet stream and ascend for 2.25 miles to a junction with a hard-to-spot use trail leading right (south) to little Grouse Lake. Jog left (north) to cross a small rise, turn east again, drop almost southward, and then descend to ford the inlet of shallow Crescent Lake, just out of sight to the south. Eastbound again, another mile of level walking brings you to the north edge of Johnson Lake (good fishing for brook and rainbow).

Over the next 0.75 mile, ascend 250 feet to a junction with the Buck Camp Trail continuing ahead (east). Turn left (north) for a 0.75-mile climb to Royal Arch Lake (8729'; 11S 278975 4161785). Fishing is good for rainbow and brook.

DAY 3 (Royal Arch Lake to Illilouette Creek Tributary, 11 miles): *(Partial Recap: Trip 68, Day 3, from Royal Arch Lake to the junction with the trail to the Chilnualna Lakes.)* Although it's long, this day's trip is mostly downhill. Begin by continuing the climb from Royal Arch Lake and passing through a large meadow before topping out at Buena Vista Pass. Descend to skirt Buena Vista Lake's north shore. Beyond the lake, you descend to a junction where the left fork goes west to the Chilnualna Lakes. Here, take the right fork generally north into Buena Vista Creek's drainage.

Leave the Day 3 route of Trip 68 and turn right to descend steeply past two ponds into Buena Vista Creek canyon. After crossing the creek a few times and then the outlet from Hart Lakes, climb over a large moraine. Beyond, the descent is steady for 2 miles through dry forest until you cross the seasonal outlet from Edson Lake between two wet meadows. Turning northeast, the grade soon steepens, and the trail descends over indistinct glacial moraines. Presently, the forest of white fir and Jeffrey pine shows sign of a fire that occurred in 1981. As the trail nears the sometimes seasonal Buena Vista Creek, you see many living trees whose trunks were barely touched by flames. But there are always variations in nature, and after you curve northwest and climb over a low ridge, you descend to cross two small creeks where stands of lodgepole pine have been completely killed.

FIRE AND TREES

The kind of damage you saw as you neared Buena Vista Creek—living trees barely touched by fire—indicates that the fire there was not very hot and burned slowly along the ground. This type of low-intensity fire is a normal event in natural coniferous forests. Such fires prevent a large buildup of dead wood, which in turn prevents fires from reaching severe intensity.

However, lodgepoles, like most pines, burn easily, and, because they have thin bark, they often die in a fire. The logical counterpart to this property is that lodgepole pines produce a dense crop of fast-growing seedlings. The new generation thrives in bright light and dry soil and outcompetes other trees in newly opened parts of a forest.

After crossing another low ridge, the trail descends along the margins of a flowery meadow to ford a larger creek, a north-flowing tributary of Illilouette Creek, beside which there's a good campsite in a stand of unburned pine and fir (6827'; 11S 276824 4172948).

DAY 4 (Illilouette Creek Tributary to Glacier Point—Panorama Trailhead, 5.1 miles): Descending northwest, you see more signs of fire, as well as massive Mt. Starr King looming in the northeast. The route passes several giant sugar pines, survivors of many fires over the centuries. After 1.3 miles, the trail reaches a signed junction near Illilouette Creek. (A short distance toward the creek is an overused campsite, but there are better ones upstream.) You go left (ahead, west) and in 50 yards reach a signed junction with a trail left (west) to Mono Meadow. Turn right (north-northwest), soon descending more steeply, and in 0.3 mile ford the creek from Mono Meadow.

From here, descend parallel to Illilouette Creek as it winds through a gorge for almost a mile. Beyond the gorge, the trail begins the challenging 1200-foot ascent to Glacier Point. Soon the trail leaves the shade of huge white firs and enters an area that burned in 1987. The ascent here is gentle, and you see fire succession in the form of black oaks that have regrown from the crown of their roots. A small, seasonal creek provides a lush rest stop before you meet the Panorama Trail coming up from Illilouette Fall, which you may want to detour to see in early season (right, northeast, downhill).

ALONG THE PANORAMA TRAIL

On this well-known trail, on a clear day, you can look across the vast chasm of the Merced River's canyon and, with the aid of binoculars, see hikers on the summit of Half Dome. Nearer at hand, you can see the work of avalanches that have thundered down from the heights, carrying rocks, trees, and soil across the trail. The fine views from just below Washburn Point include Nevada Fall, Vernal Fall, Half Dome, Mt. Starr King, and many high peaks of eastern Yosemite marching off to the southeast horizon.

At the junction with the Panorama Trail, turn left (north-northwest) and begin the exposed and hot but very scenic ascent whose views are described in the sidebar "Along the Panorama Trail" on page 240. The last half mile to Glacier Point is on switchbacks that rise to the signed trailhead on the roadend near this famous overlook (7197'; 11S 273227 4178778). If you've never visited Glacier Point, certainly do so. The short trail over to it, on your right (northeast), offers incredible views down into Yosemite Valley.

70 Yosemite Valley—Happy Isles Trailhead

Trip Data: 11S 274550 4179235; 32.7 miles; 4/1 days

see map on p.236

Topos: *Yosemite, Merced Peak, Half Dome, Mariposa Grove*

Highlights: This route traverses some of the finer forest stands in Yosemite, crosses the Buena Vista Crest, and concludes via the famous Panorama Trail and JMT into the Valley. On this trip, you get close-up views of many world-famous Yosemite landmarks.

Shuttle Directions: You can't drive to the take-out trailhead at Yosemite Valley, but you can leave a car in Curry Village and take a shuttle to and from there. Whether you drive from the west or the east, get to the junction of highways 140 and 120 in Yosemite Valley. On what is now the Yosemite Valley Road, drive east and deeper into the valley—a somewhat confusing effort, as parts of this road are one way, and you must follow signs to Curry Village. Note that private cars cannot drive the Yosemite Valley Road east beyond the big parking lot at Curry Village. That means you can't leave a car or pick someone up at the Yosemite Valley—Happy Isles Trailhead. Weary hikers will probably want to ride the free shuttlebus from the Happy Isles bus stop to their pick-up point or to Curry Village parking. Or they can walk 1 mile more generally west on paved trail to Curry Village parking.

DAY 1 (Bridalveil Creek Trailhead to Turner Meadow, 6.3 miles): *(Recap: Trip 68, Day 1.)* From the trailhead, the trail scrambles over a low dome and then winds along Bridalveil Creek's south bank. At a junction where a spur to Glacier Point Road hooks sharply left (north), you continue ahead (southeast). Beyond, the trail veers south beside one of the larger tributaries of Bridalveil Creek, fords it, and meets a lateral left (northeast) to the Ostrander Lake Trail. Go right (south), and in a half mile ford the tributary again.

Now make an easy, 400-foot climb over a ridge. From its top, the trail drops south-southeast to meet the Deer Camp Trail (right, northwest). Go ahead (southeast), climb over Turner Ridge, and descend to ford a tributary of Turner Meadow.

Continue descending until you are tracing the east side of long Turner Meadow. Just before the ford of a sizeable tributary to the meadows (7485'; 11S 270734 4164202), there's a large packer campsite on your right (southwest), and beyond the ford a short distance, there's a slender, open, sandy flat on the trail's right.

DAY 2 (Turner Meadow to Royal Arch Lake, 6.7 miles): *(Recap: Trip 68, Day 2.)* Resume your descent and soon meet the Wawona Trail (right, south). Go left (southeast) here, and in a little over 0.75 mile, meet the Chilnualna (chill-NWAHL-nah) Lakes Trail branching left (east) near a campsite. Take the right fork southward to ford swirling Chilnualna Creek (difficult in early season). From the ford, climb southeast over an eastward-rising ridge to a junction with a second lateral trail to Wawona, leading right (west). Take the left fork eastward here.

South of the ridgecrest, turn east up the valley of Grouse Lake's outlet stream and ascend for 2.25 miles to a junction with a hard-to-spot use trail leading right (south) to little Grouse Lake. Jog left (north) to cross a small rise, turn east again, drop almost southward, and then descend to ford the inlet of shallow Crescent Lake, just out of sight to the south. Eastbound again, another mile of level walking brings you to the north edge of Johnson Lake (good fishing for brook and rainbow).

Over the next 0.75 mile, ascend 250 feet to a junction with the Buck Camp Trail continuing ahead (east). Turn left (north) for a 0.75-mile climb to Royal Arch Lake (8729'; 11S 278975 4161785). Fishing is good for rainbow and brook.

DAY 3 (Royal Arch Lake to Illilouette Creek Tributary, 11 miles): *(Partial Recap: Trip 68, Day 3, from Royal Arch Lake to the junction with the trail to the Chilnualna Lakes.)* Although it's long, this day's trip is mostly downhill. Begin by continuing the climb from Royal Arch Lake and passing through a large meadow before topping out at Buena Vista Pass. Descend to skirt Buena Vista Lake's north shore. Beyond the lake, you descend to a junction where the left fork goes west to the Chilnualna Lakes. Here, take the right fork generally north into Buena Vista Creek's drainage.

Leave the Day 3 route of Trip 68 and turn right to descend steeply past two ponds into Buena Vista Creek's canyon. *(Partial Recap: Trip 69, Day 3, from the junction with the trail to Chilnualna Lakes to Illilouette Creek Tributary.)* Cross the creek a few times and then the outlet from Hart Lakes. Climb over a large moraine and maintain a steady descent for 2 miles to ford Edson Lake's seasonal outlet. Curve northeast and descend over indistinct glacial moraines. Presently, you curve northwest, climb over a low ridge, and descend to cross two small creeks. Cross another low ridge, descend along a meadow, and ford a north-flowing tributary of Illilouette Creek near a good campsite (6827'; 11S 276824 4172948).

DAY 4 (Illilouette Creek Tributary to Yosemite Valley—Happy Isles Trailhead, 8.7 miles): Descend northwest for 1.3 miles to a signed junction near Illilouette Creek, on the right. Turn sharply right (northeast) here to descend past an overused campsite. A short climb then brings you to a small clearing on red ground. Ford Illilouette Creek here as the trail curves north (difficult in high runoff). A short ascent on deeply weathered glacial deposits brings you to a dry flat and a signed junction with the Merced Pass Trail. Go left (north) here and descend through trees to cross a lovely little creek. There is a good campsite shortly before the creek.

Ascending steeply now, and then moderately through Jeffrey pine, white fir, and bracken fern, you come to a seasonal creek. Here the soil thins, as does the forest cover, and the grade steepens. This sunny slope gets hot, and you can rest while taking in the view of the burn across the canyon.

FIRE'S LASTING EFFECTS

In that burn area, you can see one reason forests vary in both tree age and species composition. This typical mosaic pattern results when a fire kills some trees entirely while barely touching others nearby.

From this slope, climb through more shady environs and reach a signed junction where you turn left (north), cross a low ridge, curve northeast, and descend switchbacks to join the aptly named Panorama Trail. Turning right (east), you soon begin descending northeast-trending switchbacks into the immense, glacially polished canyon of the Merced River. Half Dome falls behind Liberty Cap as you drop 600 feet to the JMT. At the junction with the JMT, your route to the valley turns left (west)—but first, you may want to turn right (east) to see Nevada Fall, whose roar will lead you there (try the viewpoints on the north side of the footbridge across the Merced above the fall).

(Partial Recap: Trip 50, Day 2, from the Panorama Trail/JMT junctions to Yosemite Valley—Happy Isles.) From the Panorama Trail/JMT junctions, go west (downstream and downhill) on the JMT to begin long, steep, mostly paved switchbacks. At Clark Point and a junction with the Clark Trail (on the right), continue down the JMT by going ahead (generally west).

After a long descent on switchbacks, the JMT levels out and meets a signed HORSE TRAIL coming in from the left. Avoid that and go ahead (west) on the JMT; the Mist Trail shortly joins the JMT from the right. The JMT then curves north to the Merced's south bank and crosses the river on a footbridge that offers a superb view of 317-foot Vernal Fall.

Cross the bridge to the river's north side, where the trail climbs a little before descending steeply again. The JMT presently passes above the Happy Isles (two rocky islets in the Merced) and then a gauging station and the remains of a bridge to the Happy Isles. At last, the trail levels out near its end, where it meets the road that curves through Yosemite Valley's floor at the east side of the Happy Isles Bridge (4023'; 11S 274550 4179235).

Cross the bridge westward to the Happy Isles bus stop, where you can pick up a free Valley shuttlebus to numerous Valley destinations, including Curry Village and its overnight parking lot where your car or a ride should be waiting. Or you can follow the paved path northwest beyond the bus stop for a mile to Curry Village (distance not included in this trip).

W. YOSEMITE

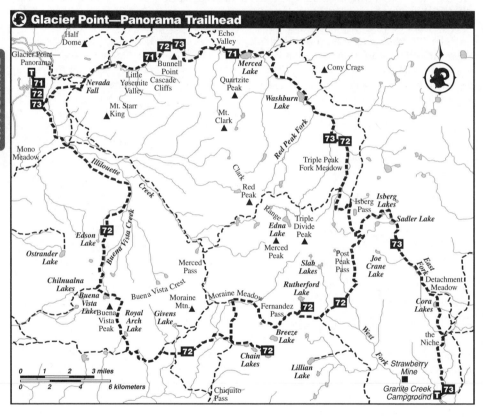

Glacier Point—Panorama Trailhead

Glacier Point—Panorama Trailhead   7197'; 11S 273227 4178778

DESTINATION/ UTM COORDINATES	TRIP TYPE	BEST SEASON	PACE (HIKING/ LAYOVER DAYS)	TOTAL MILEAGE
71 Merced Lake 11S 287918 4179565	Out & back	Early	4/1 Leisurely	31.8
72 Rutherford Lake 11S 290795 4163584	Loop	Mid or late	10/1 Moderate	71.5

73 Granite Creek
   Campground
   11S 299555 4157469
	Shuttle	Mid or late	7/1
			Leisurely
				41.1

Information and Permits: These trips enter Yosemite National Park: Yosemite Permits, PO Box 545, Yosemite National Park, CA 95389; 209-372-0740; www.nps.gov/yose/wilderness/permits.htm. Bear canisters are required; pets and firearms are prohibited.

Driving Directions: Follow Hwy. 41 to a junction near its summit, Chinquapin Junction, with the Glacier Point Road. Turn onto that road and follow it 15.5 miles generally north and then east to its end at Glacier Point. Turn right into the large, two-level parking lot. Here you'll find toilets, a snack bar, a gift shop, and knock-your-socks-off views at Glacier Point proper. These hikes begin at the Glacier Point—Panorama Trailhead, which is well signed and almost opposite the toilets.

71 Merced Lake

Trip Data: 11S 287918 4179565; 31.8 miles; 4/1 days

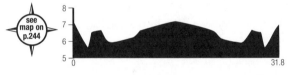
see map on p.244

Topos: *Yosemite, Merced Peak, Half Dome, Merced Peak*

Highlights: This early-season scenic excursion begins high above the Merced River's canyon, where you'll enjoy an airy view that provides a better feeling for the glacial history of the area. Mild elevation change and solid mileage make this route a fine choice for the hiker who wants to shake winter's kinks out of early-season muscles.

DAY 1 (Glacier Point—Panorama Trailhead to Little Yosemite Valley, 6.7 miles): From the signed Panorama Trailhead almost opposite the toilets, the trail begins a moderate-to-steep descent trending generally south into Illilouette Creek's gorge. Views of Half Dome and the sound of the falls filter through a forest cover that includes white fir, sugar pine, Jeffrey pine, and black oak. Manzanita, huckleberry oak, and deer brush form most of the ground cover.

After 1.6 miles, you find a junction with a trail leading right (southeast) into Illilouette Creek's canyon. You turn left (north) here and switchback down to seasonally raging Illilouette Creek. Just before the bridge, a short spur trail leads down to an airy overlook of Illilouette Fall. Beyond the impressive footbridge, the little-used trail begins an 800-foot ascent to the top of Panorama Cliff.

> **DOUGLAS FIRS**
>
> On this ascent, you see some Douglas firs at about 6500 feet. This is an unusually high elevation for them. Warm air flowing up the Merced River's canyon rises up Panorama Cliff, creating an unusually warm and favorable microclimate here.

The route traverses along the top of aptly named Panorama Cliff to a junction with a trail right (south). Here, you go left (east) to stay on the Panorama Trail, which begins the 800-foot descent to Nevada Fall. Via a long series of switchbacks, the trail descends through a dense forest of tall, water-loving Douglas firs and incense cedars to join the JMT. Turn right (east) here; staying on the JMT, you may shortly notice a junction with a use trail right (south) and back to the Panorama Trail. *(Partial Recap: Trip 67, Day 1, from the JMT/Panorama Trail junctions to Little Yosemite Valley.)* Stay on the JMT and cross the footbridge above Nevada Fall. Beyond Nevada Fall, the trail ascends past a junction with the Mist Trail, turns right (east), and switchbacks over a low bedrock ridge under Liberty Cap. After a half mile you pass a JMT cutoff going left (northeast) and take the right fork ahead (east) into Little Yosemite Valley to find its main, heavily used camping area (where the trail crosses Sunrise Creek; 6095'; 11S 278493 4179091; toilets, a ranger station, and bear boxes). There are less-crowded sites about 2 level miles farther on at the east end of Little Yosemite Valley.

DAY 2 (Little Yosemite Valley to Merced Lake, 9.2 miles): *(Recap: Trip 67, Day 2.)* Head for Little Yosemite Valley's east end, and then climb through a gorge leading to Lost Valley. At Lost Valley's east end, climb eastward to another, smaller valley. Before leaving this valley, the trail crosses one branch of the Merced via an island and a second branch on a wooden bridge. The trail soon begins climbing steeply to Echo Valley, detouring 400 feet south and traversing over open slabs where glacial erratics mark the path. Curving north, the trail descends, crosses the river on a bridge at the valley's west end, and presently arrives at a junction and a multi-bridged crossing of Echo Creek. Cross the creek and bear southeast to wind up slabs. The grade eases again in the valley containing Merced Lake. Follow the lake's north shore to its east end, where you find the camping area in conjunction with Merced Lake High Sierra Camp (7234'; 11S 287918 4179565).

DAYS 3–4 (Merced Lake to Glacier Point—Panorama Trailhead, 15.9 miles): Retrace your steps.

72 Rutherford Lake

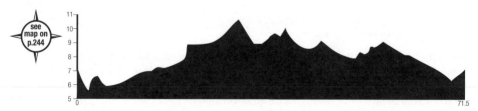

Trip Data: 11S 290795 4163584; 71.5 miles; 10/1 days

Topos: *Yosemite, Merced Peak, Half Dome, Merced Peak, Mt. Lyell, Timber Knob, Sing Peak, Mariposa Grove*

Highlights: Designed for the experienced backpacker, this trip offers a combination of excellent fishing and superlative vistas. Almost a dozen angling lakes, most of them in high-country settings, also provide swimming to alleviate the trail dust. Three major passes challenge the most ambitious hiker, and the wide variations in plants and wildlife will engage naturalists.

DAY 1 (Glacier Point—Panorama Trailhead to Little Yosemite Valley, 6.7 miles): *(Partial Recap: Trip 71, Day 1, from the Panorama Trailhead to the junction with JMT.)* From the signed Panorama Trailhead almost opposite the toilets, the trail begins a moderate-to-steep descent trending generally south into Illilouette Creek's gorge for 1.6 miles to a junction

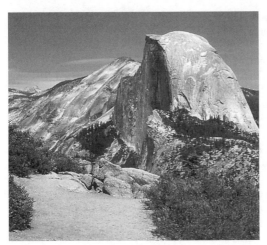

View of Half Dome from Glacier Point

with a trail leading right (southeast) into Illilouette Creek's canyon. You turn left (north) here and switchback down to Illilouette Creek. Cross the creek and begin an 800-foot ascent to the top of Panorama Cliff. Traverse the cliff-top to a junction with a trail right (south). Here, you go left (east) to stay on the Panorama Trail, which begins the 800-foot descent to Nevada Fall. Via a long series of switchbacks, the trail descends through a dense forest of tall, water-loving Douglas firs and incense cedars to join the JMT. Turn right (east) here; staying on the JMT, you may shortly notice a junction with a use trail right (south) back to the Panorama Trail.

(Partial Recap: Trip 67, Day 1, from the JMT/Panorama Trail junctions to Little Yosemite Valley.) Stay on the JMT and cross the footbridge above Nevada Fall. Beyond Nevada Fall, the trail ascends past a junction with the Mist Trail, turns right (east), and switchbacks over a low bedrock ridge under Liberty Cap. After a half mile you pass a JMT cutoff going left (northeast) and take the right fork ahead (east) into Little Yosemite Valley to find its main, heavily used camping area (where the trail crosses Sunrise Creek; 6095'; 11S 278493 4179091; toilets, a ranger station, and bear boxes). There are less-crowded sites about 2 level miles farther on at the east end of Little Yosemite Valley.

DAY 2 (Little Yosemite Valley to Merced Lake, 9.2 miles): *(Recap: Trip 67, Day 2.)* Head for Little Yosemite Valley's east end, and then climb through a gorge leading to Lost Valley. At Lost Valley's east end, climb eastward to another, smaller valley. Before leaving this valley, the trail crosses one branch of the Merced via an island and a second branch on a wooden bridge. The trail soon begins climbing steeply to Echo Valley, detouring 400 feet south and traversing over open slabs where glacial erratics mark the path. Curving north, the trail descends, crosses the river on a bridge at the valley's west end, and presently arrives at a junction and a multi-bridged crossing of Echo Creek. Cross the creek and bear southeast to wind up slabs. The grade eases again in the valley containing Merced Lake. Follow the lake's north shore to its east end, where you find the camping area in conjunction with Merced Lake High Sierra Camp (7234'; 11S 287918 4179565).

DAY 3 (Merced Lake to Lyell Fork Merced River, 5.8 miles): From Merced Lake High Sierra Camp, the trail ascends slabs to a drift fence and enters an area much used by livestock. A shaded stroll brings you to an engineered ford of multibranched Lewis Creek, a junction with the Lewis Creek Trail, and the Merced Lake Ranger Station.

(Recap in Reverse: Trip 62, Day 5, from Merced Lake Ranger Station to Lyell Fork Merced River.) From the station, continue the level stroll to a riverside drift fence. Staying closer to the river now, the trail soon begins a moderate ascent along the east canyon wall, crossing several small creeks before traversing above the outlet of Washburn Lake (7600'). Skirting the east shore of the lake, cross a small creek and pass the shaded campsites at the head of the lake. Beyond the lake, the trail ascends a dry slope and then swings over to riverside. The gentle ascent continues, and presently the Merced River flows near the trail in places along this idyllic setting. Where the Lyell Fork Merced River comes down on the left, you meet the main river, and there are good campsites near the footbridge (7897'; 11S 293022 4175251). Fishing in the river is fair to good for rainbow trout.

DAY 4 (Lyell Fork Merced River to Triple Peak Fork Meadow, 4.2 miles): *(Recap in Reverse: Trip 62, Day 5, from Lyell Fork Merced River to Triple Peak Fork Meadow.)* Cross the footbridge if you haven't already done so. Beyond it, the trail soon begins to climb south. This ascent steepens as it passes the confluence of Merced Peak Fork and Triple Peak Fork and levels momentarily where it crosses Merced Peak Fork on another footbridge. Then the trail leaves the riverside and switchbacks up the north side of Merced Peak Fork's bowl. As the ascent continues, the trail begins angling generally east into the lowest of the hanging valleys on Triple Peak Fork Merced River. Above the switchbacks, the trail ascends gently to a flat on Triple Peak Fork. After a steep, short climb, the trail ascends gradually near the river for 2 miles to the foot of mile-long Triple Peak Fork Meadow. The best campsites are at the south end of the meadow, near the junction with the westbound Red Peak Pass Trail (9094'; 11S 293186 4170519). Fishing is good for brook and rainbow trout.

DAY 5 (Triple Peak Fork Meadow to Post Creek, 7.2 miles): *(Recap in Reverse: Trip 62, Day 4, from Triple Peak Fork Meadow to the cairn that marks the junction with a trail down to Triple Peak Fork.)* Avoid the Red Peak Pass Trail that turns west out of the south end of Triple Peak Fork Meadow. Instead, go ahead (south) and make a gradually increasing climb for a long mile away from Triple Peak Fork. The trail then turns northeast and climbs almost a mile on a traverse with two short switchbacks before arriving at the rock monument at the cairned junction with the Isberg Pass Trail.

(Partial Recap: Trip 62, Day 4, from the junction with the Isberg Pass Trail to the junction with the trail to Post Peak Pass.) Turn right (south, curving south-southeast) and quickly ascend a beautiful hillside with broken, light-colored granite close on the left and the soaring Clark Range across the canyon on the right. The trail then levels off in a spectacular high bowl encircled by Triple Divide Peak, Isberg Peak, and some unnamed peaks between. After fording the unmapped, unnamed outlet of the unnamed but mapped lakes in this bowl, the trail dips into a bowl-within-the-bowl and there crosses another clear stream. Finally you ascend out of the huge meadow, cross another stream, and begin a northeastern curve before arriving at a hillside junction.

Leaving the Day 4 route of Trip 62, turn right (south) here onto the Post Peak Pass Trail, which climbs to the ridgeline north of Post Peak and then follows this ridge south to the actual pass (10,769'), which straddles the divide between the great Merced and San Joaquin rivers. The scenery from the trail—but not from the pass—is among the most outstanding in Yosemite's South Boundary Country, with views of the Clark Range to the west, the Cathedral Range to the north, and the tops of Banner Peak, Mt. Ritter, and the Minarets to the east. At the pass, this trip briefly leaves Yosemite and enters Ansel Adams Wilderness. The trail descends southwest 600 feet on steep, loose, rocky trail to campsite-less little Porphyry Lake (10,100'), where fishing is fair for brook and rainbow. Continue descending, now generally southward over tributaries to Post Creek. Pikas and marmots may appear on the rocky parts of this trail, and deer, grouse and quail in the meadowy parts. After going almost levelly for a half mile through several meadows, you enter lodgepole forest and descend moderately to the fair but mosquito-filled campsite at Post Creek (9000'; 11S 293598 4164149). Fishing along the creek is good for brook trout.

DAY 6 (Post Creek to Rutherford Lake, 3.9 miles): From Post Creek, the trail climbs southwest over a small rise, descends past two nameless lakelets (no fish), briefly curves west, and meets a primitive trail right (north-northwest) toward the Slab Lakes. Go left (ahead, southwest) at this junction, almost immediately ford the Slab Lakes' outlet (three parallel washes), and enter a small meadow along Fernandez Creek. Just past the meadow, the track splits, one fork on each bank of Fernandez Creek. Both soon meet the Fernandez Pass Trail, where your route turns right (west) on a gently ascending, densely timbered stretch that offers fine views over the shoulder to Fernandez Creek. After a long a half mile, the trail switchbacks moderately up a morainal slope, trending northwest, to a junction with the Rutherford Lake lateral.

Here the route turns right (northeast) and climbs into to the cirque nestling 28-acre Rutherford Lake (9800'), where there are fair-to-good campsites on the lake's east side a little beyond the dam on its south end (9771'; 11S 290795 4163584). Fishing is fair for brook and golden. (If you notice a junction partway to Rutherford, the left fork goes to Rutherford, the right to Anne Lake.)

DAY 7 (Rutherford Lake to Middle Chain Lake, 9.4 miles): Return to the Fernandez Pass Trail and turn right (west) toward that pass. The trail climbs generally westward, crosses a small meadow, and then ascends ledges above the headwaters of Fernandez Creek, where there are good views of the Ritter Range to the east. Veering south below the headwall of the headwaters' cirque, the trail ascends past a tree-dotted saddle before descending a little to signed Fernandez Pass (10,175') and the Yosemite boundary. Step back into Yosemite and curve southwest to drop 600 steep, rocky feet under lodgepole and western white pine and over weathered granite. Near the bottom of this descent, you find a junction with a faint trail left (south) to Breeze Lake, but you go right (northwest) on a gradual, 0.75-mile descent past a shallow, meadow-fringed lake. Soon you step over a seasonal stream and begin a 400-foot, shaded descent.

Near the end of this descent, the trail veers north to a ford of flower-lined South Fork Merced River. Beyond the ford, the trail soon curves west and continues descending gradually under lodgepole pine. The track enters Moraine Meadows and meets a signed junction with a trail left (south) to Chain Lakes (ahead, west goes to Buck Camp). You turn left toward Chain Lakes, pass some campsites, ford South Fork Merced again (wet in early season), and descend past a packer campsite on your right. The undulating trail continues its southward course over a lodgepole-covered flat, along a small watercourse, past a glacial tarn, over a low ridge, and finally descends to a junction with a trail right (southwest) to Buck Camp and left (southeast) toward Chain Lakes.

Turn left along the Chain Lakes' outlet and climb to yet another junction. Right (initially west) heads for Chiquito Pass; you go left (east) toward Chain Lakes. The trail leaves the outlet creek and swings north of Lower Chain Lake (signed CHAIN LAKES) as it heads east toward the Middle Chain Lake (also signed CHAIN LAKES). Camping is best on this lake's south side (9104'; 11S 287277 4160764). All three lakes contain rainbow, brook trout, or both. Ambitious hikers can continue east and then southeast to beautiful Upper Chain Lake.

DAY 8 (Middle Chain Lake to Royal Arch Lake, 9 miles): First, regain the trail you came in on and return past Lower Chain Lake to the junction along the Chain Lakes' outlet. Turn right (ahead, west) here and retrace your steps to the next junction, with the trail from Moraine Meadows. Instead of going back there (a right turn), turn left on long, west-trending switchbacks, roughly paralleling the Chain Lakes' outlet creek but at some distance north of it as it falls to rendezvous with the South Fork Merced River, which turned almost directly south a little west of yesterday's ford in Moraine Meadows.

Just before the South Fork is a signed lateral trail leading left (south) a quarter mile to good camping at Soda Springs. Your route, however, continues ahead (west), fords another fork of South Fork Merced, and swings southwest over a lodgepole-covered slope. The depth of the U-shaped, glacially formed slopes indicates the strength of the forces at work when the ice flow originating in the Clark Range to the north was in its heyday.

The trail crosses over a ridge trending south from Moraine Mountain before fording Givens Creek. Beyond this ford, your route meets a trail left (south) to Chiquito Pass; here, you continue ahead (generally west). Just 60 yards farther on, there's another junction where you take the well-used left (southwest) fork, not the little-used right fork, and then continue a half more mile to meet the Buck Camp/Merced Pass Trail on a ridgetop. Turning left (southwest) here, you descend through red fir forest and then climb northwest to the meadowy precincts of Buck Camp. At Buck Camp, the Park has a summer ranger station, and emergency services may be available.

From Buck Camp, the trail ascends a tough 750 feet via switchbacks before dropping 350 feet to a junction with the Royal Arch Lake Trail. Turn right (north) here.

(Partial Recap: Trip 68, Day 2, from the Buck Camp Trail junction to Royal Arch Lake.) Make a 0.75-mile climb to Royal Arch Lake and the campsites on its south shore (8729'; 11S 278975 4161785). Fishing is good for rainbow and brook.

DAY 9 (Royal Arch Lake to Illilouette Creek Tributary, 11 miles): *(Partial Recap: 69, Day 3, from Royal Arch Lake to the junction with the trail to the Chilnualna Lakes.)* This day is long but mostly downhill. Continue the northward climb from Royal Arch Lake, topping out at Buena Vista Pass. Descend to skirt Buena Vista Lake's north shore. Beyond the lake, descend to a junction where the left fork goes west to the Chilnualna Lakes. Now leave the Day 3 route of Trip 68 behind.

(Partial Recap: Trip 69, Day 3, from the junction with the trail to the Chilnualna Lakes to Illilouette Creek Tributary.) Take the right fork generally north into Buena Vista Creek's drainage. Descend steeply into Buena Vista Creek's canyon, cross the creek a few times, ford the outlet from Hart Lakes, and then climb over a large moraine. Beyond, descend steadily for 2 miles to cross Edson Lake's seasonal outlet. Turning northeast, the trail descends over indistinct moraines, passes through burn areas near the occasionally seasonal Buena Vista Creek, curves northwest to climb over a low ridge, and descends to cross two small creeks. After crossing another low ridge, the trail descends to ford a larger creek, a north-flowing tributary of Illilouette Creek, beside which there's a good campsite in a stand of unburned pine and fir (6827'; 11S 276824 4172948).

Day 10 (Illilouette Creek Tributary to Glacier Point—Panorama Trailhead, 5.1 miles): *(Recap: Trip 69, Day 4.)* Descending northwest, after 1.3 miles, the trail reaches a signed junction near Illilouette Creek, on the right. You go left (ahead, west) and in 50 yards reach a signed junction with a trail left (west) to Mono Meadow. Turn right (north-northwest) and in 0.3 mile, ford the creek from Mono Meadow. From here, descend into Illilouette Creek's gorge and parallel the creek for almost a mile. Beyond the gorge, ascend 1200 feet to Glacier Point and presently meet the Panorama Trail coming up from Illilouette Fall. At this junction, turn left (north-northwest) and continue climbing. The last half mile to Glacier Point is on switchbacks that rise to the signed trailhead on the roadend near this famous overlook (7197'; 11S 273227 4178778), where you close the loop.

73 Granite Creek Campground

Trip Data: 11S 299555 4157469; 41.1 miles; 7/1 days

see map on p.244

Topos: *Yosemite, Merced Peak, Half Dome, Merced Peak, Mt. Lyell, Timber Knob, Sing Peak*

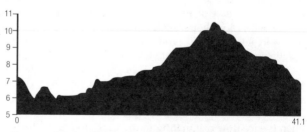

Highlights: This route traverses the very heart of Yosemite's South Boundary Country and crosses the divide of the Merced River and San Joaquin River watersheds at Isberg Pass. Fishing on the lakes and streams is fair to excellent, and the life zones range from Canadian to arctic-alpine. Remoteness and panoramic vistas invite you to take this trip.

HEADS UP! *Road 4S57 may be impossible to drive as late as early July. Note also that Forest Service road numbers tend to change, so when in doubt, follow directions to the named landmarks instead.*

Shuttle Directions: Granite Creek Campground is the most remote trailhead used in this book. Get yourself to Yosemite Forks on Hwy. 41, 3.5 miles north of Oakhurst and about 12 miles south of Yosemite National Park's Wawona entrance station. At Yosemite Forks, there's a junction with the road to popular Bass Lake. Turn east on it and drive to where the road forks at Bass Lake's northwest end. Take the left (southeast) fork around the lake's north shore to a junction with northeast-bound Beasore Road 434, which becomes Road 5S07. Turn left (north) onto Beasore Road 434 and drive 20 more miles to Globe Rock; then continue 9.8 more miles to the junction with the Minarets Road (on your right). Stay on your Road 5S07 for 1.7 more miles to Clover Meadow Ranger Station and then continue past it 0.5 mile to a junction with Road 4S57. Branch right (northeast) onto this road and follow it for 1 mile to a hikers' parking area in Granite Creek Campground.

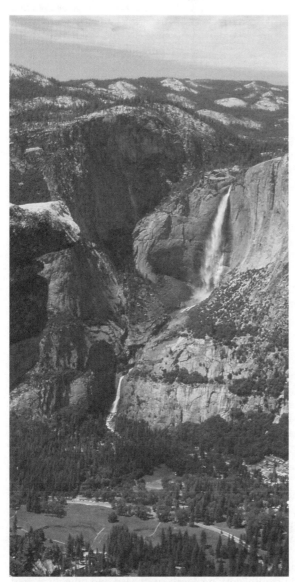

Yosemite Falls as seen from Glacier Point

DAY 1 (Glacier Point—Panorama Trailhead to Little Yosemite Valley, 6.7 miles): From the signed Panorama Trailhead almost opposite the toilets, the trail begins a moderate-to-steep descent trending generally south into Illilouette Creek's gorge for 1.6 miles to a junction with a trail leading right (southeast) into Illilouette Creek's canyon. You turn left (north) here and switchback down to seasonally raging Illilouette Creek. Cross the creek and begin an 800-foot ascent to the top of Panorama Cliff. Traverse the cliff-top to a junction with a trail right (south). Here, you go left (east) to stay on the Panorama Trail, which begins the 800-foot descent to Nevada Fall. Via a long series of switchbacks, the trail descends through a dense forest of tall, water-loving Douglas firs and incense cedars to join the JMT. Turn right (east) here; staying on the JMT, you may shortly notice a junction with a use trail right (south) back to the Panorama Trail.

(Partial Recap: Trip 67, Day 1, from the JMT/Panorama Trail junctions to Little Yosemite Valley.) Stay on the JMT and cross the footbridge above Nevada Fall. Beyond Nevada Fall, the trail ascends past a junction with the Mist Trail, turns right (east), and switchbacks over a low bedrock ridge under Liberty Cap. After a

half mile you pass a JMT cutoff going left (northeast) and take the right fork ahead (east) into Little Yosemite Valley to find its main, heavily used camping area (where the trail crosses Sunrise Creek; 6095'; 11S 278493 4179091; toilets, a ranger station, and bear boxes). There are less-crowded sites about 2 level miles farther on at the east end of Little Yosemite Valley.

DAY 2 (Little Yosemite Valley to Merced Lake, 9.2 miles): *(Recap: Trip 67, Day 2.)* Head for Little Yosemite Valley's east end, and then climb through a gorge leading to Lost Valley. At Lost Valley's east end, climb eastward to another, smaller valley. Before leaving this valley, the trail crosses one branch of the Merced via an island and a second branch on a wooden bridge. The trail soon begins climbing steeply to Echo Valley, detouring 400 feet south and traversing over open slabs where glacial erratics mark the path. Curving north, the trail descends, crosses the river on a bridge at the valley's west end, and presently arrives at a junction and a multi-bridged crossing of Echo Creek. Cross the creek and bear southeast to wind up slabs. The grade eases again in the valley containing Merced Lake. Follow the lake's north shore to its east end, where you find the camping area in conjunction with Merced Lake High Sierra Camp (7234'; 11S 287918 4179565).

DAY 3 (Merced Lake to Lyell Fork Merced River, 5.8 miles): From Merced Lake High Sierra Camp, the trail ascends slabs to a drift fence and enters an area much used by livestock. A shaded stroll brings you to an engineered ford of multibranched Lewis Creek, a junction with the Lewis Creek Trail, and the Merced Lake Ranger Station.

(Recap in Reverse: Trip 62, Day 5, from Merced Lake Ranger Station to Lyell Fork Merced River.) From the station, continue the level stroll to a riverside drift fence. Staying closer to the river now, the trail soon begins a moderate ascent along the east canyon wall, crossing several small creeks before traversing above the outlet of Washburn Lake (7600'). Skirting the east shore of the lake, cross a small creek and pass the shaded campsites at the head of the lake. Beyond the lake, the trail ascends a dry slope and then swings over to riverside. The gentle ascent continues, and presently the Merced River flows near the trail in places along this idyllic setting. Where the Lyell Fork Merced River comes down on the left, you meet the main river, and there are good campsites near the footbridge (7897'; 11S 293022 4175251). Fishing in the river is fair to good for rainbow trout.

DAY 4 (Lyell Fork Merced River to Triple Peak Fork Meadow, 4.2 miles): *(Recap in Reverse: Trip 62, Day 5, from Lyell Fork Merced River to Triple Peak Fork Meadow.)* Cross the footbridge if you haven't already done so. Beyond it, the trail soon begins to climb south. This ascent steepens as it passes the confluence of Merced Peak Fork and Triple Peak Fork and levels momentarily where it crosses Merced Peak Fork on another footbridge. Then the trail leaves the riverside and switchbacks up the north side of Merced Peak Fork's bowl. As the ascent continues, the trail begins angling generally east into the lowest of the hanging valleys on Triple Peak Fork Merced River. Above the switchbacks, the trail ascends gently to a flat on Triple Peak Fork. After a steep, short climb, the trail ascends gradually near the river for 2 miles to the foot of mile-long Triple Peak Fork Meadow. The best campsites are at the south end of the meadow, near the junction with the westbound Red Peak Pass Trail (9094'; 11S 293186 4170519). Fishing is good for brook and rainbow trout.

DAY 5 (Triple Peak Fork Meadow to Isberg Lakes, 4.9 miles): *(Recap in Reverse: Trip 62, Day 4, from Triple Peak Fork Meadow to the junction with a trail down to Triple Peak Fork.)* Avoid the Red Peak Pass Trail that turns west out of the south end of Triple Peak Fork Meadow. Instead, go ahead (south) and make a gradually increasing climb for a long mile away from Triple Peak Fork. The trail then turns northeast and climbs almost a mile on a traverse with two short switchbacks before arriving at the rock monument at the cairned junction with the Isberg Pass Trail.

(Partial Recap: Trip 62, Day 4, from the junction with Isberg Pass Trail to the junction with the trail to Post Peak Pass.) Turn right (south, curving south-southeast) and quickly ascend

a beautiful hillside with broken, light-colored granite close on the left and the soaring Clark Range across the canyon on the right. The trail then levels off in a spectacular high bowl encircled by Triple Divide Peak, Isberg Peak, and some unnamed peaks between. After fording the unmapped, unnamed outlet of the unnamed but mapped lakes in this bowl, the trail dips into a bowl-within-the-bowl and crosses another clear stream. Finally, you ascend out of the huge meadow, cross another stream, and begin a northeastern curve before arriving at a hillside junction.

Leaving the Day 4 route of Trip 62, turn left (northeast) here toward Isberg Pass and climb steadily among large blocks of talus. The views north and west, which already have been excellent, become even better as the route switchbacks farther up the ridge, as high as the pass you are approaching. Then the tread goes more or less level to signed ISBERG PASS (10,500'). At last, this trail leaves Yosemite, enters Ansel Adams Wilderness, and continues to weave sinuously along the crest beyond Isberg Pass. It passes through a tiny defile between two stunted whitebark pines that frame a very dramatic view of the Ritter Range a few miles east. In the distance to the right of this dark range, much of the northern High Sierra is visible, and hikers who have rambled among its summits will spy some of their favorite monuments. From this pass between the Merced River and the San Joaquin River watersheds, the trail descends by switchbacks to rocky Upper Isberg Lake and then more gradually to Lower Isberg Lake. Fishing in these lakes is fair to good for brook and some rainbow. There are a few fair campsites at Lower Isberg (north shore; 9832'; 11S 296065 4169455).

DAY 6 (Isberg Lakes to Middle Cora Lake, 5.7 miles): After rejoining the Isberg Pass Trail, head east into forest cover, cross a small creek, and swing south. Soon the lodgepole-shaded trail becomes steep as it winds down to the meadowed fringes of trout-filled Sadler Lake (9345'). Camping is legal only on the south and west sides of this popular lake. Rounding the east side of the lake brings you to the outlet and then to a junction with the trail right to McClure Lake.

At this junction, go left (southeast) as the trail descends moderately under lodgepole pines and then through a stretch of avalanche-downed trees before fording East Fork Granite Creek. Descending more gently now, the trail follows the orange bedrock channel for a half mile before veering away from the creek and passing a junction on the right with the Timber Creek Trail. Go left again (southeast) here as the trail continues to descend, crossing several small creeks before it levels off in the cow-infested environs of East Fork Granite Creek. Then the trail crosses to the east side of the creek (wet in early season), skirts a number of meadows, and swings south-southeast away from the creek to cross a low bedrock ridge. Over a mile from the ford, you reach a junction with a lateral left (southeast) toward Chetwood Creek. Take the right fork (also southeast) at this junction. From here, it is an easy half mile over a low moraine down to the shaded east shore of Middle Cora Lake (southwest shore; 8351'; 11S 299357 4163236). Check for posted regulations regarding any camping restrictions here.

DAY 7 (Middle Cora Lake to Granite Creek Campground, 4.6 miles): Return to the trail and, if you haven't done so already, ford Middle Cora Lake's outlet. From here, the trail heads south through lodgepole forest, fords a tributary of East Fork Granite Creek, and, 1.25 miles from Middle Cora Lake's outlet, fords East Fork Granite Creek for the last time (wet in early season). Immediately beyond is a junction with a trail right (west), but you go left (southeast) to another junction, this one with a lateral going left (northeast) back across the creek. Go right (south-southwest), staying on the creek's west side. The trail descends the west bank for a half mile to the Niche, west of Green Mountain, and then it passes through the Niche and swings west to leave Ansel Adams Wilderness.

Soon you turn south again, and the descent steepens as the trail winds down a ravine, crossing and recrossing its tiny creek, under red fir, lodgepole pine, and Jeffrey pine. The grade eases and the trail briefly swings near East Fork Granite Creek before the last, dusty descent brings you to a trailhead parking lot on the east side of West Fork Granite Creek. A bridge downstream takes you to the east end of Granite Creek Campground (6978'; 11S 299555 4157469).

US HIGHWAY 395 TRIPS

Whether you come from the north or the south, Hwy. 395 is a scenic delight. Better yet, it offers easy access to trailheads from which you can explore the wonder and beauty of, for this book, Carson-Iceberg and Hoover wildernesses and northern Yosemite National Park. We invite you to enjoy Sierra adventures from three major trailheads: Corral Valley, Twin Lakes, and Green Creek Roadend.

At the Corral Valley Trailhead, diverse topography awaits backpackers embarking from the east side of the 160,000-acre Carson-Iceberg Wilderness, where fellow travelers are few and far between.

Few trailheads that aren't already *in* Yosemite National Park offer such fine access to the spectacular backcountry of northern Yosemite as does the Twin Lakes Trailhead out of Bridgeport. This trailhead offers seven irresistible trips in Hoover Wilderness and Yosemite's northern backcountry.

The Green Creek drainage is an eastside gem, less crowded than the more popular trailheads out of Twin Lakes to the north and than Tuolumne Meadows to the south. The trips out of Green Creek Roadend Trailhead showcase the surrounding peaks, plus easy access to the northern Yosemite backcountry. All three trips get a gentle start in a rocky, aspen-filled canyon, making the already colorful trail even more spectacular in early autumn. Hikers interested in the next trailhead to the south, Virginia Lakes, will find the second and third Green Creek trips easy to adapt for Virginia Lakes.

TRAILHEADS: Corral Valley
Twin Lakes
Green Creek Roadend

HWY 395

Corral Valley Trailhead

8210'; 11S 277105 4266262

DESTINATION/ UTM COORDINATES	TRIP TYPE	BEST SEASON	PACE (HIKING/ LAYOVER DAYS)	TOTAL MILEAGE
74 Lower Fish Valley 11S 271915 4261518	Semiloop	Mid or late	2/1 Leisurely	14
75 Ebbetts Pass 11S 255501 4270384 (field)	Shuttle	Mid	3/1 Leisurely	26.5
76 Lake Alpine–Silver Valley 11S 239528 4263335 (field)	Shuttle	Mid or late	5/2 Moderate	41.5

Information and Permits: Responsibility for Carson-Iceberg Wilderness is split between Stanislaus and Humboldt-Toiyabe national forests. For trips from the Corral Valley Trailhead out of Rodriguez Flat, get information from Humboldt-Toiyabe National Forest's Carson Ranger District: 1536 S. Carson Street, Carson City, NV 89701; 775-882-7766; www.fs.fed.us/r4/htnf/r4/htnf/. Wilderness permits are required, but there are no quotas, and permits can be self-issued at the information bulletin boards near the trailhead. Note that for trail information, the USDA/USFS Carson-Iceberg Wilderness Map is generally more accurate than the topos.

Driving Directions: From the junction of highways 395 and 89, travel 5.5 miles south on Hwy. 395 to Coleville and continue another 2.2 miles to a road heading west, signed MILL CANYON ROAD (for northbound motorists this junction is 15.5 miles north of the Hwy. 395/Hwy. 108 junction, about 2.5 miles north of Walker). Take the Mill Canyon Road west and, following signs for Little Antelope Pack Station, proceed up the dirt road 0.3 mile to a fork and veer right. Continue another 5.7 miles to a mountain-crest road junction at broad, open Rodriguez Flat. Turn left (south), following signed directions for the Corral Valley Trailhead, and drive a rocky 0.4 mile to the end of the road and the signed trailhead.

HWY 395

74 Lower Fish Valley

Trip Data: 11S 271915 4261518; 14 miles; 2/1 days

Topos: *Coleville, Lost Cannon Peak*

Highlights: A fine weekend selection, this two-day trip visits five subalpine valleys. The country contains some of the largest Sierra junipers to be found anywhere. In addition, more than a half dozen side trips can be made from the Silver Creek Trail.

see map on p.258

DAY 1 (Corral Valley Trailhead to Lower Fish Valley, 7.5 miles): On the Corral Valley Trail, make a moderate climb southwest, shortly reaching a trail on the right from the Little Antelope Pack Station and almost immediately entering signed Carson-Iceberg Wilderness. Go ahead (southwest) to stay on the Corral Valley Trail. A forest cover of white firs, western white pines, and lodgepole pines persists for the next 0.3 mile of stiff ascent, and then yields to sagebrush where the old, metamorphosed sediments of Rodriguez Flat give way to much younger volcanic rocks. The view here is quite spectacular on clear days, with desert ranges visible in the northeast well beyond Rodriguez Flat.

The short, open ascent soon curves around the base of a volcanic hill to provide new views of Slinkard Valley in the north and the Sierra Crest in the northwest. A traverse south-southwest across broad, gentle, sagebrush-covered slopes leads to a signed junction, where the trail to Long Valley forks right (southwest; tomorrow's return route).

Veer left (south) at the junction, remaining on the Corral Valley Trail, and descend moderately through sagebrush and bitterbrush to the well-used grazing lands of Corral Valley

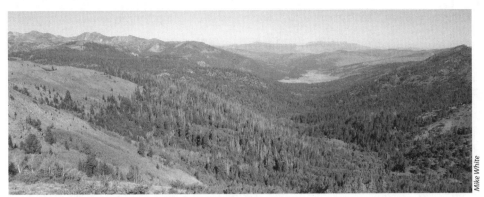

Mike White

View north to Slinkard Valley from the Corral Valley Trail

Creek. On the valley floor, the trail crosses two branches of Corral Valley Creek. Paiute trout, an endangered and protected species, live in Corral Valley Creek, as well as in Silver King Creek and Coyote Valley Creek, so no fishing!

Beyond Corral Valley Creek, the southbound trail heads into forest, curves west, parallels the valley for a short distance, and then climbs an ever-increasing slope to a dry saddle. From here, the descent into Coyote Valley is steep, made slightly easier by the cushioning effect of the deep gravel. Near the bottom of a gully, the trail crosses a seasonal creek and continues a short distance southwest before encountering an enormous, twin-trunked juniper. Beyond, the trail winds south down toward Coyote Valley, reaching the sagebrush-covered floor beside a large, 5-foot diameter lodgepole pine (a key landmark for northbound hikers).

Hike a level quarter mile across the valley floor to an easy ford of Coyote Valley Creek. Beyond the ford, the trail veers away from the creek and gradually climbs south. Near the crest above Upper Fish Valley, the forest becomes more dense and aspens more dominant. Pass through a fence gate at the crest's broad saddle and descend steeply to Upper Fish Valley. On the floor of the valley, near an orange snow-depth marker, reach a signed junction with a lateral left (southwest) to Whitecliff Lake. Go right (north) about 300 yards past the junction to a meeting of three fences, each with a gate. Go through the north gate and follow the path that parallels the west side of the north-northeast-trending fence. The trail soon curves northwest, climbs over a low moraine, and then comes to within earshot of unseen Llewellyn Falls, just a short distance southwest. A short walk leads to the significant 20-foot cascade of Llewellyn Falls.

HWY 395

WHAT'S FISHY ABOUT LLEWELLYN FALLS

Biologists speculate that as a giant glacier slowly retreated up Silver King Canyon, perhaps 50,000 years ago, cutthroat trout followed its path. The fish were able to swim into Upper Fish Valley and beyond before Silver King Creek eroded away bedrock to form Llewellyn Falls. Once isolated, the trout evolved into a subspecies known as Paiute cutthroat trout (*Salmo clarki seleniris*), or simply Paiute trout. Ironically, these fish became endangered not because of overfishing but rather through the introduction of Lahontan cutthroats and rainbows, which bred with the Paiutes to produce hybrids. Once this miscegenation was discovered, Department of Fish and Game workers removed the purebreds and, in 1964, treated Silver King Creek with rotenone to kill the hybrids. After the purebreds were reintroduced to the stream above the falls, their numbers grew from approximately 150 in the late 1960s to about 600 in the early 1970s. By 1975, the population stabilized, but fishing is strictly prohibited, as the Paiute could easily be fished out of existence.

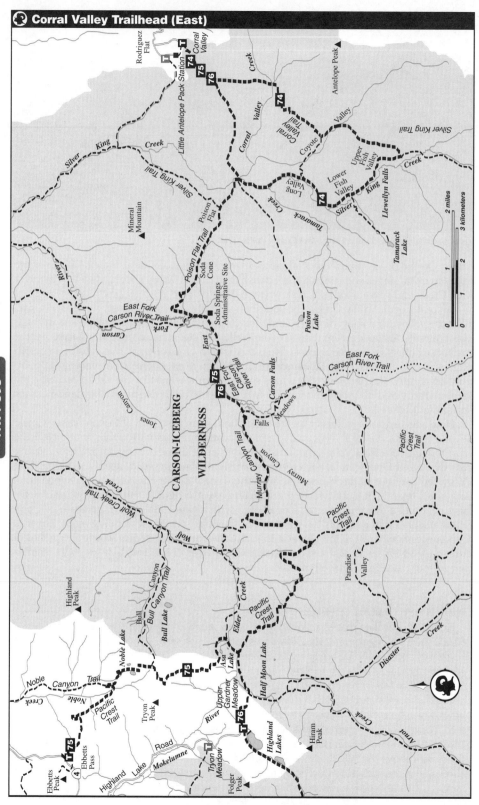

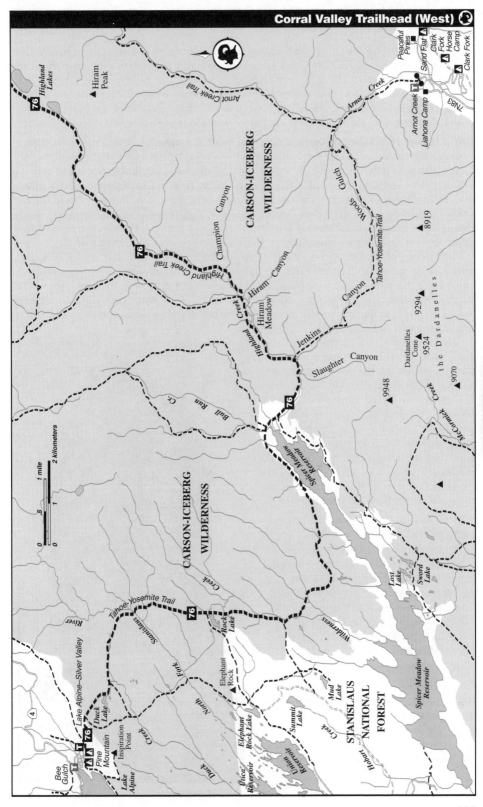

Highland
Lakes

▲ Hiram
Peak

Arnot Creek Trail

Arnot Creek

Peaceful
Pines

Sand Flat

Clark
Fork
Horse
Camp

Clark Fork

Arnot Creek Camp
Liahona Camp

7N83

CARSON-ICEBERG
WILDERNESS

Champion Canyon

Highland Creek Trail

Woods

Gulch

Tahoe-Yosemite Trail

8919

Highland Creek

Hiram Canyon

Hiram
Meadow

Jenkins

Canyon

9294

Dardanelles
Cone

the Dardanelles

9524

Slaughter Canyon

9070

McConnick Creek

76

9948

Bull Run Cr.

Spicer Meadow
Reservoir

HWY 395

1 mile

2 kilometers

.5

1

0

0

CARSON-ICEBERG
WILDERNESS

Creek

Lost
Lake

Sword
Lake

Tahoe-Yosemite Trail

River

76

Rock
Lake

Wilderness

Spicer Meadow Reservoir

Stanislaus

North

Fork

Elephant
Rock

Lake Alpine–Silver Valley

Duck
Lake

76

Pine
Mountain

Inspiration
Point

Duck

Creek

Elephant
Rock Lake

Utica
Reservoir

Union
Reservoir

Summit
Lake

Mud
Lake

Creek

Hobart

STANISLAUS
NATIONAL
FOREST

Bee
Gulch

Lake
Alpine

4

259

From Llewellyn Falls gorge, the trail descends briefly northeast into Lower Fish Valley. The trail approaches Silver King Creek several times before crossing the stream at the north end of this grassland. Although tree-shaded campsites are nearby (7950'; 11S 271915 4261518), they may be less than desirable if people and cattle have left too much of a mess. Fishing along Silver King Creek below Llewellyn Falls may yield rainbow, Paiute, or rainbow-Paiute hybrids. But beware, taking Paiute purebreds is prohibited.

DAY 2 (Lower Fish Valley to Corral Valley Trailhead, 6.5 miles): Continuing downstream, walk northwest toward a low ridge that hides the forested, little-visited valley of Tamarack Creek. The path leaves Lower Fish Valley, turns northeast, and climbs over a low granitic saddle before entering the south end of Long Valley. To avoid springs and boggy meadows, follow the trail that circles around the east side of the valley. Partway down the flat valley, the trails rejoin and then approach Silver King Creek, which meanders lazily through the glacial sediments that buried the canyon's bedrock floor long ago. The trail approaches several of these meanders before exiting the valley at the north end.

Following Silver King Creek, the trail passes the confluence of Tamarack Creek and, after an easy half mile of shaded descent, leads to a ford of the stream where granite outcrops force the path to the west bank. Anticipate a wet ford in early season. About 200 yards downstream is a junction with multiple trails: Your route goes right (northeast) across the creek; to the left (north), the trail you've been on for a while climbs a sandy slope to meet the trail to Poison Lake.

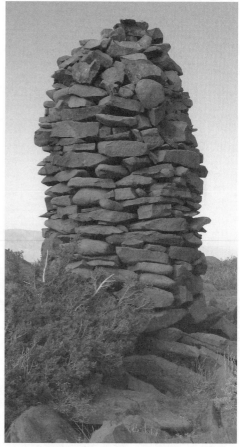

Heading right, now on the Long Valley Trail, make another wet ford of the creek (last water late in the season) and begin ascending a largely unshaded slope above the creek on long, gentle-to-moderate switchbacks through chaparral. When the switchbacks end, the dusty trail bears generally east and then northeast across the sunstruck hillside on a gentle, occasionally moderate, grade. As you approach the next junction, you'll see an unusual monument, an *arri mutillak*, on your left.

ARRI MUTILLAK

An *arri mutillak* is a large stone cairn—this one is said to be 7 feet high—built to pass the time by lonely Basque sheepherders who once tended flocks in this area. You can make your way through the chaparral to take a closer look, but don't alter the *arri mutillak*, which means "stone boy" in Basque.

Shortly beyond the *arri mutillak*, you reach the junction with the Corral Valley Trail, onto which you turned on Day 1. Here, 2.5 hot, dusty miles from your last crossing of Silver King Creek, you close the loop and turn left (north-northeast) to retrace your steps to the trailhead.

The *arri mutillak*

75 Ebbetts Pass

Trip Data: 11S 255501 4270384;
26.5 miles; 3/1 days

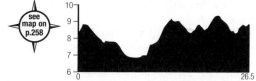

Topos: *Coleville, Lost Cannon Peak,*
Wolf Creek. Disaster Peak,
Dardanelles Cone, Ebbetts Pass

Highlights: Ridges and canyons east of the Sierra
Crest wait to be explored along this scenic route. Backpackers will encounter mammoth
junipers, soda and carbonate springs, diverse scenery, and good fishing. The last 11 miles
are along the famous, ridge-hugging PCT.

HEADS UP! *The mile-long southerly connector linking the Poison Flat Trail with the Soda Springs
Administrative Site that is shown on both the USGS* Wolf Creek *7.5' quadrangle and the USFS* Carson-
Iceberg Wilderness *maps no longer exists on the ground—and probably never did. Unfortunately,
the only existing route of the Poison Flat Trail, which intersects the East Fork Carson River Trail and
then proceeds south to Soda Springs, is nearly 0.75 mile longer.*

Shuttle Directions: The PCT crosses Hwy. 4 a mere 0.1 mile east of Ebbetts Pass, the highest point on the highway. The signed turnoff for the official PCT trailhead parking lot,
where this trip ends, is another 0.3 mile east down a short access road.

DAY 1 (Corral Valley Trailhead to Murray Canyon Trail Junction, 9.5 miles): *(Partial Recap:
Trip 74, Day 1.)* On the Corral Valley Trail, make a moderate climb southwest, avoiding a
trail on the right to the pack station and continuing ahead to enter Carson-Iceberg
Wilderness. Continue climbing to the high point and its excellent views. At the signed Y-
junction, 1.1 mile from the trailhead, take the right fork southwest.

(Recap in Reverse: Trip 74, Day 2, from the junction near the **arri mutillak** *to the junction
with the Silver King Trail.)* Descend past the *arri mutillak* and down the sunstruck slope
before switchbacking down to ford Silver King Creek (may be the last water before East
Fork Carson River). On the creek's west bank, you go ahead about 80 yards, through a gate
in a drift fence, to a junction with the Silver King Trail.

Now leave the Day 2 route of Trip 74 and turn right (north) to climb steeply through
another gate to a junction with the Poison Lake Trail (left, southwest).

*(Recap in Reverse: Trip 27, Day 2, from Wilver King/Poison Lake Trail junction to Soda
Springs.)* From here, go right (north) to stay on the Silver King Trail and pass through an
aspen grove before climbing steeply over a ridge and dropping to the eastern outskirts of
attractive Poison Flat and its multilobed meadow.

Past a third gate, the trail heads generally north, then generally west, skirting the
meadow's left (west or south) side. Reach a signed junction about one third of the way
along the meadow, where the Silver King and Poison Flat trails part company.

From the junction, proceed ahead (left, west) on the Poison Flat Trail, cutting across a
lobe of the meadow. From here to the end of the meadow, the tread will periodically fade
and then shortly reappear again. At a barely discernible rise, the trail angles across to the
right (north) side of the meadow.

At the meadow's end, the trail makes a stony westbound descent and passes the Soda
Cone (see page 113), which lies across a small gully from the trail. The open descent continues moderately down to a broad, granitic ridge.

Curving northwest, the trail makes a moderate descent on very long switchbacks
toward the canyon floor. Proceed to the crossing of a seasonal stream and wind southward
down the east wall of the canyon for a half mile to a junction with the East Fork Carson
River Trail at expansive Dumonts Meadows.

Turn left (south) at the junction and follow the East Fork Carson River Trail to cross the first of as many as a half dozen distributaries of Poison Creek. Continue upstream and meet the fenced-in compound around Soda Springs Administrative Site: Observe posted regulations here.

(Recap: Trip 25, Day 2, from Soda Springs to Murray Canyon Trail junction.) Leaving the shady administrative site, hike west on a jeep trail and after 0.3 mile cross a spring-fed stream. Just beyond is a well-used campsite 20 yards downslope. Immediately below this campsite is a trail coming from a large meander of the river (westward, this trail parallels the jeep trail before dying out in a grassy meadow). An easy, half-mile route along the jeep trail passes through sagebrush before dying out in the same meadow as the trail. The jeep tracks quickly reappear at the northwest end of the meadow and continue 200 yards northwest to a wide ford of East Fork Carson River. After fording the river, which may be difficult in early season, follow the trail northwest to an unsigned junction with a path that heads right (east). Here, you go ahead (southwest) to stay on the East Fork Carson River Trail as it curves southwest for the next 1.5 miles, tending to stay away from the river on a gentle ascent. The canyon bends south; beyond, the trail reaches Falls Meadow. On the northwest side of the meadow, about 50 yards beyond the ford of Murray Creek, is a signed junction with the Murray Canyon Trail. There are campsites nearby (6923'; 11S 265768 4264430). Both the creek and the river offer fair-to-good fishing.

DAY 2 (Murray Canyon Trail Junction to Asa Lake, 10 miles): *(Partial Recap: Trip 25, Day 2, from Murray Canyon Trail junction to the junction a few hundred yards northwest of the actual crest.)* At the signed junction for Murray Canyon Trail, face toward the forks and take the right fork generally westward, leaving the East Fork Carson River Trail, and climb, steeply at times, into Murray Canyon. From the top of the switchbacks, the trail leads to a ford of Murray Canyon Creek, and after 100 steep yards, a moderate grade resumes. Pass through the gate of a cattle fence 0.3 mile from the ford, and continue upward. Where the canyon splits, the trail forks; go right (generally west) and climb steeply west up the canyon. About a quarter mile up from the junction, ford a perennial creek and then ford another stream a quarter mile farther. Next, climb a few short switchbacks up a granitic slope and into a small gully. Beyond this gully, climb steadily north for a half mile to a crest saddle and a junction a few hundred yards northwest of the actual crest.

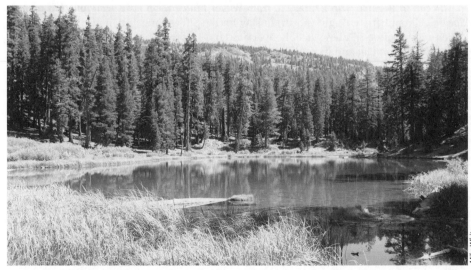

Asa Lake, Day 2's destination

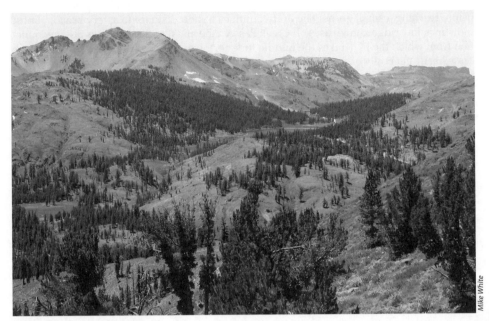

Mike White

View of Highland Lakes on Day 3

From the junction, you leave the Day 2 route for Trip 25 and take the left fork south-southwest, cross a pebbly flat, and then return to the crest. Follow the crest for a short distance, where, through the thinning forest, Highland Peak and other volcanic summits are visible in the northwest, along with the volcanic cliffs of Arnot Peak in the southwest. The trail soon leaves the crest to contour a half mile south across a brushy slope to a saddle just north of a low knoll. Cross the saddle, descend southeast, and then gradually curve southwest through lodgepole forest to a grassy meadow south of the knoll. The trail disappears at the south end of this meadow but reappears near the west end. From there, a vague route heads southwest across a large, open bowl, contours south just below the edge of the forest, and then climbs southeast toward a saddle on the southwest side of a very prominent summit of highly broken volcanic rock. Just before the saddle, reach a junction with the PCT.

From the junction, head right (north-northwest) on the PCT and descend the west side of the bowl. As the bowl gives way to steeper slopes, the trail circles west around a ridge, descends southwest, and momentarily enters and then leaves a small but deep side canyon before reaching the slightly cloudy east fork of Wolf Creek, flowing down a wide and rocky wash. A 0.3-mile traverse past caves and fingers of a cliff leads to the wide, silty, middle fork of Wolf Creek.

Leaving the stream, the trail curves west briefly, then climbs steadily northwest across several branches of the west fork of Wolf Creek. The PCT climbs north up a slope just beyond the main, east-flowing branch, switchbacks west, and climbs more steeply through thinning forest. Rather than traversing west to a forested saddle, the trail continues to climb northwest above the saddle's east end—a route designed to avoid cattle-grazing lands on the other side.

After reaching the west slopes of Peak 8982, the PCT heads diagonally northwest down those slopes and then follows a curving descent to a small, flat saddle that lies at the base of the summit's northwest ridge. From here, the trail doesn't continue north and cross the saddle but heads west down a small gully and then parallels a low ridge, remaining on the southwest side. A large cow meadow soon appears below, and the trail nearly meets it just before reaching a small gorge. The PCT continues a short distance to a very broad, almost indistinct, low ridge known as Wolf Creek Pass. In the midst of this "pass" is a signed junction from which the PCT takes the middle fork northward. (The right fork, the Wolf Creek Trail, heads generally east up Elder Creek, while the left fork goes west toward Highland Lakes.)

Staying on the PCT, climb roughly north along rocky slopes above the boggy pasture-lands of fenced Lower Gardner Meadow. Pass through a gate and immediately encounter a junction with the signed lateral to Asa Lake. Turn left (north) on this lateral and make a steep but short climb to the south shore of the tiny, tree-rimmed Asa Lake (8540'; 11S 258409 4265244), which is continually fed by clear water from the refreshing springs above the east shore. Red fir-shaded campsites lie on the northeast side. Brook trout await the angler.

DAY 3 (Asa Lake to Ebbetts Pass, 7 miles): From Asa Lake, retrace your steps to rejoin the PCT and head north, passing through mixed forest to ford Asa Lake's outlet. Climb moderately to steeply around a ridge, and then pass through a small nook shaded by red firs. Climb out of the nook through hemlocks and pines that give way to sagebrush along an open traverse northwest toward a saddle. Tryon Peak looms ahead, and, in the southwest, the popular Highland Lakes stand out clearly in their broad, glaciated canyon. Reaching the usually windy saddle (9300'), you observe clusters of whitebark pines, which, unlike most other conifers, are able to tolerate the harsh conditions. Still on the PCT, you cross a dilapidated crestline fence and follow a descending path that heads diagonally through tight clusters of whitebark pines and mountain hemlocks before breaking out into open terrain. Cross numerous willow-and-flower-lined meltwater streams on the way to a junction with the lightly used Bull Canyon Trail, which goes right (southeast).

At this junction, you go ahead (north) on the PCT, which skirts above the east edge of a lush, flower-filled meadow and descends gradually southwest. The tread falters a bit in a patch of meadow grass but soon reappears on the far side and reaches a bench above the south end of Noble Lake, where a copse of lodgepole pines shades a couple of fair campsites. Head past a pair of small ponds just above Noble Lake and continue high above the willow-covered shoreline to the north end of the lake.

Beyond the lake, the PCT makes a steep descent through a gully that carries the lake's willow-lined outlet stream. From the gully, the trail switchbacks down a bizarre landscape of eroded *aa*, which is able to support only a few hardy junipers. Hop across the outlet and then head west briefly to a ridge of glacial sediments. Follow this ridge a quarter mile north to a marked junction just east of the ridge's crest, where the Noble Canyon Trail leaves the PCT to go right (north) down the canyon. Staying on the PCT, you take the left fork briefly north before curving around the ridge's nose and descending the side of the ridge south toward the boulder-littered main arm of Noble Creek. From the creek, begin a northwest traverse in and out of scattered-to-light, mixed forest. After 0.3 mile, start climbing in earnest. After attaining the crest, the trail curves around a couple of these knobs before a winding traverse leads west along the base of some impressive, deeply eroded volcanic cliffs above a wildflower-covered, sloping meadow. To the northeast, across Noble Canyon, is 10,774-foot Silver Peak, site of a flurry of mining activity that began in 1863.

Beyond the meadow, head back into the trees and make a brief climb north to the top of another northeast-trending ridge. A short descent southwest leads to a junction where the PCT goes left and winds 0.3 mile west to a crossing of Hwy. 4, only 200 yards north of Ebbetts Pass, before continuing toward Kinney Lakes. To reach the Ebbetts Pass PCT parking area, veer right at the junction and travel north a quarter mile on a spur trail to the lot (8683'; 11S 255501 4270384 (field)).

76 Lake Alpine–Silver Valley

Trip Data:
11S 239528
4263335;
41.5 miles;
5/2 days

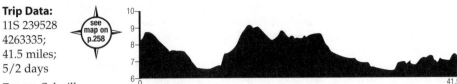

Topos: *Coleville,*
Lost Cannon Peak, Wolf Creek, Disaster Peak, Dardanelles Cone, Pacific Valley,
Spicer Meadows Reservoir

Highlights: This exciting route traverses major Sierra ridges along its westward course. As you progress west, the vegetation changes dramatically, with sagebrush and juniper giving way to dense forests of pine and fir. You hike sections of two famous trails along this route: first, a section of the 2600-mile PCT, and second, a section of the 186-mile TYT.

HEADS UP! *The mile-long connector linking the Poison Flat Trail with the Soda Spring Administrative Site that is shown on both the USGS Wolf Creek 7.5' quadrangle and the USFS Carson-Iceberg Wilderness maps no longer exists.*

Shuttle Directions: Lake Alpine is about 50 miles east of Angels Camp and 16.4 miles west from Ebbetts Pass on Hwy. 4. Near the east end of Lake Alpine, turn south on East Shore Road and go 0.3 mile more to the Silver Valley Campground entrance and the Silver Valley Trailhead. Along the East Shore Road, you will find a backpackers' campground near Hwy. 4, Pine Marten Campground to the west, and Silver Valley Campground just west of the trailhead. There is no parking lot; park along the shoulder as best you can.

DAY 1 (Corral Valley Trailhead to Murray Canyon Trail Junction, 9.5 miles): *(Partial Recap: Trip 74, Day 1.)* On the Corral Valley Trail, make a moderate climb southwest, avoiding a trail on the right to the pack station and continuing ahead to enter Carson-Iceberg Wilderness. Continue climbing to the high point and its excellent views. At the signed Y-junction, 1.1 mile from the trailhead, take the right fork southwest.

(Recap in Reverse: Trip 74, Day 2, from the junction near the **arri mutillak** *to the junction with the Silver King Trail.)* Descend past the *arri mutillak* and down the sunstruck slope before switchbacking down to ford Silver King Creek (may be the last water before East Fork Carson River). On the creek's west bank, you go ahead about 80 yards, through a gate in a drift fence, to a junction with the Silver King Trail.

Now leave the Day 2 route of Trip 74 and turn right (north) to climb steeply through another gate to a junction with the Poison Lake Trail (left, southwest). From here, go right (north) to stay on the Silver King Trail and pass through an aspen grove before climbing steeply over a ridge and dropping to the eastern outskirts of attractive Poison Flat and its multilobed meadow. Past a third gate, the trail heads generally north, then generally west, skirting the meadow's left (west or south) side. Reach a signed junction about one third of the way along the meadow, where the Silver King and Poison Flat trails part company.

From the junction, proceed ahead (left, west) on the Poison Flat Trail, cutting across a lobe of the meadow. From here to the end of the meadow, the tread will periodically fade and then shortly reappear again. At a barely discernible rise, the trail angles across to the right (north) side of the meadow.

At the meadow's end, the trail makes a stony westbound descent and passes the Soda Cone, which lies across a small gully from the trail. The open descent continues moderately down to a broad, granitic ridge.

Curving northwest, the trail makes a moderate descent on very long switchbacks toward the canyon floor. Proceed to the crossing of a seasonal stream and wind southward down the east wall of the canyon for a half mile to a junction with the East Fork Carson River Trail at expansive Dumonts Meadows.

Turn left (south) at the junction and follow the East Fork Carson River Trail to cross the first of as many as a half dozen distributaries of Poison Creek. Continue upstream and meet the fenced-in compound around Soda Springs Administrative Site: Observe posted regulations here.

(Recap: Trip 25, Day 2, from Soda Springs to Murray Canyon Trail junction.) Leaving the shady administrative site, hike west on a jeep trail and after 0.3 mile cross a spring-fed stream. Just beyond is a well-used campsite 20 yards downslope. Immediately below this campsite is a trail coming from a large meander of the river (westward, this trail parallels the jeep trail before dying out in a grassy meadow). An easy, half-mile route along the jeep trail passes through sagebrush before dying out in the same meadow as the trail. The jeep tracks quickly reappear at the northwest end of the meadow and continue 200 yards northwest to a wide ford of the East Fork Carson River. After fording the river, which may be difficult in early season, follow the trail northwest to an unsigned junction with a path that heads right (east). Here, you go ahead (southwest) to stay on the East Fork Carson River Trail as it curves southwest for the next 1.5 miles, tending to stay away from the river on a gentle ascent. The canyon bends south; beyond, the trail reaches Falls Meadow. On the northwest side of the meadow, about 50 yards beyond the ford of Murray Creek, is a signed junction with the Murray Canyon Trail. There are campsites nearby (6923'; 11S 265768 4264430). Both the creek and the river offer fair-to-good fishing.

DAY 2 (Murray Canyon Trail Junction to Asa Lake, 10 miles): *(Partial Recap: Trip 25, Day 2, from Murray Canyon Trail junction to the junction a few hundred yards northwest of the actual crest.)* At the signed junction for Murray Canyon Trail, face toward the forks and take the right fork generally westward, leaving the East Fork Carson River Trail, and climb, steeply at times, into Murray Canyon. From the top of the switchbacks, the trail leads to a ford of Murray Canyon Creek, and after 100 steep yards, a moderate grade resumes. Pass through the gate of a cattle fence 0.3 mile from the ford, and continue upward. Where the canyon splits, the trail forks; go right (generally west) and climb steeply west up the canyon. About a quarter mile up from the junction, ford a perennial creek and then ford another stream a quarter mile farther. Next, climb a few short switchbacks up a granitic slope and into a small gully. Beyond this gully, climb steadily north for a half mile to a crest saddle and a junction a few hundred yards northwest of the actual crest.

From the junction, you leave the Day 2 route for Trip 25 and take the left fork south-southwest, cross a pebbly flat, and then return to the crest. Follow the crest for a short distance, where, through the thinning forest, Highland Peak and other volcanic summits are visible in the northwest, along with the volcanic cliffs of Arnot Peak in the southwest. The trail soon leaves the crest to contour a half mile south across a brushy slope to a saddle just north of a low knoll. Cross the saddle, descend southeast, and then gradually curve southwest through lodgepole forest to a grassy meadow south of the knoll. The trail disappears at the south end of this meadow but reappears near the west end. From there, a vague route heads southwest across a large, open bowl, contours south just below the edge of the forest, and then climbs southeast toward a saddle on the southwest side of a very prominent summit of highly broken volcanic rock. Just before the saddle, reach a junction with the PCT.

From the junction, head right (north-northwest) on the PCT and descend the west side of the bowl. As the bowl gives way to steeper slopes, the trail circles west around a ridge, descends southwest, and momentarily enters and then leaves a small but deep side canyon before reaching the slightly cloudy east fork of Wolf Creek, flowing down a wide and rocky wash. A 0.3-mile traverse past caves and fingers of a cliff leads to the middle fork of Wolf Creek.

Leaving the stream, the trail curves west briefly, then climbs steadily northwest across several branches of the west fork of Wolf Creek. The PCT climbs north up a slope just beyond the main, east-flowing branch, switchbacks west, and climbs more steeply through thinning forest. Rather than traversing west to a forested saddle, the trail continues to climb northwest above the saddle's east end.

After reaching the west slopes of Peak 8982, the PCT heads diagonally northwest down those slopes and then follows a curving descent to a small, flat saddle that lies at the base of the summit's northwest ridge. From here, the trail doesn't continue north and cross the saddle but heads west down a small gully and then parallels a low ridge, remaining on the southwest side. A large cow meadow soon appears below, and the trail nearly meets it just before reaching a small gorge. The PCT continues a short distance to a very broad, almost indistinct, low ridge known as Wolf Creek Pass. In the midst of this "pass" is a signed junction from which the PCT takes the middle fork northward.

Staying on the PCT, climb roughly north along rocky slopes above the boggy pasturelands of fenced Lower Gardner Meadow. Pass through a gate and immediately encounter a junction with the signed lateral to Asa Lake. Turn left (north) on this lateral to Asa Lake (8540'; 11S 258409 4265244). Brook trout await the angler.

DAY 3 (Asa Lake to Hiram Meadow, 9 miles): From Asa Lake, retrace your steps to the PCT and continue retracing them on the PCT to the junction at Wolf Creek Pass. At the junction, leave the PCT by turning right (west) onto a track that follows a stream through spacious Lower Gardner Meadow. Beyond the meadow, proceed on an undulating traverse southwest across forested terrain to cross a creek in a small, flower- and grass-filled meadow. After a short climb to the top of a hill, you reach a signed junction with a trail left (south) to Arnot and Disaster creeks and the Carson-Iceberg Wilderness boundary.

At this junction, turn right (briefly north) and pass through open to lightly forested terrain with a fine midsummer display of wildflowers, including lupine, daisy, buttercup, columbine, aster, monkeyflower, corn lily, rock fringe, yarrow, mountain bluebells, pennyroyal, and cow parsnip. A short climb out of this canyon leads to a willow-and-flower-lined crossing of North Fork Mokelumne River, which drains Lower Highland Lake—a wet ford in early season. You see a parking lot on the creek's west bank here; head for it to walk on a road that curves westward for 100 yards to the Highland Lakes Road.

Turn left (southwest) onto wide, level Highland Lakes Road and follow it as it contours around the west shore of Lower Highland Lake, which is popular with anglers in search of the resident brook trout. Beyond the lake, the road climbs gradually to Highland Lakes Campground, just north of the upper lake. The campground is divided into two camps; backpackers will usually find quieter sites in the camp at the end of a short, eastbound spur road.

At the southwest end of Lower Highland Lake, you pick up a trail along the lake's outlet, which is Highland Creek. The trail descends steeply southwest before gently curving west-southwest, roughly paralleling the westbound creek's north bank for about a mile.

Ford the creek to its south side near a small knoll on its south bank. Beyond here, the trail leaves the creek to angle southwest, and you presently ford Highland Creek again, this time to its west bank, as the creek has turned southwest. The trail stays on the creek's west side for nearly 2 miles, crossing an intermittent tributary before angling south and fording Highland Creek for the third time.

Now on Highland Creek's east bank, the trail continues south to a point where it may seem to fork; if so, you can take either fork, as they rejoin after fording the creek draining Champion Canyon. At first you stay close to Champion Canyon's creek as it swings west, but where that creek joins Highland Creek, your trail bears southwest and then south to ford Highland Creek a fourth time and reach a junction with the trail right (north) up Weiser Creek. You take the left fork west-southwest to Hiram Meadow, where you may find campsites (7121'; 11S 250042 4258939).

Day 4 (Hiram Meadow to Rock Lake, 8.5 miles): The trip continues through wide, flat Hiram Meadow before re-entering lodgepole forest. Beyond cabin ruins, the trail turns southwest to meet Highland Creek again and then crosses some low knolls. One mile southwest of Hiram Meadow, the trail briefly climbs away from the creek where it turns south to cascade down a sizeable gorge. Descending steeply, the trail meets the creek again near the junction with a trail heading left (south-southeast) across the creek and up Jenkins Canyon (the route of the TYT).

(Recap in Reverse: Trip 22, Day 2.) Go right (southwest and then west) on the TYT along Highland Creek and below Point 7635. This section of trail isn't correctly shown on the topo, which doesn't show greatly expanded Spicer Meadow Reservoir and its drowning of Gabbot Meadow, either. (The *Carson-Iceberg Wilderness* map is much more accurate here.)

Now the trail begins to curve around the northeast end of largely unseen Spicer Meadow Reservoir. Soon after the trail leaves Highland Creek (in late season, may be the last chance for water before Rock Lake), you reach a junction with a trail left (southwest) to Sword Lake. Take the right-hand trail (northwest and then southwest) over an unnamed creek to continue traversing above the reservoir.

More junctions and creek crossings await you on this traverse, including the nearly immediate crossing of Bull Run Creek. The next junction, perhaps hard to spot, is with an unmaintained track bearing right (north-northwest) and steeply upward toward Bull Run Peak. Veer left (west-southwest) above the reservoir and shortly step over a trail that runs left (south) to the reservoir and right (north and also steeply up) to meet Bull Run Creek. Your trail continues southwest, high above the reservoir and over two intermittent creeks about a mile apart.

At last the trail angles west-southwest, climbing away from the reservoir and over a pair of small gaps (the tread may be a little hard to follow here) to curve southwest and then northwest around Point 7502.

Descending, the trail crosses two forks (dry by late season) of Wilderness Creek and presently descends to ford the creek's main fork (difficult in early season but may be dry by late season). Shortly beyond the ford is a junction with a trail left (west) to Summit Lake. Go right (northeast and then north) toward the east end of pretty Rock Lake (7315', 11S 242683 4260034; good fishing for brook trout).

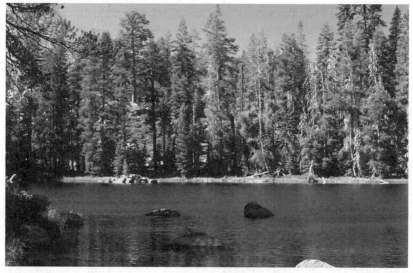

Rock Lake

DAY 5 (Rock Lake to Lake Alpine–Silver Valley, 4.5 miles): Return to the east end of Rock Lake and pick up the main trail you came in on. Bear left (north-northwest) and, just out of sight of the lake, turn northeast and follow a granitic ridge. Then, from the slightly higher main ridge, curve north, cross a small dry wash, and descend to a flat a quarter mile east of North Fork Stanislaus River. A short climb north, followed by a steep descent, leads to a ford of the river, which is difficult in early season.

Beyond the ford, climb steeply northwest to cross a ridge and then wind a half mile down glacier-polished slabs to a large, forested flat with a trail junction not shown on the 7.5' topo. The left fork, the old trail on the topo, goes west to a huge meadow and to Duck Lake. You turn right (northwest) on the newer trail (not on the topo), immediately cross a creek, and wind west along the north edge of this forested flat. When the trail reaches a point about 200 yards north of Duck Lake, the path abruptly turns north and climbs up a ridge. After 300 yards, the trail turns abruptly west and then climbs more moderately 0.3 mile west up to a switchback in the now closed jeep road that ascends northward from the Duck Lake basin.

On this closed road, climb west briefly up to a saddle, pass through a gate, follow the crest southwest, and then descend a half mile to the trailhead, signed SILVER VALLEY TRAIL-HEAD, at the east end of Lake Alpine's Silver Valley Campground (7386'; 11S 239528 4263335 (field)).

HWY 395

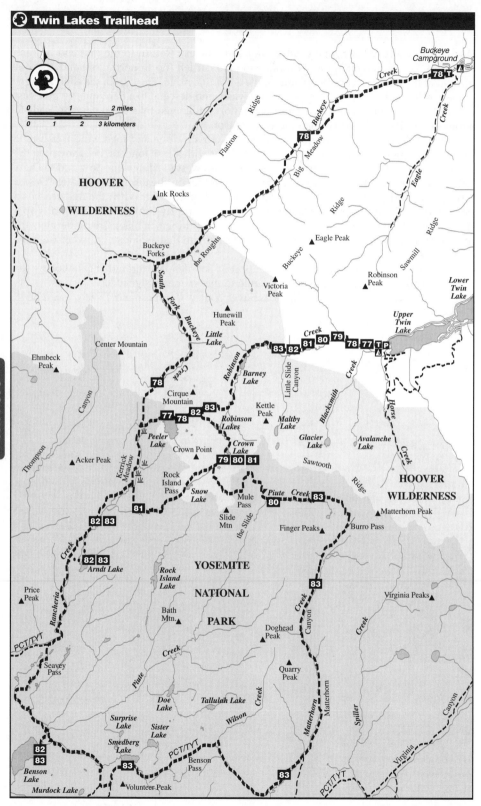

Twin Lakes Trailhead

7098'; 11S 291659 4224870

DESTINATION/ UTM COORDINATES	TRIP TYPE	BEST SEASON	PACE (HIKING/ LAYOVER DAYS)	TOTAL MILEAGE
77 Peeler Lake 11S 283674 4222462	Out & back	Mid or late	2/1 Moderate	16
78 Buckeye Forks 11S 283366 4227850	Shuttle	Mid or late	3/1 Moderate	22.4
79 Crown Lake 11S 285715 4221307	Out & back	Mid or late	2/1 Moderate	16
80 Upper Piute Creek 11S 288102 4219393	Out & back	Mid or late	4/1 Moderate	23
81 Peeler Lake via Kerrick Meadow 11S 283674 4222462	Semiloop	Mid or late	3/1 Moderate	22
82 Benson Lake 11S 278374 4211043	Out & back	Mid or late	6/1 Moderate, part cross-country	37.2
83 Smedberg Lake 11S 281748 4210078	Semiloop	Mid or late	8/3 Leisurely, part cross-country	49.6

Information and Permits: This trailhead is in Humboldt-Toiyabe National Forest's Bridgeport Ranger District. Wilderness permits are required for overnight stays, and a trail quota is in place from late June through mid-September. Contact: Bridgeport Ranger District, HCR 1 Box 1000, Bridgeport, CA; 760-932-7070; www.fs.fed.us.r4/htnf. Bear canisters are not required but are highly recommended.

Driving Directions: From the north end of the town of Bridgeport on Hwy. 395, find a junction with the Twin Lakes Road. Turn west onto Twin Lakes Road, toward the Sierra, and drive 13.5 miles past the Twin Lakes to the road's end at Mono Village Resort (lodging, campground, store, café, marina). There's limited public parking near the resort's marina, so continue into the resort to the kiosk at the entrance to the campground and ask the person on duty there to direct you to the currently designated parking lot.

The official trail begins west of the campground, so ask for directions to the Barney Lake Trail, which you will find by heading westward along a confusing snarl of little dirt roads through the forested campground on a poorly signed route for BARNEY LAKE. In a little less than a quarter mile, you walk around a road closure at the campground's west end. The Barney Lake Trail begins here. (If you get to a trail signed for HORSETAIL FALLS, backtrack; that's *not* your trail.)

77 Peeler Lake

Trip Data: 11S 283674 4222462; 16 miles; 2/1 days

Topos: *Buckeye Ridge, Matterhorn Peak*

Highlights: Beautiful Peeler Lake is a delightful and unique Sierra destination: You camp literally on the Sierra Crest, for this lake pours its waters down both sides of the Sierra. It's an excellent destination for a long weekend.

see map on p.270

HEADS UP! Get an early start: This trip requires a stiff, 2500-foot climb to its destination. Campfires are prohibited at Barney and Peeler lakes. If you camp farther west than Peeler's west shore, you'll be in Yosemite, where bear canisters are required and pets and firearms are prohibited.

DAY 1 (Twin Lakes Trailhead to Peeler Lake, 8 miles): Beyond the campground, the sandy trail winds through a moderate-to-dense forest of Jeffrey pine, juniper, lodgepole pine, aspen, and cottonwood along Robinson Creek. Crossing several small tributaries, the trail then ascends gently and within 0.75 mile encounters the first fir trees. But the forest cover soon gives way to a sagebrush-covered, gently sloping bench from which you can see the great headwall of the valley in the west.

As you make your way up this open bench through thigh-high sagebrush, rabbit brush, chamise, and mule ears, you have unobstructed views of Victoria, Hunewill, and Robinson peaks on the right (north), and some ragged teeth of Sawtooth Ridge on the left. Ignore use trails left (south) to unseen Robinson Creek.

> **NATURAL HISTORY AND VIEWS**
>
> About halfway up this bench, the trail passes a "ghost forest" of drowned trees caused by beaver dams downstream. Beavers still share this fine Sierra stream. On the right (north), look for marmots dozing among the piles of scree that flow from the feet of the avalanche chute scarring Victoria Peak; on the left (south), the dramatic, unbroken granite wall of Blacksmith Peak at the top of Little Slide Canyon dominates the view.

About 2 miles from the start, you enter Hoover Wilderness. About a half mile into the wilderness, the trail rises more steeply on switchbacks, fording several small tributaries that support monkeyflower, monkshood, red columbine, swamp onion, shooting star, and bracken fern. Drier stretches of trail feature colorful patches of Indian paintbrush, mariposa lily, scarlet gilia, yarrow, whorled penstemon, pussypaws, streptanthus, and goldenrod. After the ascent levels out, the trail veers south, fords another tributary, and arrives at the outlet of overused Barney Lake (8258'), where camping is poor because most former campsites are now closed. Fishing is fair to good for eastern brook and rainbow. Given the serious climb ahead, don't linger here.

The rocky trail initially skirts Barney's west shore before switchbacking up to a long traverse above the lake and then above the extensive meadow on its inlet. Well up the meadow stretch, the trail zigs upward, crosses some springs, and then zags down to the meadow's head. Just before a ford of Robinson Creek, a use trail veers right to a fair campsite in the aspens—probably the last legal campsite with reliable water before Peeler Lake

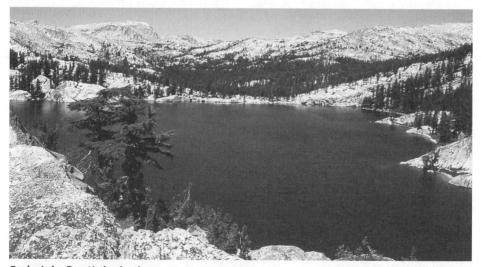

Peeler Lake, Day 1's destination

or Crown Lake. Lavender swamp onion, red columbine, orange tiger lily, and yellow mon-keyflower brighten the willow-lined stream. The trail now climbs more steeply along Robinson Creek through a moderate forest cover that shows the increasing elevation by including hemlock and some western white pine. About a quarter mile upstream, the trail fords Robinson Creek again and then fords the outlet creek from Peeler Lake just above its confluence with Robinson Creek. This is your last chance to easily refill your water bottles by late season or in a dry year.

Now the trail rises by a long series of gradual-to-moderate switchbacks, pausing briefly on a campsite-less bench. Rising again, it reaches another bench with a junction: left (initially southwest) to Crown Lake; right (northwest) to Peeler Lake.

Go right and climb moderately for about a half mile to a small bench at 9300 feet where the trail crosses Peeler Lake's east outlet twice. Next, the trail ascends very steeply up the draw just northeast of the lake to a point well above the outlet. From here, a faint cross-country route climbs south through a gap and then drops very steeply on loose terrain to good campsites on the lake's east shore. Continuing on the trail, you descend abruptly to cross the outlet and then make an up-and-down traverse of Peeler's rocky north shore, passing a few poor-to-fair campsites (about midway along north shore; 9549'; 11S 283674 4222462). Many former sites are closed due to overuse. Look farther afield for good sites. Just beyond the lake's west shore is the signed Yosemite-Hoover Wilderness boundary. Fishing for eastern brook and rainbow trout is sometimes good.

DAY 2 (Peeler Lake to Twin Lakes Trailhead, 8 miles): Retrace your steps.

78 Buckeye Forks

Trip Data: 11S 283366 4227850;
22.4 miles; 3/1 days

Topos: *Buckeye Ridge, Matterhorn Peak*

Highlights: This trip around Buckeye Ridge visits a surprising range of Sierran environments, from the sagebrush-scrub of the east side, to subalpine Kerrick Meadow, past water-loving clumps of quaking aspen, and through windblown, gnarled whitebark pine. Its variety makes it an everything trip for everyone.

HEADS UP! Get an early start: This trip requires a stiff, 2500-foot climb to Day 1's destination. Campfires are prohibited at Barney and Peeler lakes. When you enter Yosemite, bear canisters are required and pets and firearms are prohibited.

Shuttle Directions: To access the take-out site at Buckeye Campground from Hwy. 395 in Bridgeport, turn toward the Sierra on Twin Lakes Road near the town's north end. Follow that road for 7 miles (avoiding a turnoff left to Hunewill Guest Ranch) to a junction signed BUCKEYE CAMPGROUND. Turn right (north) on the dirt road here and pass Doc and Al's Resort as you go 4 more miles to a T-junction with the dirt road just beyond Buckeye Creek. Turn left (west) here and go 1.1 miles, passing through a USFS campground, to the end of the road. Alternatively, you could drive 3.8 miles north of Bridgeport on Hwy. 395 and then turn left (west) on signed, dirt Buckeye Road. Drive 6 miles, avoiding a dirt road on the right as you negotiate a hairpin turn, through the campground to the road's end.

DAY 1 (Twin Lakes Trailhead to Peeler Lake, 8 miles): *(Recap: Trip 77, Day 1.)* Beyond the campground, head generally west across the bench through which Robinson Creek flows, usually out of sight. Climb switchbacks and curve southwest to Barney Lake, then traverse above that lake and the long meadow on its inlet. Ford Robinson Creek and begin climbing along it to another ford and then to a ford of Peeler Lake's outlet (last easy-to-get water by late season or in a dry year). Continue climbing switchbacks, eventually veering away from Robinson Creek, to a bench with a junction: left (initially southwest) to Crown Lake; right (northwest) to Peeler Lake. Go right to Peeler Lake, ford its eastern outlet twice on a small bench, and ascend very steeply up a draw northeast of the lake to a point well above the lake. Descend abruptly to cross the outlet and traverse Peeler's rocky north shore (about midway along north shore; 9549'; 11S 283674 4222462), where most former campsites are closed due to overuse (seek sites farther afield). Just beyond the lake's west shore is the signed Yosemite-Hoover Wilderness boundary. Fishing for eastern brook and rainbow trout is sometimes good.

DAY 2 (Peeler Lake to Buckeye Forks, 5 miles): Regain the trail and head west as the trail descends along the lake's west outlet, crossing and recrossing it and entering Yosemite National Park. You soon meet the Kerrick Canyon Trail in Upper Kerrick Meadow. At this junction, turn right (north) on the Kerrick Canyon Trail and climb to Buckeye Pass (9572') on sand-and-duff trail through a moderate forest cover of mostly pines to Buckeye Pass on the park boundary. Leaving the park, the duff trail drops northeast down the pass's north side and soon fords infant South Fork Buckeye Creek. From here to the next ford, this descent skirts a series of charmingly meadowed and richly flowered steps on the northwest side of the creek.

A LITTLE ORNITHOLOGY

Owls hunt these meadows at night. Keep a lookout for large groups of agitated birds. At the core of such gatherings, frequently, is a large owl seeking protection in dense foliage.

The series of meadows ends at a ford; cross, and about a quarter mile beyond the ford, find a junction with an unmaintained trail over the ridge to Barney Lake. Stay on your main trail northeastward and, for the next half mile, descend moderately through an area full of avalanche-smashed trees. You presently jump across an unnamed tributary from Hunewill Peak and, in another half mile, reach the first of several fair and good campsites at places where the trail touches the stream. A steep descent and then a couple of less steep descents bring you to a flat and the nearby confluence Buckeye Creek's north and south forks. Ford the south fork here and 200 yards farther on, ford the north fork. There are good campsites (8423'; 11S 283366 4227850) near a snow-survey cabin here, and a junction with trail from the West Walker River watershed is just beyond (see Trip 45). Fishing for rainbow and brook is good.

DAY 3 (Buckeye Forks to Buckeye Roadend, 9.4 miles): *(Recap: Trip 45, Day 5.)* From the cabin, the trail continues to descend steadily. The canyon narrows and the trail curves northeast as it enters the Roughs (some good campsites). You presently climb steeply to a juniper-topped saddle on the Hoover Wilderness boundary. A few hundred steep yards down from the saddle, you ford a vigorous creek and then make a long, rocky traverse. Beyond the traverse, the rest of the walk is over long, gradual slopes. Eventually, you reach Big Meadow, a 2-mile-long grassland. You pass through a gate in a fence at the bottom of the meadow and immediately head right, downhill, to ford Buckeye Creek (difficult in early season). From the creek, the trail leads up a small ridge and then undulates over several more ridges, traverses a hillside, crosses two little rills, and skirts another large meadow. About a half mile farther, you cross an unmapped stream. Soon the trail becomes an abandoned, two-track road, and you stroll through alternating green meadows and gray sagebrush fields. Past one last meadow, you come to a fence, pass through, and go one more mile to the roadend parking lot at Buckeye Campground's west end (7230'; 11S 294180 4234456).

79 Crown Lake

Trip Data: 11S 285715 4221307; 16 miles; 2/1 days

Topos: *Buckeye Ridge, Matterhorn Peak*

Highlights: This route follows Robinson Creek all the way to Crown Lake. Along the way, you see some of the finest east-side scenery available anywhere along

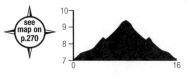

the Sierra. Lovely Crown Lake itself is set near the Sierra Crest and "crowned" with rugged peaks and green forests. This is another excellent choice for a long weekend trip.

HEADS UP! *Get an early start: This trip requires a stiff, climb to Day 1's destination. Campfires are prohibited at Barney Lake.*

DAY 1 (Twin Lakes Trailhead to Crown Lake, 8 miles): *(Partial Recap: Trip 77, Day 1, to the Peeler Lake-Crown Lake junction.)* Beyond the campground, head generally west across the bench through which Robinson Creek flows, usually out of sight. Climb switchbacks and curve southwest to Barney Lake, then traverse above that lake and the long meadow on its inlet. Ford Robinson Creek and begin climbing along it to another ford and then to a ford of Peeler Lake's outlet (last easy-to-get water by late season or in a dry year). Continue climbing switchbacks, eventually veering away from Robinson Creek, to a bench with a junction: left (initially southwest) to Crown Lake; right (northwest) to Peeler Lake.

Leaving the Day 1 route of Trip 77, turn left toward Crown Lake and head generally southeast, undulating gently between large outcroppings of glacially polished granite. As the trail ascends moderately below Robinson Lakes, it winds through one near-pure stand of hemlock—unusual for this part of the Sierra. Just before you reach Robinson Lakes, you wind through huge boulders and pass an inviting, natural, deep pool that is colored bright aqua. Alas, from this pool past the Robinson Lakes, any "campsite" you can see from the trail is almost certainly illegal, and you must scramble up into the surrounding rocks to find legal sites. Continuing, you find Robinson Lakes, two small, shallow, placid lakes with a sparse forest cover of lodgepole pine, western white pine, and hemlock, separated by an isthmus. The larger Robinson Lake is rockbound.

The trail crosses the isthmus between the Robinson Lakes, rounds the south side of the larger Robinson Lake, fords Robinson Creek, and turns south on a steady ascent. Just below Crown Lake, you ford the creek again, pass a use trail right (north) to an excellent campsite, and then switchback up to the good campsites just downstream from the lake along the outlet (9482'; 11S 285715 4221307), where there are excellent views of Kettle Peak and Crown Point. Fishing for rainbow and some eastern brook is fair. A use trail that crosses the outlet leads to another campsite.

DAY 2 (Crown Lake to Twin Lakes Trailhead, 8 miles): Retrace your steps.

80 Upper Piute Creek

Trip Data: 11S 288102 4219393; 23 miles; 4/1 days

Topos: *Buckeye Ridge, Matterhorn Peak*

Highlights: Following Robinson Creek nearly to the crest of the Sierra, this route circles the west end of the Sawtooth Ridge and then

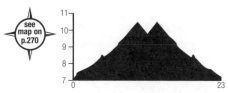

drops down into the scenic upper reaches of Piute Creek. Those who appreciate spectacular alpine scenery should consider this trip a must.

see map on p.270

HWY 395

HEADS UP! Get an early start: This trip requires a stiff, climb to Day 1's destination. Campfires are prohibited at Barney Lake. When you enter Yosemite, bear canisters are required and pets and firearms are prohibited.

DAY 1 (Twin Lakes Trailhead to Crown Lake, 8 miles): *(Partial Recap: Trip 77, Day 1, to the Peeler Lake-Crown Lake junction.)* Beyond the campground, head generally west across the bench through which Robinson Creek flows, usually out of sight. Climb switchbacks and curve southwest to Barney Lake, then traverse above that lake and the long meadow on its inlet. Ford Robinson Creek and begin climbing along it to another ford and then to a ford of Peeler Lake's outlet (last easy-to-get water by late season or in a dry year). Continue climbing switchbacks, eventually veering away from Robinson Creek, to a bench with a junction: left (initially southwest) to Crown Lake, right (northwest) to Peeler Lake.

(Recap: Trip 79, Day 1, from the Peeler-Crown junction to Crown Lake.) Leaving the Day 1 route of Trip 77, turn left toward Crown Lake and head generally southeast, undulating gently between large outcroppings of glacially polished granite. Just before you reach Robinson Lakes, you wind through huge boulders and pass an inviting, aqua-tinted pool. From here past the Robinson Lakes, any "campsite" you can see from the trail is almost certainly illegal, and you must scramble up into the surrounding rocks to find legal sites. Continuing, you find Robinson Lakes, two small, shallow, placid lakes separated by an isthmus. The larger Robinson Lake is rockbound.

Cross the isthmus, round the south side of the larger Robinson Lake, ford Robinson Creek, and turn south on a steady ascent. Just below Crown Lake, ford the creek again, pass a use trail right (north) to an excellent campsite, and then switchback up to the good campsites along the lake's outlet (9482'; 11S 285715 4221307). Fishing for rainbow and some eastern brook is fair.

DAY 2 (Crown Lake to Upper Piute Creek, 3.5 miles): From Crown Lake's outlet, the trail ascends along the west side, offering fine views of the meadowed inlet. The ascent soon steepens as the trail begins a series of short, rocky switchbacks that end just east of Crown Point. Here, the trail levels out in a willowed, meadowy area with several small lakelets, and it meets a junction just beyond: right (southwest) to Snow Lake and Rock Island Pass; left (south-southeast) to Mule Pass and Upper Piute Creek. The route turns left, fords the stream draining Snow Lake, and climbs over an easy talus-and-scree pile. This rocky ascent levels briefly within sight of another small lakelet, then the trail cuts across a bench and climbs steeply by rocky switchbacks. In most years, there is a large snowbank across this slope well into summer—be cautious here. After one more bench, this climb terminates at a tundra-topped saddle, Mule Pass, on the divide north of Slide Mountain and the Hoover Wilderness-Yosemite National Park boundary.

From this pass, the trail enters the park and switchbacks down through a series of sandy tundra pockets, winding its way north and then east before beginning the long traverse down to Upper Piute Creek. This traverse strikes timberline just below the cross-country turnoff to Ice and Maltby lakes, which is at the ford of the stream draining the swale that gives access to Ice Lake. (The excellent fishing for eastern brook in these two lakes is worth the side trip.)

HISTORICAL NOTE

The lodgepoles and hemlocks that line the trail are marked with the historic T-blaze typical of the older trails in Yosemite National Park. These signs were emblazoned on these trails by the US Cavalry in the early part of the 20th Century when it was their responsibility to patrol the Park.

This hiking day ends at the campsites upstream from the turnoff to the cross-country route down Slide Canyon, located on Upper Piute Creek along the first half mile after the trail comes within sight of the creek (at about half mile: 9618'; 11S 288102 4219393). Fishing for eastern brook is fair.

DAYS 3–4 (Upper Piute Creek to Twin Lakes Trailhead, 11.5 miles): Retrace your steps.

81 Peeler Lake via Kerrick Meadow

Trip Data: 11S 283674 4222462; 22 miles; 3/1 days

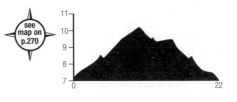

Topos: *Buckeye Ridge, Matterhorn Peak*

Highlights: Embracing both Crown and Peeler lakes, this semiloop takes in the fine scenery on those trips and adds the idyllic beauty of subalpine Kerrick Meadow.

HEADS UP! *Get an early start: This trip requires a stiff, climb to Day 1's destination. Campfires are prohibited at Barney Lake. When you enter Yosemite, bear canisters are required and pets and firearms are prohibited.*

DAY 1 (Twin Lakes Trailhead to Crown Lake, 8 miles): *(Partial Recap: Trip 77, Day 1, to the Peeler Lake-Crown Lake junction.)* Beyond the campground, head generally west across the bench through which Robinson Creek flows, usually out of sight. Climb switchbacks and curve southwest to Barney Lake, then traverse above that lake and the long meadow on its inlet. Ford Robinson Creek and begin climbing along it to another ford and then to a ford of Peeler Lake's outlet (last easy-to-get water by late season or in a dry year). Continue climbing switchbacks, eventually veering away from Robinson Creek, to a bench with a junction: left (initially southwest) to Crown Lake; right (northwest) to Peeler Lake.

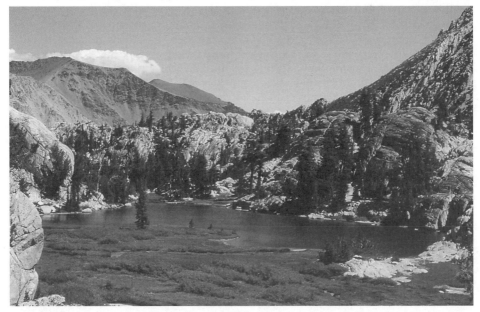

Crown Lake

(Recap: Trip 79, Day 1, from the Peeler-Crown junction to Crown Lake.) Leaving the Day 1 route of Trip 77, turn left toward Crown Lake and head generally southeast, undulating gently between large outcroppings of glacially polished granite. Just before you reach Robinson Lakes, you wind through huge boulders and pass an inviting, aqua-tinted pool. From here past the Robinson Lakes, any "campsite" you can see from the trail is almost certainly illegal, and you must scramble up into the surrounding rocks to find legal sites. Continuing, you find Robinson Lakes, two small, shallow, placid lakes separated by an isthmus. The larger Robinson Lake is rockbound.

Cross the isthmus, round the south side of the larger Robinson Lake, ford Robinson Creek, and turn south on a steady ascent. Just below Crown Lake, ford the creek again, pass a use trail right (north) to an excellent campsite, and then switchback up to the good campsites along the lake's outlet (9482'; 11S 285715 4221307). Fishing for rainbow and some eastern brook is fair.

DAY 2 (Crown Lake to Peeler Lake, 6 miles): *(Partial Recap: Trip 80, Day 2, from Crown Lake to the Rock Island Pass-Mule Pass junction.)* From Crown Lake's outlet, the trail ascends along the lake's west side and steepens as it begins switchbacks that end just east of Crown Point. Here, the trail levels out in a meadowy area and meets a junction just beyond: right (southwest) to Snow Lake and Rock Island Pass; left (south-southeast) to Mule Pass and Upper Piute Creek.

Leave the Day 2 route for Trip 80 and go right here. Begin a long, steadily traversing climb toward Snow Lake. This traverse gives way to switchbacks midway up the hill and jogs southwest under Crown Point before resuming its southward course steeply on more switchbacks by a little stream. Looking back from the top of this climb, you have fine views to the east of the soldier-tipped summit of Kettle Peak and the west end of the Sawtooth Ridge (called Blacksmith Peak). Snow Lake itself, like Peeler Lake to the north, is perched atop a divide, but anglers know it best for its golden trout. As the trail traverses high above the rocky north edge of the lake, you see the meadowy lake fringes, which are most extensive at the southwest end. Here, the meadows extend from the lake's edge to the indistinct saddle called Rock Island Pass (10,240'). There are campsites in the rocks above the head of this lake and the meadows, though it may be a long walk back to water. Snow Lake may be the last water before Rancheria Creek in a dry year.

At Rock Island Pass, you step out of Hoover Wilderness and into Yosemite National Park. The poor, stony, faint trail descends into the Rancheria Creek drainage through sparse whitebark pine at the top to a mixed forest of lodgepole, hemlock, and western white pine. After traversing above a sandy meadow, the T-blazed trail rises sharply over a sandy ridge and then drops moderately on switchbacks through dense forest to idyllic Kerrick Meadow, passing a campsite on the left just before the meadow. Partway across the meadow is a ford of Rancheria Creek. The trail fades out almost completely on the other side of the ford, but just bear straight across the meadow to intersect the Kerrick Canyon Trail.

At the junction with the Kerrick Canyon Trail, turn right (northeast) and stroll gradually up Kerrick Meadow. Rancheria Creek meanders through these sandy grasslands, leaving behind the large accumulations of sand you see when it changes channels. The meadow bottlenecks briefly where the creek tumbles over a silver cascade and then opens into a beautiful, open, wetter section near the headwaters. In the middle of this marshy section, the trail fords one arm of the creek and then continues to meet the signed Peeler Lake Trail at the meadow's head, where the route turns right (east; left would take you to Buckeye Pass).

From this junction, the trail crosses the open meadow and winds through a broken, moderate forest cover of lodgepole. This route crisscrosses Peeler Lake's west outlet and arrives at the lake's west shore. Continuing, you step out of Yosemite and back into Hoover

Wilderness as the trail begins a traverse of the lake's north shore. Look for campsites at Peeler (about midway along the north shore; 9549'; 11S 283674 4222462).

DAY 3 (Peeler Lake to Twin Lakes Trailhead, 8 miles): *(Recap in Reverse: Trip 72, Day 1.)* Skirt Peeler's north shore, ford its east outlet, and climb steeply but briefly to a point well above the lake (from which a faint cross-country route leads to good campsites on the east shore). Now make a very steep descent of a draw northeast of the lake to a bench where you ford the east outlet twice. Beyond, you soon find the junction with the trails to Crown Lake (right, southeast) and back to Twin Lakes (left, northeast). The loop closes here. Turn left and continue your descent to Twin Lakes, reversing the first half of Day 1 of this trip.

82 Benson Lake

Trip Data: 11S 278374 4211043; 37.2 miles; 6/1 days

see map on p.270

Topos: *Buckeye Ridge, Matterhorn Peak, Piute Mountain*

Highlights: This long trip leads to the heart of northern Yosemite, reaching Benson Lake with its "Benson Riviera"—a long, wide, sandy beach at the lake's northeast end. Because the lake is just off the main trail and is relatively warm, it's quite popular; you'll have company here.

HEADS UP! *Get an early start: This trip requires a stiff, 2500-foot climb to Day 1's destination. Campfires are prohibited at Barney and Peeler lakes. When you enter Yosemite, bear canisters are required and pets and firearms are prohibited. The brief cross-country leg to Arndt Lake is very easy.*

DAY 1 (Twin Lakes Trailhead to Peeler Lake, 8 miles): *(Recap: Trip 77, Day 1.)* Beyond the campground, head generally west across the bench through which Robinson Creek flows, usually out of sight. Climb switchbacks and curve southwest to Barney Lake, then traverse above that lake and the long meadow on its inlet. Ford Robinson Creek and begin climbing along it to another ford and then to a ford of Peeler Lake's outlet (last easy-to-get water by late season or in a dry year). Continue climbing switchbacks, eventually veering away from Robinson Creek, to a bench with a junction: left (initially southwest) to Crown Lake; right (northwest) to Peeler Lake. Go right to Peeler Lake, ford its eastern outlet twice on a small bench, and ascend very steeply up a draw northeast of the lake to a point well above the lake. Descend abruptly to cross the outlet and traverse Peeler's rocky north shore (about midway along north shore; 9549'; 11S 283674 4222462), where most former campsites are closed due to overuse (seek sites farther afield). Just beyond the lake's west shore is the signed Yosemite-Hoover Wilderness boundary. Fishing for eastern brook and rainbow trout is sometimes good.

DAY 2 (Peeler Lake to Arndt Lake, 5 miles, part cross-country): *(Recap in Reverse: Trip 81, Day 2, from Peeler Lake to the junction with the Kerrick Canyon Trail-Rock Island Pass junction.)* Regain the trail and, assuming you camped somewhere along Peeler's north shore, head west, cross into Yosemite while crisscrossing the lake's west outlet, enter Kerrick Meadow's north end, and meet a junction with the Kerrick Canyon Trail. Turn left (south) and stroll gradually down Kerrick Canyon with Rancheria Creek on the east (your left). In 1.3 miles, at a junction with the trail across the meadow toward Rock Island Pass and Crown Lake, continue ahead (now southwest).

Leaving the Day 2 route of Trip 81, continue your easy descent out of the meadow and into forest. This brief stretch of hemlock and lodgepole pine opens to yet another long meadow that is flanked on the southwest by Price Peak. The canyon starts to narrow, and where the trail starts a gentle 200-yard ascent, your route leaves the trail for an obvious swale ahead to the south and slightly to the left, and separated from the main canyon by a prominent hill. Your short, very easy, cross-country segment strikes southward, fords Rancheria Creek, and ascends the swale beside the tundra-lined outlet of Arndt Lake. A good route to the north shore of hidden Arndt Lake is via the forested saddle in the granite just west of where the outlet leaves the lake—just keep going along the outlet as it hooks east toward the lake. Don't be fooled by an unmapped channel draining the knolls ahead, to the south. There are good campsites around the north shore of pretty Arndt Lake (9251'; 11S 280239 4217333).

DAY 3 (Arndt Lake to Benson Lake, 5.6 miles, part cross-country): From Arndt Lake, retrace your steps cross-country to the Kerrick Canyon Trail. Turn left (south) on that trail and continue down through a narrow, rocky canyon. The unseamed white granite canyon walls in this narrows show the glacial polish, smoothing and sculpting that reflect the geologic history of the canyon. Rancheria Creek on the left bumps and splashes down through a series of fine potholes offering swimming and fishing spots.

The sparse-to-moderate forest cover of mountain hemlock and whitebark and lodgepole pine in the narrows gives way to another meadow as the trail continues to descend. This meadow is surrounded by several magnificent examples of glacial domes. Near the meadow's foot, the trail fords to the east side of Rancheria Creek, where it hugs the sheer, water-stained granite wall. Both the trail and the creek make an exaggerated Z before straightening out on a westward course and reaching the PCT/TYT.

At this junction, it's left (southwest) to Benson Lake on the PCT/TYT and ahead (right, west) to continue down Kerrick Canyon. Go left on the PCT/TYT and climb steeply under a moderate forest cover of hemlock, through two beautiful gaps that should be Seavey Pass but aren't. Approaching a tarn in the first gap, the trail veers abruptly away to climb steeply to the second and highest gap, passing a pair of tarns and then a sandy campsite overlooking a little meadow. As the forest grows increasingly sparse, the trail drops to the little meadow before attacking the third gap, beyond which is Seavey Pass (9150'), 30 feet lower than the second gap before it.

From Seavey Pass, the trail drops past another tarn and finally plummets down Piute Mountain's east slopes. The track is steep and rocky as it drops along a riotous, unnamed stream that feeds Benson Lake's beach, which is an alluvial fan. It's a tough descent, but the scenery is fine. After the trail levels out on the valley floor, it soon grows faint in rank growth. Benson Lake offers the only good camping in the area, and the best route to it branches right (south) at a signed junction just before the ford of Piute Creek. This lateral winds along the northwest bank of Piute Creek through fields of corn lily and bracken fern to the sandy, seasonally buggy campsites on the lake's east shore (7581'; 11S 278374 4211043). Fishing is good for rainbow and eastern brook trout.

DAYS 4–6 (Benson Lake to Twin Lakes Trailhead, 18.6 miles): Retrace your steps.

OPTIONAL SEMILOOP

You could easily add a little loop to this trip on your way back: In lower Kerrick Meadow, at the Kerrick Canyon Trail-Rock Island Pass junction, turn right (east over Rancheria Creek and then south) toward Crown Lake and reverse Trip 81, Days 2 and 1, from the Kerrick Canyon Trail-Rock Island Pass junction to the Peeler-Crown junction. From there, reverse the rest of Day 1 of this trip.

83 Smedberg Lake

Trip Data:
11S 281748
4210078;
49.6 miles;
8/3 days

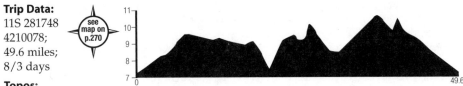

Topos:
*Buckeye Ridge,
Matterhorn Peak, Piute Mountain*

Highlights: Making a grand semiloop through northern Yosemite, this trip traces three major watersheds, visits six major lakes, and views the finest scenery in the region. There are plenty of opportunities for rewarding side trips on layover days.

HEADS UP! *Get an early start: This trip requires a stiff, 2500-foot climb to Day 1's destination. Campfires are prohibited at Barney and Peeler lakes. When you enter Yosemite, bear are required and pets and firearms are prohibited. The brief cross-country leg to Arndt Lake is very easy. However, this is a long and demanding trip overall, so take one or more easier trips before tackling this one.*

DAY 1 (Twin Lakes Trailhead to Peeler Lake, 8 miles): *(Recap: Trip 77, Day 1.)* Beyond the campground, head generally west across the bench through which Robinson Creek flows, usually out of sight. Climb switchbacks and curve southwest to Barney Lake, then traverse above that lake and the long meadow on its inlet. Ford Robinson Creek and begin climbing along it to another ford and then to a ford of Peeler Lake's outlet (last easy-to-get water by late season or in a dry year). Continue climbing switchbacks, eventually veering away from Robinson Creek, to a bench with a junction: left (initially southwest) to Crown Lake; right (northwest) to Peeler Lake. Go right to Peeler Lake, ford its eastern outlet twice on a small bench, and ascend very steeply up a draw northeast of the lake to a point well above the lake. Descend abruptly to cross the outlet and traverse Peeler's rocky north shore (about midway along north shore; 9549'; 11S 283674 4222462), where most former campsites are closed due to overuse (seek sites farther afield). Just beyond the lake's west shore is the signed Yosemite-Hoover Wilderness boundary. Fishing for eastern brook and rainbow trout is sometimes good.

DAY 2 (Peeler Lake to Arndt Lake, 5 miles, part cross-country): *(Recap in Reverse: Trip 81, Day 2, from Peeler Lake to the junction with the Kerrick Canyon Trail-Rock Island Pass junction.)* Regain the trail and, assuming you camped somewhere along Peeler's north shore, head west, cross into Yosemite while crisscrossing the lake's west outlet, enter Kerrick Meadow's north end, and meet a junction with the Kerrick Canyon Trail. Turn left (south) and stroll gradually down Kerrick Canyon with Rancheria Creek on the east (your left). In 1.3 miles, at a junction with the trail across the meadow toward Rock Island Pass and Crown Lake, continue ahead (now southwest).

*(**Recap: Trip 82, Day 2, from the Kerrick Canyon Trail-Rock Island Pass junction.**)* Leaving the Day 2 route of Trip 81, continue your descent through a forested patch to yet another long meadow. Where the trail starts a 200-yard ascent, your route leaves the trail for an obvious swale ahead to the south and slightly to the left, and separated from the main canyon by a prominent hill. Strike southward, ford Rancheria Creek, and ascend the swale beside Arndt Lake's outlet. Keep going along the outlet as it hooks east toward the lake. Don't be fooled by an unmapped channel draining the knolls ahead, to the south. There are good campsites around the north shore of pretty Arndt Lake (9251'; 11S 280239 4217333).

DAY 3 (Arndt Lake to Benson Lake, 5.6 miles, part cross-country): *(Recap: Trip 82, Day 3.)* From Arndt Lake, retrace your steps cross-country to the Kerrick Canyon Trail. Turn left (south) on that trail and continue down through a narrow, rocky canyon.

see map on p.270

The canyon presently widens into another meadow. Near the meadow's foot, the trail fords to the east side of Rancheria Creek. Both the trail and the creek make an exaggerated Z before straightening out on a westward course and reaching the PCT/TYT. At this junction, it's left (southwest) to Benson Lake on the PCT/TYT and ahead (right, west) to continue down Kerrick Canyon.

(Partial Recap: Trip 40, Day 6, PCT/TYT junction in Kerrick Canyon to Benson Lake.) Go left on the PCT/TYT and climb steeply under a moderate forest cover of hemlock, through two gaps that should be Seavey Pass but aren't. The third gap is Seavey Pass (9150'), 30 feet lower than the second gap before it.

From Seavey Pass, the trail makes a long drop down Piute Mountain's east slopes. After the trail levels out on the valley floor, it soon grows faint in rank growth. The best route to Benson Lake branches right (south) at a signed junction just before the ford of Piute Creek. This lateral winds along the northwest bank of Piute Creek through fields of corn lily and bracken fern to the sandy, seasonally buggy campsites on the lake's east shore (7581'; 11S 278374 4211043). Fishing is good for rainbow and eastern brook trout.

DAY 4 (Benson Lake to Smedberg Lake, 4.5 miles): *(Recap: Trip 40, Day 7.)* Return to the main trail and turn right (southeast). Soon the PCT/TYT fords Piute Creek (difficult in early season) and starts a 1900-foot ascent over the next 3 miles. The first pitch takes hikers to a saddle, then descends 0.3 mile to a ford of Smedberg Lake's outlet creek (difficult in early season). The next leg switchbacks up over metamorphic rock to another, easier stream crossing. The following leg is a steady, moderate 1-mile ascent to an easy ford, followed by switchbacks southward up to a meadowed area and a junction with a trail to Murdock Lake. Go left (west) on the PCT/TYT toward Smedberg Lake.

In a quarter mile, the PCT/TYT meets a trail right (south) to Rodgers Lake; go left (northeast) here to curve around Volunteer Peak, plunge down a canyon, climb up a ridge, and descend to the south shore of lovely Smedberg Lake (9219'; 11S 281748 4210078) and its campsites.

DAY 5 (Smedberg Lake to Matterhorn Canyon, 6.5 miles): *(Recap: Trip 40, Day 8.)* Follow the PCT/TYT up its steep, rocky course toward Benson Pass (10,139'). From Benson Pass, the PCT/TYT drops to splashing Wilson Creek (campsites), fords it, and winds down through dense forest cover. After fording Wilson Creek for the third time, the trail plunges steeply 500 feet down to the floor of Matterhorn Canyon. The trail turns north and follows the canyon's meandering stream a mile to several good campsites. Ford the creek to more good campsites a little downstream (8480' at the ford; 11S 288137 4210225). Fishing for eastern brook and rainbow trout is good.

DAY 6 (Matterhorn Canyon to Upper Piute Creek, 8.5 miles): If you haven't done so already, ford the creek (difficult in early season) and meet the Matterhorn Canyon Trail (left, north-northeast) in about 80 yards. Turn left on that trail, leaving the PCT/TYT, and ascend moderately through alternately sandy and rocky sections on Matterhorn Creek's east side. On

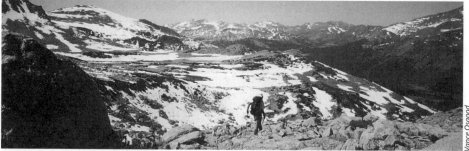

Matterhorn Canyon in early season

both sides of the canyon, glaciated gray granite shoulders with eerie patterns of water stains drop to the valley floor. In a wet, muddy section where the trail fords several small tributaries, it winds through lupine, elephant heads, monkeyflower, paintbrush, golden-rod, aster, and mariposa lily. Ford and reford the creek and then, about a half mile above a meadow, ford back to the west side again.

From this ford, the trail keeps to the west side of the creek, winding through meadow and tundra sections on a moderate ascent. Ahead, the pointed tops of Finger Peaks come into view and, later, the massive granite of Whorl Mountain and Matterhorn Peak. Scattered lodgepole and hemlock trees dot the trail as it rises to the meadows of the upper basin. Clumps of trees in protected areas (possible campsites) alternate with stretches of grassland laced with sagebrush and willow.

Now the trail passes the last stand of trees and ascends steadily on a long, northeast-ward traverse below Finger Peaks. Views across the barren upper basin of Whorl Mountain are awesome as you near Burro Pass through delicate wildflowers: primrose, scarlet penstemon, wallflower, and Douglas phlox. The final climb, on rocky switchbacks, ends at Burro Pass (10,560'), where there are fine views of both the Matterhorn and Piute Creek canyons and of the Sawtooth Ridge to the north.

HISTORICAL NOTE

The first recorded crossing of this pass was made by Lt. N.F. McClure in 1894. Today's travel-ers can compare their observations of the pass and its surroundings with those of McClure, who said, "The route now led for 5 miles through little meadows on each side of the stream, until a comparatively low saddle was seen to the left of you and near the head of the canyon. Investigating this, I found it was a natural pass. The scenery here was truly sublime. I doubt if any part of the main chain of the Sierra presents a greater ruggedness... ."

As the trail descends the north side of the pass along the infant Piute Creek, curving westward, there are fine views of the tiny, barren lakes at the foot of Finger Peaks. This area is usually wet and sometimes snow covered. Belding squirrels pipe in the tundra stretch-es, and marmots on the nearby scree whistle as you make the gentle descent into a mod-erate forest cover of lodgepole and hemlock. This day ends at the good campsites along that stretch of Piute Creek where the trail touches the creek banks northeast of Finger Peaks (9618'; 11S 288102 4219393). Fishing for eastern brook is fair.

DAY 7 (Upper Piute Creek to Crown Lake, 3.5 miles): (Recap in Reverse: Trip 80, Day 2.) Continue downstream along Piute Creek's north bank until the trail curves northwest and north away from the creek, climbing switchbacks and eventually fording a stream drain-ing Ice and Maltby lakes (cross-country up the stream). Still rising, the trail follows an indi-rect arc across the ridge separating the Piute Creek and Robinson Creek watersheds. Finally, it crosses the ridge at Mule Pass and descends, sometimes steeply, on rocky switch-backs and over a bench. Beware of a slope below this bench that holds a large snow bank well into summer. Beyond this slope, the track crosses a bench with a lakelet. Then the trail crosses an easy talus-and-scree pile, fords Snow Lake's outlet, and meets the trail to Rock Island Pass and Crown Lake. Turn right (northeast) through meadow, past lakelets, and down rocky switchbacks to Crown Lake and the campsites along its outlet (9482'; 11S 285715 4221307).

DAY 8 (Crown Lake to Twin Lakes Trailhead, 8 miles): (Recap in Reverse: Trip 79, Day 1, to the Peeler Lake-Crown Lake junction.) Regain the main trail and descend on it southward and then northwestward past the Robinson Lakes and the aqua pool to the junction with the trail to Peeler Lake and Twin Lakes. The loop closes here.

Turn right (northeast) and continue your descent to Twin Lakes, reversing the first leg of Day 1 of this trip.

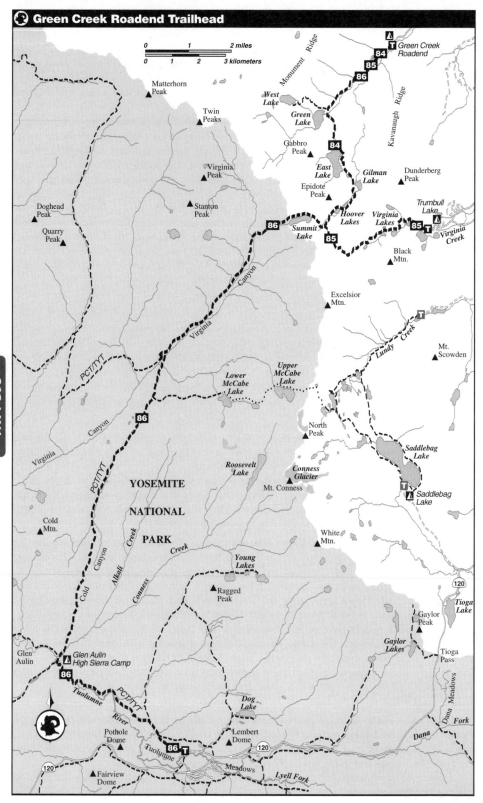

HWY 395

84 Green Creek Roadend

85
86

West Lake

Green Lake

Monument Ridge

Kavanaugh Ridge

Matterhorn Peak

Twin Peaks

Virginia Peak

Gabbro Peak

84

East Lake

Gilman Lake

Dunderberg Peak

Epidote Peak

Doghead Peak

Stanton Peak

86 Summit Lake

Hoover Lakes

Virginia Lakes

Trumbull Lake

85 T

Virginia Creek

Quarry Peak

85

Black Mtn.

Excelsior Mtn.

Virginia

Canyon

Lundy Creek

T

Mt. Scowden

PCT/TYT

Upper McCabe Lake

Lower McCabe Lake

North Peak

Canyon

86

Saddlebag Lake

Virginia

PCT/TYT

Roosevelt Lake

Conness Glacier

Mt. Conness

T

Saddlebag Lake

Cold Mtn.

YOSEMITE

NATIONAL

Creek

Alkali Creek

Conness

White Mtn.

PARK

Cold Canyon Creek

120

Young Lakes

Tioga Lake

Ragged Peak

Gaylor Peak

Gaylor Lakes

Glen Aulin

Glen Aulin High Sierra Camp

86

Tioga Pass

Dana Meadows

PCT/TYT

Tuolumne River

Dog Lake

Lembert Dome

Dana Fork

Pothole Dome

86 T

Tuolumne

120

Meadows

Lyell Fork

120

Fairview Dome

284

Green Creek Roadend Trailhead

8060'; 11S 300175 4220350

DESTINATION/ UTM COORDINATES	TRIP TYPE	BEST SEASON	PACE (HIKING/ LAYOVER DAYS)	TOTAL MILEAGE
84 East Lake 11S 298053 4216826	Out & back	Early to late	2/0 Leisurely	8
85 Virginia Lakes Campground 11S 301604 4213709	Shuttle	Mid or late	2/1 Leisurely	10.5
86 Tuolumne Meadows 11S 292557 4195059	Shuttle	Mid or late	4/1 Leisurely	26.7

Information and Permits: This trailhead is in Humboldt-Toiyabe National Forest's Bridgeport Ranger District. Wilderness permits are required for overnight stays, and a trail quota is in place from late June through mid-September. Contact: Bridgeport Ranger District, HCR 1 Box 1000, Bridgeport, CA; 760-932-7200; www.fs.fed.us.r4/htnf. Bear canisters are not required but are highly recommended.

Driving Directions: From Hwy. 395, 3.8 miles south of Bridgeport and just north of the intersection with Hwy. 270, turn west on signed, unpaved Green Creek Road (USFS Road 142). Drive for 1 mile to a junction with Summit Meadow Road and go left, continuing for another 2.5 miles to a junction with a spur road southbound for Virginia Lakes. Go right here and continue 5.2 more miles, veering right to a parking loop at the trailhead (left goes to Green Creek Campground), where you'll find toilets and water.

84 East Lake

Trip Data: 11S 298053 4216826; 8 miles; 2/0 days

Topos: *Dunderberg Peak*

Highlights: This is a fine beginner's weekend hike. East Lake's scenery includes three colorful peaks, Gabbro, Page, and Epidote, each of which are composed of rocks varying in hue from vermilion reds to ochre, and set in metavolcanic blacks for contrast. Nearby Nutter, Gilman, and Hoover lakes offer good fishing to supplement the angling in East Lake, and the wide-ranging scenery along the way rivals any found on longer backpack trips.

DAY 1 (Green Creek Roadend Trailhead to East Lake, 4 miles): Head southwest on a dusty trail through patchy to moderate Jeffrey pine forest and cross a creeklet after about a quarter of a mile. In a little more than a half mile, you descend to meet the road coming in on the left from the campground. Continue ahead (southwest) here. At 0.6 mile, you meet Green Creek on your left, near a former trailhead. Continue southwest, ignoring an unmapped, gated spur road on your right at a little over 0.75 mile. The trail shortly crosses a creek, beyond which the trail dwindles to a footpath. A ground cover of sagebrush, mule ears, serviceberry, western blueberry, wild lilac, lupine, wallflower, paintbrush, pennyroyal, and buckwheat lines the trail in the initial, drier stretches. Along the wetter spots, you may find tiger lily, penstemon, shooting star, monkshood, monkeyflower, columbine, rein-orchid, and aster.

The ascent then becomes steeper as it crosses a rocky ridge, finally beginning a long series of easy switchbacks. Crossing several intermittent runoff tributaries coming down from Monument Ridge, the trail keeps to the northwest side of West Fork Green Creek. Ahead, on the left, is Gabbro Peak, and on the right is the stream that falls from the hanging valley containing West Lake. Added to the wildflowers to be seen along the trail here are iris, corn lily, cow parsnip, stickseed, gooseberry, Douglas phlox, and pussypaws.

The trail then climbs another dry slope by moderately ascending switchbacks to a signed junction (11S 297878 4218185) just shy of Green Lake. Take the left (south) fork to descend to a deep ford of West Fork Green Creek just below Green Lake (8945', 11S 297695 4217935). This crossing can be very difficult in early season; an easier crossing might be found by following a use trail up to the lake's half-ruined, low dam. Large (50-acre) Green Lake is surrounded by mixed forest cover, with very limited camping just below it and on its east shore; restrictions are posted.

After fording the creek, the trail switchbacks up to the first ford of the vigorous outlet stream from East Lake. Next, the trail ascends generally south on small switchbacks and then fords East

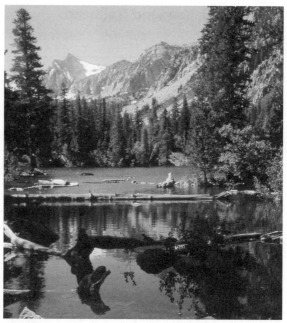

Green Lake

Lake's outlet a second time. Beyond, the trail ascends by long, gradual switchbacks as it continues on to ford the two meadowed outlets of East Lake (9458'; 11S 298053 4216826), just below the lake. There is a fair campsite between the outlets, and fair-to-good campsites are east of the trail as it rounds the lake's east shore and on the north shore. Fishing for rainbow trout on this 75-acre lake is good. This lake makes a fine basecamp for forays to nearby Nutter, Gilman, and Hoover lakes.

DAY 2 (East Lake to Green Creek Roadend Trailhead, 4 miles): Retrace your steps.

85 Virginia Lakes Campground

Trip Data: 11S 301604 4213709l; 10.5 miles; 2/1 days

Topos: *Dunderberg Peak*

Highlights: This U-shaped trip circles around Kavanaugh Ridge and Dunderberg Peak and touches 14 lakes. Scenery along this route is mostly alpine, and the route is a fine sampling of the majestic Sierra Crest. This trip is an excellent choice for a weekend excursion.

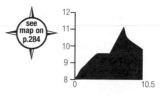

HEADS UP! *As a dayhike, this is probably easier to do in reverse, starting higher from Virginia Lakes to the lower elevation Green Creek Roadend Trailhead.*

Shuttle Directions: To get to the Virginia Lakes Campground, take Hwy. 395 to Conway Summit, the highway's highest point, located between Bridgeport and Lee Vining. From there, take Virginia Lakes Road west 5 miles to trailhead parking.

DAY 1 (Green Creek Roadend Trailhead to East Lake, 4 miles): *(Recap: Trip 84, Day 1.)* Head southwest and, in a little over a half mile, descend to meet the road coming in on the left from the campground. Continue ahead (southwest) here. At 0.6 mile, you meet Green

Creek on your left, near a former trailhead. Continue southwest, ignoring an unmapped, gated spur road on your right at a little over 0.75 mile. The trail shortly crosses a creek and dwindles to a footpath. Sometimes on switchbacks, the trail climbs along the northwest side of West Fork Green Creek. At a signed junction (11S 297878 4218185) just shy of Green Lake, take the left (south) fork to ford West Fork Green Creek (an easier crossing might be found by following a use trail up to the lake's half-ruined, low dam).

After fording the creek, the trail switchbacks up to the first ford of East Lake's outlet. Next, the trail switchbacks up and generally south to ford East Lake's outlet a second time. Beyond, the trail rises on easier switchbacks and finally fords two meadowed outlets of East Lake just below the lake (9458'; 11S 298053 4216826).

DAY 2 (East Lake to Virginia Lakes Campground, 6.5 miles): From the outlet of East Lake, the trail skirts the east side of the lake, veering away from it on an ascending traverse before descending to Nutter Lake. The trail then climbs above the west shore of beautiful Gilman Lake (9486'), passing a lateral trail left and down to it. Going ahead (south) from the Gilman Lake lateral, your main trail ascends to the Hoover Lakes (9819'), fords the stream connecting the two lakes, and then fords the inlet of Upper Hoover Lake. From the ford, the trail zigzags up to a small bench where it meets the Virginia Lakes Trail.

At this junction, turn left (southeast) on the Virginia Lakes Trail and climb steeply up a series of switchbacks that overlook the Hoover Lakes in the valley of East Creek below and Summit Lake to the west. After reaching an often snow-filled bowl, climb more switchbacks and cross two streams. The way grows steeper, and, at frequent rest stops, you can see the small, white petals of Douglas phlox and the purple trumpets of Davidson's penstemon. There are even a few specimens of a yellow flower hardly ever found below 10,000 feet: alpine gold. Finally you cross the divide at 11,119 feet at an unnamed pass where the red rocks of the crest on the right contrast with the somber dark grays of Black Mountain straight ahead.

Your descent begins with a fairly tame series of switchbacks that crosses a lingering snowfield before you reach the Frog Lakes (fair fishing for eastern brook and rainbow trout here and in the stream below). You splash across the stream linking two of the lakes, reach the lowest of them, ford its outlet, and descend to lovely Cooney Lake (better fishing than the Frog Lakes). Continuing the moderate descent over a rocky ledge system, the trail winds down through sparse clumps of whitebark pine and past a tiny, ruined cabin, and then fords the willowed outlet stream of Moat Lake. Now the trail angles down a rocky tra-

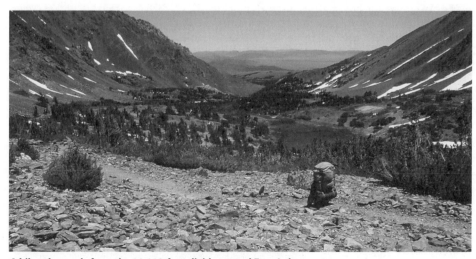

A hiker descends from the 11,119-foot divide toward Frog Lakes.

verse to skirt the north shore of Blue Lake. Leave Hoover Wilderness, pass a couple of ponds, curve south around a patch of forest, and ignore a stock trail on the left. As you come into sight of Upper Virginia Lake, ignore use trails to the lake, cross an open slope and descend southeastward to the trailhead parking next to a restroom (9760'; 11S 301604 4213709).

86 Tuolumne Meadows

Trip Data: 11S 292557 4195059;
26.7 miles; 4/1 days

Topos: *Tuolumne Meadows, Dunderberg Peak, Matterhorn Peak, Falls Ridge, Tioga Pass*

Highlights: The middle section of this scenic route travels through relatively remote sections of Yosemite National Park that see few dayhikers. Upper Virginia Canyon offers solitude, and the trip as a whole is an angler's delight.

HEADS UP! *This trip starts in Hoover Wilderness and ends in Yosemite National Park. All Yosemite rules and regulations (e.g., bear canisters required; pets and firearms prohibited) apply once you cross the park boundary.*

Shuttle Directions: To reach the Tuolumne Meadows take-out trailhead at Lembert Dome, take Hwy. 120 (Tioga Road) in Yosemite National Park 7 miles west of Tioga Pass. At Lembert Dome, turn west onto a road and drive past the parking lot at the dome's west base. Look for legal parking along that road, up to a gate across it (from which a spur road with more parking turns right to Tuolumne Stables). Your trip ends at that gate.

DAY 1 (Green Creek Roadend Trailhead to East Lake, 4 miles): *(Recap: Trip 84, Day 1.)* Head southwest and in a little over a half mile, descend to meet the road coming in on the left from the campground. Continue ahead (southwest) here. At 0.6 mile, you meet Green Creek on your left, near a former trailhead. Continue southwest, ignoring an unmapped, gated spur road on your right at a little over 0.75 mile. The trail shortly crosses a creek and dwindles to a footpath. Sometimes on switchbacks, the trail climbs along the northwest side of West Fork Green Creek. At a signed junction (11S 297878 4218185) just shy of Green Lake, take the left (south) fork to ford West Fork Green Creek (an easier crossing might be found by following a use trail up to the lake's half-ruined, low dam).

After fording the creek, the trail switchbacks up to the first ford of East Lake's outlet. Next, the trail switchbacks up and generally south to ford East Lake's outlet a second time. Beyond, the trail rises on easier switchbacks and finally fords two meadowed outlets of East Lake just below the lake (9458'; 11S 298053 4216826).

DAY 2 (East Lake to Lower Virginia Canyon, 9 miles): *(Partial Recap: Trip 85, Day 2, from East Lake to the Virginia Lakes Trail-Summit Lake junction.)* From the outlet of East Lake, skirt the lake's east side before veering away from it on an ascending traverse and then descending to Nutter Lake. Climb past Gilman Lake, avoiding the lateral left (east) and down to it, ascend to the Hoover Lakes, ford the stream connecting the two lakes, and finally ford the upper lake's inlet. From the ford, the trail zigzags up to a small bench where it meets the Virginia Lakes Trail (10,114'; 11S 297607 4213854).

Leaving the Day 2 route of Trip 85, turn right (northwest) toward Summit Lake, ford the Hoover Lakes' inlet again, and ascend to aptly named Summit Lake (10,183'). Dramatic Summit Lake sits atop the Sierra Crest and has outlets on both sides of the range. There are a few exposed and overused campsites here—better to continue to fine camping in Virginia Canyon below.

The trail skirts the north side of Summit Lake, enters Yosemite National Park, and then switchbacks steeply down Virginia Canyon's east wall on the west side of the range. Across the cirque basin of upper Virginia Canyon, the rounded Grey Butte and the tops of Virginia and Stanton peaks dominate the views to the west. The trail levels out before it fords Return Creek, the stream draining Virginia Canyon, and it continues down-canyon. There is excellent camping here at the ford and also downstream. Farther along, avalanches have made obvious incursions into the sparse forest cover of lodgepole, aspen, and occasional red fir and hemlock.

The trail crosses several tributary streams as it keeps to the west side of Return Creek on a long, moderate descent to a junction with the PCT/TYT (11S 291367 4209208). At this junction, you turn left (heading south after a brief jog north) on the PCT/TYT, ford Return Creek (very difficult in early season, and may be difficult throughout the season), and arrive at some good campsites (8600') in the granite ledge system on the east side of the creek. Fishing for eastern brook and rainbow is fair to good, and the pools in the splashing stream are inviting. (If the PCT/TYT ford is too intimidating, backtrack about a quarter mile upstream to find a wider but easier ford—where campsites are nearby in the rocks above—and follow a use trail downstream to the PCT/TYT ford.)

DAY 3 (Lower Virginia Canyon to Glen Aulin High Sierra Camp, 8 miles): *(Partial Recap: Trip 40, Day 10, from the Return Creek ford to Glen Aulin.)* The trail hooks south and descends to ford smaller McCabe Creek. This may be the last water before Glen Aulin in late season. Next, the trail climbs switchbacks to a junction with the trail left (northeast) up McCabe Creek. You go right (southwest) into Cold Canyon for a long, gentle descent; when there's water in Cold Canyon, you may be able to camp in the occasional dry, forested patch. Continuing the Cold Canyon descent, the trail passes through long, broad meadows that are usually dry by late season. Then the trail climbs over a saddle and gently descends for about a half mile. Over the next mile, always near Cold Canyon's creek (mostly dry in late season), the path passes a few possible campsites.

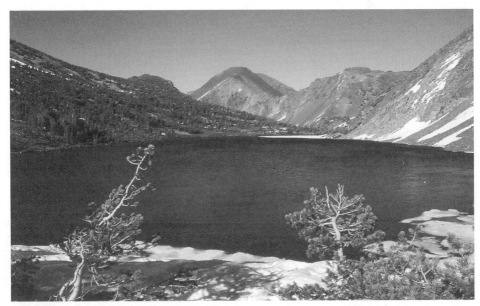

Summit Lake

From here, the trail leaves the creek and descends about halfway to the Tuolumne River. Within sight of Glen Aulin High Sierra Camp, you reach a junction with the Tuolumne River Trail right (northwest; poor, unsafe camping), and in 15 more yards, you come to a spur trail that goes left (east) to cross Conness Creek on a footbridge to Glen Aulin High Sierra Camp (7910'; 11S 287493 4198572) with its backpackers' campground. Camping along the PCT/TYT is prohibited between Glen Aulin and the TYT's end at Tuolumne Meadows.

DAY 4 (Glen Aulin High Sierra Camp to Tuolumne Meadows, 5.7 miles): *(Recap: Trip 40, Day 11.)* From Glen Aulin, cross Conness Creek back to the PCT/TYT, turn left (south) on the that trail, and shortly cross the Tuolumne River on a footbridge just below the White Cascade. Now turning southeast, the PCT/TYT climbs to a junction with a trail right (southwest) to McGee and May lakes; here, you go ahead (southeast) on the PCT/TYT and climb past Tuolumne Falls. You cross the river on one last footbridge before beginning a ducked route over slabs along the river.

After the PCT/TYT's tread resumes, the river gradually curves away from the trail, which presently crosses the three branches of Dingley Creek. In a half mile, you meet the Young Lakes Trail going left (north), while you go ahead (south-southeast) on the PCT/TYT toward Tuolumne Meadows. Stay on the PCT/TYT at any more junctions as you touch the northwest edge of Tuolumne Meadows, cross three branches of Delaney Creek, ascend and cross a long, sandy ridge, and finally descend to pass Soda Springs. Remain on the PCT/TYT as it becomes an eastbound dirt road and reaches a locked gate (8590'; 11S 292581 4194990) with a road leading ahead to Hwy. 120, the Tioga Road (the right fork at this gate leads to the stables). Your trip ends here, and your car or pick-up ride should be along the road.

INDEX

MAP INDEX

ABOUT THE AUTHORS

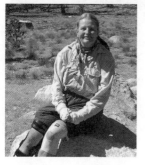

Kathy Morey

The backpacking bug hit Kathy Morey hard in the 1970s and hasn't let go yet. In 1990 she abandoned an aerospace career to write for Wilderness Press, authoring four hiking guides on Hawaii, *Hot Showers, Soft Beds, and Dayhikes in the Sierra*, and *Guide to the John Muir Trail*. She was a co-author of several previous editions of *Sierra North* and *Sierra South*. For the 9th edition of *Sierra North*, Kathy served as lead author. Kathy lives in Mammoth Lakes, California.

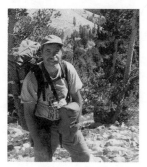

Mike White

Mike White was born and raised in Oregon and learned to hike in the Cascades. In the early 1990s, he began writing about the outdoors full time, and he has since written or contributed to almost a dozen Wilderness Press books, including *Kings Canyon National Park*, *Sequoia National Park*, and *Top Trails Lake Tahoe*. He also has written for *Sunset* and *Backpacker* magazines and the *Reno Gazette-Journal*. Mike lives in Reno and teaches backpacking and snowshoeing at Truckee Meadows Community College.

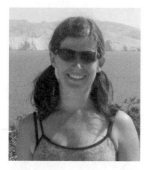

Stacy Corless

Stacy Corless is a hiker, trail runner, and writer in Mammoth Lakes, California. Since trading the Berkeley Hills for the Eastern Sierra seven years ago, Stacy has logged hundreds of miles in the backcountry that, conveniently, is her backyard.

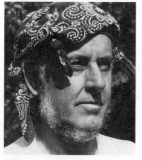

Thomas Winnett

Thomas Winnett founded Wilderness Press in 1967 with the publishing of *Sierra North*, his first guidebook. During his more than 30 years as publisher, he also wrote numerous books on how to backpack and where to hike in the wild areas of the western United States. He is now retired and lives with his wife, Lu, in Berkeley, California.

Books to the Sierra Nevada from Wilderness Press

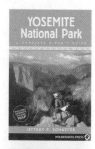

Yosemite National Park

Called the "Cadillac" of Yosemite books by the National Park Service. It details 83 trips, from dayhikes to extended backpacks and includes a foldout 4-color topographic map of the entire park.
ISBN 0-89997-383-3

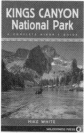

Kings Canyon National Park

An information-packed guide to the peaks and gorges of the majestic apex of the Sierra Nevada. Includes detailed maps, comprehensive trail descriptions, and enlightening background chapters.
ISBN 978-0-89997-335-7

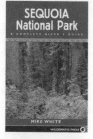

Sequoia National Park

A comprehensive hiker's guide to 62 trips in the national park, plus information on campgrounds, outfitters, and facilities in the park and its surrounding areas.
ISBN 0-89997-327-2

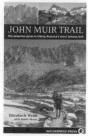

Guide to the John Muir Trail

The best guide to the legendary trail that runs from Yosemite Valley to Mt. Whitney. Written for both northbound and southbound hikers and includes updated 2-color maps from Tom Harrison.
ISBN 978-0-89997-436-1

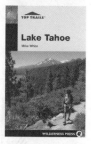

Top Trails Lake Tahoe

Forty-two "must do" hikes, strolls, runs, and bike rides in the Lake Tahoe Basin. Highly visual easy-access format to help you choose your trail and get going.
ISBN 978-0-89997-349-4

For ordering information, contact your local bookseller or Wilderness Press www.wildernesspress.com